Back-Alley Abortion

HEALTH COMMUNICATION

The Health Communication series features rhetorical, critical, and qualitative studies projects exploring the discourses that constitute major health issues of today and the past. Books in the series provide a comprehensive illustration of how health and medicine are communicated to, with, and through diverse individuals and populations.

Back-Alley Abortion

A RHETORICAL HISTORY

Emily Winderman

Johns Hopkins University Press
Baltimore

Printed in the United States of America on acid-free paper

2 4 6 8 9 7 5 3 1

Johns Hopkins University Press
2715 North Charles Street
Baltimore, Maryland 21218
www.press.jhu.edu

Library of Congress Cataloging-in-Publication Data is available.
A catalog record for this book is available from the British Library.

ISBN 978-1-4214-5228-9 (hardcover)
ISBN 978-1-4214-5229-6 (ebook)

EU GPSR Authorized Representative
LOGOS EUROPE, 9 rue Nicolas Poussin, 17000, La Rochelle, France
E-mail: Contact@logoseurope.eu

For my family
and the reproductive justice activists who work tirelessly
for a better tomorrow

CONTENTS

ACKNOWLEDGMENTS

One of my favorite things to do when I begin reading a book is to dive into its author's acknowledgments. Noticing the webs of love and care that contributed to a book that often has only one author's name printed on the spine reminds me that we consistently work in a community.

Seeds for this project were first sown in my doctoral work, supervised by Celeste Condit at the University of Georgia. I could not have asked for a better PhD advisor, one who was always fiercely encouraging and supportive. Celeste, thank you for modeling academic humility and reminding me to prioritize relational maintenance. I greatly benefited from an outstanding rhetorical education at UGA from incredible thinkers and committee members like Carolina Acosta-Alzuru, Barbara Biesecker, Kelly Happe, and Belinda Stillion Southard. Thank you for the time and energy you each put into my writing and into teaching me how to read and think carefully. I am also so grateful for my training from Roger Stahl and Thomas Lessl. Nate Stormer deserves credit for inadvertently spawning this entire project at least eight years ago.

I thank Robin Jensen for her mentorship and support for this project as the editor of the Health Communication series for Johns Hopkins University Press. To know Robin is to be consistently showered in unwavering enthusiasm, good humor, and incisive feedback. I always hope to model your capacity for bringing joy to all scholarly encounters. Thank you for your patience, support, encouragement, and assistance with obtaining travel funding to support this project. I offer profound gratitude to the two anonymous reviewers of this book for their feedback and support of this project. I also want to thank the incredible people at JHUP: Matthew McAdam for his support of this project and patience when it was interrupted by a global pandemic; Phoebe Peter Oathout, whose tireless effort resulted in the high-quality images that appear in this book; and Robert

Brown and Carrie Watterson's careful copyediting. Any errors that may appear in the published book are mine alone.

This book has been supported by several institutions: the University of Minnesota, Twin Cities, helped to nurture this project. In 2019 I received a UMN Library Research Sprint—a full week of the most outstanding librarians and archivists helping me pinpoint coordinates for a project that felt like tracking a needle in a haystack. Specifically, thank you to Lois Hendrickson, Shanda Hunt, Linnea Anderson, Kim Clark, Alicia Kubicek, and Cody Hennessey for such a productive week around a conference table. I wish also to thank Natalie Nachsheim, Molly Muth, and Natalie Gardner for their terrific research assistance during the spring and summer of 2019 in helping me process such immense amounts of material. UMN also provided a single-semester leave and fellowship opportunity with the Institute for Advanced Study. At the IAS, I was fortunate enough to share virtual pandemic space with some of the most wonderful people, who made academic life grand. Thank you to Jennifer Gunn, Susannah Smith, Joanne Richardson, Laurie Moberg, Juliet Burba, and Abby Travis. I thank Leslie J. Reagan for providing helpful feedback on an early version of chapter 3 during an IAS workshop. I am grateful for a travel grant from Harvard University's Schlesinger Library to complete a bulk of this book's archival research.

Thank you to members of UMN's Department of Communication Studies, past and present, for providing an important space to think, teach, and grow. Particularly, I benefited from support and encouragement from Mary Vavrus, Catherine Squires, Laurie Ouelette, Kate Lockwood Harris, Michael Lechuga, Rachel Presley, Elaine Hsieh, Ron Greene, Deborah Yoon, Zornitsa Keremidchieva, Wendy Anderson, and Atilla Hallsby. Office staff over the years, including Carmen Sims, Mark Usem, Tucker Marks, Jada Pulley, and Jo-Ellyn Pilarski, have always made life easier and more joyful. I've been blown away by the brilliance of graduate scholars in this space. I am grateful for my spring 2024 rhetorical criticism students as well as Brittany Knutson's scholarly companionship and Kristen Einertson's meticulous citational work. Natalie Warren, Bill Heinze, and Emma Newton are also beacons of joy. Lauren Ruhrold, Adam Negri, and Clare Frances Kennedy have been lovely recent scholarly additions to my life in the Healthcare under Crisis oral history project. For the scholarly community and friends I never knew I needed so badly, thank you to Maggie Hennefeld, Sonali Pahwa, Jennie Row, Sugi Ganeshananthan, Ainsley Boe, Candace Moore, Stacey Burns, Vivian Choi, and Danielle Dadras for always providing a pressure-release valve. Molly Kessler, for unwavering camaraderie, thank you.

At North Carolina State University, I am so grateful for Victoria Gallagher's mentorship and friendship. Kenneth Zagacki was always a lovely interlocutor. Chris Ingraham was a supportive friend and reader of my work. I also thank Nick Taylor, Elizabeth Nelson, Elizabeth Craig, Grant Bollmer, Steve Wiley, Jean Goodwin, Carolyn Miller, Katherine Guinness, Lynsey Romo, Kami Kosenko, Ryan Hurley, Sarah Stein, and Nicole Lee. Brandon Rogers's research assistance shaped the arc of chapter 1. Chandra Maldonado, Krystin Gollihue, Chen Chen, Max Renner, Abigail Browning, Megan Fletcher Weiner, and the late Adele Hite were joys to work with in various capacities. Undergraduate students that will forever stay with me include Abby Pugh, Renesha Miles, Pat Henry, Aditi Dholakia, and Chase Colborn. Raleigh friends who shaped me include Alecia McAlister, Monica Shannon, Ty Harrell, Cheryl Kirk-Duggan, Diana Hardy, and Tiffany Ingersoll.

I became a thinker, scholar, and teacher at Eastern Michigan University due in no small part to the influences of Michael Tew, Doris Fields, Kathy Stacey, Dennis O'Grady, Ray Quiel, Lee Stille, and the late Gary "Doc" Evans and Judy Sturgis-Hill.

This manuscript is not only stronger for, but exists at *all* thanks to, the encouragement and readers of the long-standing LDP writing group: Caitlin Frances Bruce, Kimberly Singletary, Michaela Frischherz, Lisa Silvestri, and Heather Suzanne Woods. I am grateful for the friendship and scholarly companionship of Shui-yin Sharon Yam and Natalie Fixmer-Oraiz. Allison Prasch and Stephanie Larson each deserve so much gratitude for reading probably *every* chapter of this book and being encouraging in each iteration. Allie Rowland and Jen Malkowski are true lights to my life who have also read this work. Belinda Stillion Southard and Lisa Corrigan are profound models of scholarly excellence and generosity, whose mentorship I've been so fortunate to receive. Marina Levina has always been encouraging, honest, and caring of my entire self. Grad school writing dates with Megan Fitzmaurice got me to where I am today. Thank you also to Jeff Bennett, Robert Mejia, Heather Brook Adams, Diana Isabel Martinez, Kim Harper, James Wynn, John Lynch, Ashley Mack, Lisa Keränen, Jenell Johnson, Blake Scott, Lauren Cagle, Kenny Walker, Torrie Fields, Ariel Seay-Howard, Sarah Idzik, and Nate Johnson.

I am profoundly grateful to the 2019 Rhetoric Society of America seminar "Medical Rhetoric in the Archives" for teaching me how to be comfortable in archival spaces. Robin Jensen and Jordynn Jack were terrific leaders. There, I was fortunate to incubate ideas with Madison Krall, Berkley Conner, Ryan Mitchell,

Sammi Rippetoe, and Aya Farhat. I am grateful for Barbara Heiffron, Berkley Conner, Heather Brook Adams, and Heather Voorhies, who read early drafts of chapter 1 during the height of pandemic lockdown.

I must express gratitude to the Lake Superior Group Chat: Heather Woods, Natalie Pennington, and Nikki Marcotte. Alex McVey always helps me "commit to the bit." I am grateful for the friendship of Nick Romerhausen, Coy Hernandez, Meghann Craig, Haley DeGrella, Melissa Mantei, Malisa Hinderliter, Cara Jurado, Emily Mariner, Carl Mariner, Nina Brennan, Jessica P'Simer, Jeremy Grossman, Dustin Greenwalt, Brittany Leach, Nate Ford, Amanda Ford, Ashley Mack, Bryan McCann, Paul Johnson, Megan Foley, Raquel Robvais, and Erin O'Daniel. Thank you to Justine Temke and Ale Falco for their companionship through the birth journey and helping me remember my power. Celia Napton has provided first-rate childcare, which can never be appreciated enough. I dearly love Iris L. Davis for introducing me to Buddhism and the wisdom of the Lotus Sutra.

My family has been an unwavering source of inspiration and support throughout my entire career. I am so grateful for Eden and Wayne Winderman for a level of parental love that is virtually unmatched. They deserve five pages of acknowledgement of their own. My brother, Eli Winderman, is a brave, talented, and loving soul. Allison Kodan, Genghis Hallsby, Rachel Cortez Hallsby, and Karl and Tomas Hallsby are bonus siblings that have always provided laughs, distractions, love, and care. My sweet nephew, Lil G. Annette Giorgios, and Mimi Ernay, Eve Fitzsimmons, Lynne DeBerry, Terry Fitzsimmons, Ronnie Winderman, Harry Winderman, Emily Schmetterer, Nina and David Schmetterer, Gillian and Garry Davis, and the late Mark Winderman and Jerry Schmetterer have shaped me in important ways. I also thank my puppies, Millie and the late Murray, for their many years of affective labor.

May Atilla Hallsby collect his flowers for the many, many roles he takes in our family. From serving as a perpetual sounding board to providing editing assistance, you have read and encouraged every word. More importantly, to the love of my life, I cherish our adventures together—the best of those has been parenting our children, Isidore and Alvin. Izzy and Alvie: thank you for coming into our lives and gifting us much-needed perspective, joy, and unconditional love.

Back-Alley Abortion

INTRODUCTION

"We All Heard the Stories"

> I had an illegal abortion in September 1968. I had heard many horror stories of back-alley abortions. I was determined to do it in a way that would keep me safe.[1] —*Phyllis*

> She took me to her bathroom. It was neat and clean, but it was just an ordinary bathroom in an ordinary row house. She filled the sink with water and added some Lysol. She washed her hands in this and dipped a long rubber tubing, which I later learned was a catheter, into the same sink water. I was terrified. I had never seen this woman before. I had heard horror stories of back-alley abortions, and I really had no idea what to expect. I knew absolutely nothing about her qualifications to be doing this and I didn't care. I was only grateful that she was going to help me and that she was kind.[2] —*Eleanor*

On January 21, 2018, Senator Elizabeth Warren (D-MA) commemorated the forty-fifth anniversary of *Roe v. Wade* with a *Time* magazine editorial titled "America Can Never Go Back to the Era of Back-Alley Abortions." Warren recalled, "When I was a girl growing up in Oklahoma, women got abortions. But because those procedures were illegal, many of them ended up with back alley butchers. And we all heard the stories: women who bled to death or died from an infection."[3] Framing the era of back-alley abortion as an archaic specter of US history, Warren warned that, should *Roe* be overturned, we should expect the horrors of a criminalized past to return. Her closing brought the past to bear upon the future of abortion rights: "I lived in a world of back alley butchers and wrecked lives. We're not going back—not now, not ever."

In 2019, congressional representatives Barbara Lee (D-CA), Ayanna Pressley (D-MA), and Alexandria Ocasio-Cortez (D-NY) filmed an exclusive video for the *Root* commemorating the devastating anniversary of the Hyde Amendment. As an annually reauthorized policy rider dating back to 1977, the Hyde Amendment blocks federal Medicaid funding for abortions. Representative Lee recalled:

> As a young staffer, I was furious . . . Because I knew exactly what [Hyde] would do and that would be to deny low-income women and women of color access to the full range of reproductive rights—including abortion. . . . I was determined when I was elected to Congress in '98 that I didn't care what happened; I was going to fight to repeal the Hyde Amendment. Because I remember the days of back-alley abortions very well. Before *Roe v. Wade,* I had to go to Mexico for an abortion. That was horrible.[4]

Lee described her political career as animated by her experience crossing the US-Mexico border for abortion care that was illegal at home. Juxtaposing these narratives reveal two insights: first, back-alley abortion can refer to an individual's recollection of receiving "horrible" abortion care. Second, the stories of back-alley abortion also circulate detached from personal experiences. Much like the vignettes featured in this chapter's epigraph, *public* invocations of back-alley abortion crafted the expectations about the criminalized care they might receive. Despite these differences, Representative Lee and Senator Warren spoke to an underlying unity: should abortion become criminalized or remain financially inaccessible to low-income people, the destination would undoubtedly be abortion's "back-alley." There, they would likely encounter unscrupulous, untrained, and uncaring providers operating in an unsanitary space.

Three years after Representative Lee filmed that video, the landscape of abortion jurisprudence was upended. The US Supreme Court issued its *Dobbs v. Jackson Women's Health Services* decision in June 2022, overturning *Roe v. Wade.* In response, Representative Lee returned to her story: "I survived that back-alley abortion. More women, especially Black women, did not. . . . And so here we are 50 years later. . . . I really worry about the return to unsafe abortions."[5] Since the *Dobbs* decision, Lee and many others have recalled their experiences navigating the pre-*Roe* terrain of criminalized abortion as "back-alley" abortions. These repeated refrains raise essential questions as activists, providers, and scholars orient to the needs of the post-*Dobbs* era: How common were the butchers of pre-*Roe* history? Was it typical to procure abortions in the narrow, unseen, unsanitary spaces between city buildings? To what or where are we "returning"?

Leading historians of criminalized abortion agree that although reproductive injustice in the United States has been well documented and legal restrictions have been a forceful driver of abortion-related morbidity and mortality, "back-alley butchers" were not nearly as pervasive as popular framings would lead us to believe. Carole E. Joffe writes, "The coat hanger and the butcher are certainly not invented symbols. . . . . But butchers and coat hangers were only partial aspects of a more complex reality that formed the culture of illegal abortion before *Roe*."[6] Leslie J. Reagan concurs: focusing on "back alley butchers" obfuscates a more nuanced history of how medical professionals actively helped pregnant people procure illegal abortions, even under threat of state penalty.[7] Rickie Solinger similarly critiques the wide circulation of and preoccupation with the figure of the back-alley abortion provider, noting how "focusing on the butcher stops far short of a woman's rights argument" and justifies violence against abortion providers.[8] Lina-Maria Murillo illuminates how a long-standing racial formation that associated Mexicans with filth and immorality nourished back-alley narratives in the United States, even as "firsthand accounts of patients and doctors reveal that Mexican providers were not necessarily back-alley butchers."[9] In short, there are excellent historical and deliberative reasons to distance ourselves from the back-alley to describe who performed illegal abortion before *Roe* and where these procedures transpired.

These historians of illegal abortion rightly critique the framing of "back-alley butchers" as reductive and dangerous to the well-being of abortion providers. At the same time, *appeals* to back-alley abortion have endured. In *Living a Feminist Life*, Sara Ahmed argues that "words surround us, thick with meaning and intensity."[10] Solinger recognizes that intensity and acknowledges the back-alley butcher remains "a vibrant cultural icon—and perhaps the most widely accepted justification for granting reproductive choice."[11] Importantly, she speaks to the back-alley's adaptive capacities, that it has been "capacious enough to absorb and reflect meanings, one after another."[12] Bringing Solinger's observation about the power of the back-alley into conversation with rhetorical critic Celeste Michelle Condit's *Decoding Abortion Rhetoric: Communicating Social Change* begins to reveal why. Tales of abortion bore "strong emotional force" in pre–*Roe v. Wade* days of abortion rights advocacy, narrating harrowing experiences obtaining criminalized reproductive care.[13] Although the back-alley offers a reductive representation of historical complexity, it is also an affectively potent, widely circulating rhetoric with sustained cultural impact. By juxtaposing Senator Warren's statement, "And we all heard the stories . . ." to Representative Lee's self-defined experience of "back-alley abortion," we begin to untangle how the label "back-alley abortion" can be viscerally resonant for some who experienced abortion before *Roe* and persuasive to those more detached from those experiences.

A core argument of this book affirms that back-alley abortion is a rhetoric whose meaning is often distorted with respect to historical reality. For this and many other reasons, criticisms of back-alley abortion as historically inaccurate resemble rhetoric's own history and how it has long signified a deceptive deviation from the truth. If we conceive of rhetoric as a deception, then "back-alley abortion" is rhetoric because it is an anachronism, imagining encounters that existed in a much different form than are often remembered. If we conceive of rhetoric as Plato did—a form of "mere cookery" that satisfied the senses but did not heal the body—then "back-alley abortion" may signify something similar: a diminished version of medicine's "true" art. Both rhetorical perspectives easily speak to existing critiques of the back-alley butcher.

However, if we view rhetoric—and back-alley abortion rhetoric in particular—with contemporary rhetorical theory's rich affordances, then we open ourselves to a nuanced understanding of how this term shaped not only abortion politics but facets of racialized medical legitimacy writ large. In her rhetorical history of lobotomy, rhetorical critic Jenell Johnson argues, "Stories—even wrong stories—are formidable cultural forces, and they thus are well worth our critical attention. Wrong stories, that is to say, those narratives stricken from the archive as fictive, unverifiable, unreliable, invented, polemical, mythical, imaginative, or symbolic are valuable for what they reveal about the culture that created them."[14] *Back-Alley Abortion: A Rhetorical History* has much in common with Johnson's treatment of lobotomy. Both account for sensationalized procedures that have largely been represented inaccurately. Both had a tremendous cultural force in the history of health and medicine. Both remain exemplary rhetorical objects beyond the limited scope of a medical encounter. Like lobotomy, the rhetorical life of back-alley abortion has far exceeded its technical correctness. Contemporary rhetorical theory presumes that public discussions have a constitutive role in molding subjectivity, social reality, and shared public feelings.[15] While back-alley abortion certainly "absorbs and reflects" meanings, as Solinger puts it, back-alley rhetoric also *constructs* racialized material realities that present enduring constraints to providers, patients, and the activists who care about them both. Dwelling in these tensions between the rhetoric of back-alley abortion and history of criminalized abortion is productive as it reveals crucial racialized, classed, and gendered assumptions that have long undergirded US abortion politics. Beyond the scope of abortion, contextualizing the sustained emergence, circulation, and contemporary durability of back-alley abortion also clarifies values embedded in US health care provision writ large, such as sanitary clinical space, caring providers, and effective techniques.

Back-Alley Abortion: A Rhetorical History traces how a complex and heterogeneous field of criminalized abortion became condensed into the simplified phrase "back-alley abortion," giving way to assumptions that most, if not all, illegal abortions were performed in disgusting surroundings with cruel practitioners using inept techniques. A series of deceptively simple questions have guided this project from the start: If not a historically accurate framing, then precisely what *is* back-alley abortion? Who used the phrase? How has it figured into US abortion politics? What types of relationships between patients, care providers, and clinical spaces did the phrase organize? To answer these questions, I dove into dozens of available archival collections to find elusive needles in haystacks and locate appeals to back-alley abortion as they were made visible in public and technical discourses. My findings were often surprising: even as activists, physicians, and social reformers discussed the problem of criminalized abortion, the precise phrasing "back-alley abortion" did not figure into this framing with regularity until the late 1960s—as the United States began to repeal some of its older prohibitions. Although the phrase "back-alley" had a long rhetorical life of its own before ever referring to pregnancy termination and although similar monikers like "backstreet abortion" were prevalent throughout the twentieth century, back-alley abortion *as such* emerged rather late in the pre-*Roe* history of criminalized abortion and experienced its most profound circulation after *Roe*.

Back-Alley Abortion: A Rhetorical History critically analyzes the rhetorical and cultural contours of back-alley rhetoric, both before and after its mid-twentieth-century articulation to abortion care. I argue that back-alley abortion rhetoric mediates relationships between individual embodied experiences, history, and public memory. Back-alley abortion rhetoric organizes and circulates a suite of viscerally resonant public feelings around stigmatized reproductive health care, such as horror, disgust, fear, shame, pity, and outrage. Of course, people seeking to end pregnancies encountered abhorrent conditions and questionable practitioners. Without dismissing this truth, *Back-Alley Abortion: A Rhetorical History* considers how public discussions of "back-alley" abortion spaces and practitioners have been leveraged across the US political spectrum to enable *and constrain* reproductive justice writ large. Back-alley abortion is a racializing rhetoric that was implicated in how sanitary clinical space was understood, how provider ethos was framed, and how people seeking criminalized abortions were represented.

As a deeply US-centric rhetoric, appeals to back-alley abortion have functioned as a collective barometer of how far the nation has—or has not—"evolved" in relationship to border nations, like Mexico. Back-alley abortion therefore serves as a visceral reservoir of public memory prone to anti-abortion uptake. Highlighting the rhetorical aspects of back-alley abortion recognizes this phrase's power, potency, and longevity. It reminds us that the world is, at least in part, a product of the words that make it up—for better and worse.[16]

This introductory chapter proceeds with three movements: First, I narrate a brief history of criminalized abortion, highlighting the confluence of medical, legal, and journalistic discourses in shaping that landscape. Second, I describe the analytic equipment guiding my subsequent analysis of back-alley abortion rhetoric, grounded in the theoretical and methodological affordances of reproductive justice, rhetorical studies, and affect theory. Last, I preview the chapters to come.

When Abortion Was a Crime

More than a century before "back-alley abortion" was a common phrase, legal, medical, and popular discourses mutually affected one another to mold the law, suture the racialized and gendered boundaries of medicine, and create visceral stories for public consumption. The title of this section reflects a profound intellectual indebtedness to Reagan's germinal work that traced the entire pre-*Roe* criminal abortion epoch, a task that I could not hope to replicate here. Reagan helpfully delineates this epoch (1880–1973) into four sometimes overlapping periods roughly based upon where criminalized abortions were performed, their relative availability despite criminalization, who performed them, and who regulated them.[17] Because my goal is to outline historical antecedents contributing to the mid-twentieth century emergence of explicit back-alley abortion rhetoric, I draw on but precede this periodization to identify contextual coordinates between medical, legal, and public discourse that, even before the illegal epoch, influenced the rhetorical formation of "back-alley abortion." This section unfolds in three stages: the first, abortion in the nineteenth century, explores the different communicative means through which the culture of criminal abortion materialized. The second, on the role of the American Medical Association, details how the organization espoused a racializing rhetoric that sought to control not only abortion but specific practitioners and knowledge that threatened the expertise of medical professionals. The third introduces criminalized abortion in the twentieth century, the period most centered in this book because it covers the context surrounding the emergence of phrases including "back-alley" and "back-alley abortion" as quotidian terms.

Abortion in the Nineteenth-Century United States

In the early nineteenth century, there was "legal silence" regarding abortion in the United States.[18] This legal silence did not mean the United States lacked public concern about reproduction or knowledge of pregnancy termination. Botanical contraceptives and abortifacients were common knowledge in the eighteenth-century.[19] While white women's reproduction was considered crucial for reproducing the nascent national body politic, their duties were framed more through generative ideologies of republican motherhood than restrictive statutes that criminalized pregnancy termination.[20] As Linda Kerber observes, "The tangled and complex role of the republican mother offered one among many structures and contents in which women might define the civic culture and their responsibilities to the state."[21] While republican motherhood ideologies granted a provisional sense of belonging, purpose, and morally grounded citizenship for white women excluded from voting and other forms of public civic participation, this formulation of civic inclusion existed alongside practices of profound colonial violence, including the simultaneous land dispossession and slaughter of Indigenous people and systemic reproductive control of enslaved Africans to sustain chattel slavery.[22] After the United States banned the import of enslaved humans in 1808, slavery was sustained by Black women's reproduction, which included devastating practices of rape, forced marriage, and family separation. As a way "to produce and transmit property across generations," sexual violence and forced reproduction carried a high economic incentive.[23] Loretta J. Ross describes how abortion was one significant way that Black and Indigenous people actively resisted these dehumanizing state-sponsored regimes of reproductive injustice.[24]

The United States initially followed British Common Law when regulating abortion, which until 1803, "did not formally recognize the existence of a fetus in criminal cases until it had quickened."[25] Occurring within what we would today consider the fourth and fifth months of gestation, quickening—the embodied flutter of fetal movement—separated pregnancy from other possible maladies according to the medical etiologies of the time. Kristin Luker notes, "Early in the century, a dominant therapeutic model saw the human body as an 'intake-outflow' system and disease as the result of some disturbance in the regular production of secretions."[26] Janet Farrell Brodie elaborates that "taking poisons to kill the invading ill humor causing an illness was an established part of medical theory in the eighteenth and nineteenth centuries, so it should not be surprising that women tried such dangerous poisons."[27] Within this medical framework, absent menses did not necessarily translate to pregnancy. A missed cycle could be explained through many other root causes and thus warranted herbal, chemical, or mechanical interventions to restore the regular menstrual cycle. Without contemporary pregnancy testing technologies, visceral, embodied feelings held a crucial and definitive role in the boundary of reproductive criminality.

Between 1821 and 1841, what James Mohr calls the "first wave of abortion legislation," laws targeted herbal and chemical tools of pregnancy termination. These laws often took the form of poison control, implicating those administering abortions—not necessarily the people who would procure them. The May 1821 Connecticut General Assembly had an unprecedented revision to its "crimes and punishments" section to render pregnancy termination after quickening a crime. Connecticut's 1830 regulation of herbal remedies targeted apothecaries and physicians "who the state could presume should know better than to seek profit by selling preparations that were only marginally effective as abortifacients, but demonstrably dangerous as poisons."[28] States such as Missouri, Illinois, and New York passed statutes between Connecticut's first and second iterations. By targeting what was seen as inappropriate *means* of abortions, these early statutes laid provisional rhetorical groundwork for the back-alley butcher by connecting abortion techniques to providers' moral characters.

Despite emerging legal prohibitions, abortifacient information circulated in penny papers.[29] As urban population growth and industrial printing exploded, new channels of advertising appeared "with the development of the penny papers in the 1830s, and their frequent willingness to accept advertising from virtually all comers with few questions asked."[30] The most (in)famous advertiser of them all was Ann Lohman. Known more colloquially as Madame Restell, Lohman began selling abortifacients and performing abortions in 1837. By the 1840s, Lohman expanded her New York business to include satellite offices in Boston and Philadelphia, remaining open for twelve hours daily to meet demand. Lohman was a target of public ire, and her public persona was characterized by appeals to greed and a lack of medical skill. Dr. Gunning Bedford called her a "monster, who speculates with human life with as much cruelness as if she were engaged in a game of chance."[31] Explicit invocations of monstrosity painted Lohman as reckless and unconcerned with the well-being of those who sought her wares, dissociating her from the boundaries of legitimate medicine.

Abortifacient advertising was not all one could find in penny papers. Cautionary tales simultaneously sowed fear surrounding the possibility of dying from an abortion. Penny papers trafficked in visceral sensationalism to grow their markets and compete with one another.[32] The 1833 public cases of white Rhode Island residents Sally Burdick and Sarah Maria Cornell were marked by body rhetorics that would warrant criminal statutes and build the foundation of back-alley rhetoric. Regarding Sally Burdick's death, the physician's vividly penned autopsy enjoyed wide circulation. According to Tanfer Emin Tunç, the trial report detailing Burdick's autopsy "established the tenor of invasive investigations . . . and graphic accounts that would accompany criminal abortion narratives over the century."[33] The power of the trial report largely came through Dr. Cyrus James's vivid descriptions of Burdick's body: "Gory even by contemporary standards, the trial report is an example of gothic 'body-horror,' a writing style that 'fully exposed the process by which murder victims' bodies were damaged, dismembered, and medically disemboweled."[34] James's testimony contributed to the abortion provider's conviction and changes to Rhode Island laws, "clearly suggesting the burgeoning power of the medical profession to shape public opinion, the course of official proceedings, and the legal code itself."[35] In addition to consolidating the public rhetorical power of the medical profession, this case seeded a recurring feature of post-*Roe* back-alley abortion rhetoric: how a vulnerable woman's harmed internal viscera could be externalized for public deliberation and consumption.

While Burdick's public death was significant for its instantiation of voyeuristic medical expertise, Sarah Maria Cornell's death received profoundly moralizing media coverage and literary translation in Catherine Read Arnold Williams's 1833 *Fall River: An Authentic Narrative*. Cornell, a mill worker, had a sexual relationship with Methodist pastor Ephraim Kingsbury Avery. After learning she was pregnant, Avery allegedly killed Cornell by striking her in the abdomen, covering up his actions by staging a suicide. Avery was ultimately acquitted of murder after attorneys painted Cornell as a morally fallen woman. The trial relied on the expert testimony of physicians who "not only provided information concerning Cornell's pregnancy, autopsy, and sexual history, but also medicalized her speech and behavior, which were unlike that of an 'ordinary woman' serving as 'evidence' of her moral turpitude."[36]

A nineteenth-century exemplar that linked forensic journalism, popular literature, and police surveillance was the 1841 case of Mary Cecilia Rogers. Perhaps the most storied confluence of medical, legal, and novelistic discourse, this New York case resulted in the prosecution of Ann Lohman and solidified the literary genre of criminal abortion narratives.[37] Mary Rogers worked in a cigar shop and died after procuring an abortion. Her body was left in a river in July

1841. Amy Gilman Srebnick deftly traces how, emerging in parallel with penny papers, Rogers's rhetorical life far exceeded her cause of death: "Mary Rogers' life and death became a text, or many texts really, of this new urban print culture. Through her story, urban journalists and fiction writers invented complex tales of urban life figured around the violent death of a beautiful young woman. . . . Mary's beaux, her sexual history, and even her mutilated body—became legitimate information, even 'newsworthy.'"[38] According to Daniel Stashower, "The drama of Mary Rogers would be one of the earliest and most significant murder cases to play out in the pages of the American press, laying the groundwork for every 'crime of the century' to follow."[39] Edgar Allan Poe, often credited with inventing detective fiction with his three-part series featuring Auguste Dupin, inaugurated the genre with a fictionalized account of Mary Rogers by employing the thinly veiled pseudonym Marie Roget.

The Rogers coverage intensified the monstrous qualities attributed to the "evil" abortion provider and influenced city-specific reforms and statewide statutes in abortion law and the policing system. Although Ann Lohman had no role in Rogers's death, the "Madame Restell" character became notorious because of the rhetorical connection the press made between her and Mary Rogers. During the 1840s, as urban populations grew and more married white women turned to abortion, "many Americans no doubt saw in Restellism one more confirmation of their suspicions that cities were sinful centers where people went to live unnatural lives."[40] The incorrect, but popular, assumption that Rogers was sexually assaulted and murdered was an inflection point for an already brewing "crisis" about urban social decay, sexual danger, and the insufficiencies of the existing policing system. The rhetorical power of Mary Rogers's death even exceeded the scope of abortion: coverage served as a profound public warrant to modernize, organize, and amplify social and political surveillance.[41] Illustrating how structures of abortion criminalization and reproductive surveillance developed together, the Rogers case contributed a sense of public urgency to pass two powerful pieces of legislation: a stricter abortion law and the 1845 New York City Police Reform Act, which restructured the police force.[42] Thus, the more distant impact of the Rogers case included statewide statutes that went beyond criminalizing abortifacient compounds and providers to warrant a transformation of criminal surveillance in toto.

Much like the shifting dynamics of life brought on by industrialization, urbanization, and westward colonial expansion between 1840 and 1860, anti-abortion statutes were likewise "transitional," even as pregnancy termination became bigger business—and bigger journalistic fodder.[43] Aligning with Mary Rogers's death and New York's 1845 Police Reform Act, the *National Police Gazette* published weekly missives targeting abortion providers. Not only did the *Gazette*—a proto-tabloid paper[44]—attribute a profit motive to the provision of abortions itself, but it also nurtured perceptions of monstrosity by attributing malicious and greedy intentions to abortion providers. The *Gazette* held that abortion providers were looking to enrich themselves by selling the corpses of their victims to "the midnight lectures of secret surgical techniques." This accusation largely overshadowed the horrifying reality that, at the time, the corpses of enslaved Africans were being stolen and sold to medical schools throughout the United States for anatomical education and dissection.[45] The public denigration of abortion providers' characters and capacity shifted attention away from these and other profound injustices that built the foundation of "legitimate" medical education.

The Role of the American Medical Association

Mid-nineteenth-century abortion criminalization efforts were led not by legislators or religious leaders but by the American Medical Association (AMA). Newly formed in 1847, the AMA sought to weed out "irregular" practitioners.[46] Dovetailing with an American status quo of Southern enslavement and Northern racial oppression, the AMA, "an exclusionary, segregated organization that banned African Americans from membership,"[47] specifically targeted Black practitioners and suppressed medical knowledge concerning abortion and reproductive care. Before the AMA, midwives were a strong presence throughout the antebellum United States. Many were enslaved on Southern plantations and delivered babies for white families.[48] With an encyclopedic understanding of the herbs and techniques required to prevent and end pregnancies and a decided spiritual calling, their knowledge was considered dangerous to reproducing the system of slavery after the transatlantic trade ended.[49] Ross recounts that physicians in the mid-nineteenth century were "certain that slave women were aborting either by 'medicine, violent exercise, or by external and internal manipulations.' "[50] Demonizing the competence of midwife practitioners was a sustained practice throughout the nineteenth and early twentieth centuries that performed racialized medical boundary work.

As medical reform movements shifted the terrains of power, "irregulars" consisted not only of midwives but could include "homeopaths, hydropaths, botanical physicians, eclectics, all highly critical of the European-trained urban and aristocratic physician."[51] The unfettered circulation of abortifacient advertising threatened the business prospects of allopathic physicians: "As more and more irregulars began to advertise abortion services openly, especially after 1840, regular physicians grew more and more nervous about losing their practices to healers who would provide a service that more and more American women after 1840 began to want."[52] Nathan Stormer observes that the AMA used abortion as "a litmus test of quackery."[53] By allowing abortion providers to constitute medicine's "internal enemy," the AMA used abortion to concretize professional hierarchy. Although they would never use the precise phrasing of the "back-alley," I agree with Alicia Gutierrez-Romine's assertion that the AMA's anti-abortion campaign set some of the rhetorical foundations for the "stereotype of the back-alley abortionist."[54]

By labeling providers "irregulars" and "quacks," the AMA's production of professional ethos targeted abortion through appeals to nineteenth-century racial anxieties of "declining civilization." With plunging birth rates of white Anglo-Saxon women and rising rates of immigration, "race suicide" rhetorics proliferated: "Not only did a woman seem to carry the fate of her kin in her womb, she seemed to carry the fate of an entire class, ethnicity, race, and nation."[55] As enslavement and Indigenous dispossession were justified by appeals to "civilization," AMA physicians like Horatio R. Storer juxtaposed the so-called civilized nature of white Anglo-Saxon Protestants against the alleged "barbarism" of the enslaved, Indigenous populations, Irish immigrants, and others.[56] As Stormer aptly summarizes, "In nineteenth-century medicine, morality and monstrosity were deeply imbricated in practice because 'health' and 'morality' were almost interchangeable terms. The good woman bearing children was well."[57]

Much like the precedent set by penny papers decades prior, the circulation of newspaper stories and fictional literature complemented AMA's efforts to jolt public sentiment about abortion.[58] Between 1850 and 1870, "there was a veritable explosion of 'criminal abortion narratives,' and sensational 'true crime' novels and novellas."[59] Fictional genres constituted the "problem" of abortion while news outlets influenced anti-abortion legislative action by reporting on significant stories. For instance, in January 1863, the *New York Times* printed gripping stories of abortion deaths.[60] In other cases, journalists attempted to catch criminal practitioners in action. Later, throughout July 1871, reporter Augustus St. Clair and a woman claiming to be pregnant visited abortion providers in the city. As the team went from office to office, they recorded their experiences and published the exposé "The Evil of the Age."

Stories of untimely deaths received plentiful page space. As Mohr tracks, "Through 1870 and the first half of 1871, the *Times* gave extensive, featured coverage to a series of lurid abortifacient homicide cases."[61] Carrying echoes of the Mary Rogers story, the *New York Times*' coverage of the August 1871 trunk mystery sparked public frenzy. A train porter noticed a "fetid smell emanating from a small trunk." The exposé vividly narrated the woman's corpse and tied those discussions to fears of dangerous and "foreign" practitioners, making "explicit ties among anti-abortion sentiments, racism, and life politics" by denigrating Dr. Jacob Rosenzweig, a Jewish practitioner. "The *New York Times* contributed to an emerging campaign in the United States to criminalize abortion while associating the practice with foreigners and so-called dysgenic individuals who threatened the welfare of white, middle-class Americans."[62] Lurid public stories have long been part of a rhetorical ecology of abortion criminality.

Even as some efforts to abrogate abortion were spurred by logics of exposure, other attempts at restriction relied on legal repression to limit what could be said about abortion in public. Weary of white women's declining birth rate and the availability of so-called lewd material, moral reformers sought to staunch the flow of literature, pornography, and sexual education materials. Anthony Comstock led these efforts with the New York Society for the Suppression of Vice (NYSSV). He and likeminded colleagues believed that what appeared to be the moral degradation of the body politic was attributable to "obscene" literature available in urban environments and the failure of white Anglo-Saxon Protestant women to meet their nation-building duties of moral motherhood. The NYSSV lobbied the federal government for anti-vice laws and was profoundly successful with the 1873 Comstock Act, which criminalized the circulation of any information about contraception and abortifacients. Despite abortion's increased criminalization and gags on speech brought on by the Comstock Act, abortion was widely accepted, considered an "open secret," and practiced by doctors and midwives alike.[63]

By 1880, state statutes had accomplished nationwide criminalization, and despite the Comstock Act's prohibitions, newspapers continued to materialize the sanitary and moral dangers of abortion in the late nineteenth century. Articles both reinforced the xenophobic AMA campaigns against midwives and singled out physicians' unprofessional double standards. Aligning with the first period of the illegal abortion epoch, Reagan traces one exemplary series published in the *Chicago Times* from December 1888 to January 1889 that not only resulted in the deft displacement of the quickening doctrine from public discourse but also turned the tide on punishing women for abortions rather than providers. Posing as a couple, two journalists aimed to simultaneously expose the "social cesspool" of the underworld and the "respectable physicians" who would perform abortions anyway.[64] Vividly detailing "the appearance of midwives and their homes, their cleanliness or lack thereof, and their accents," the twenty-five-part series revealed how rhetorical appeals to sanitation and morality could stage a racializing location to denigrate practitioners while attracting tremendous readership and profit in the process.[65]

Detailing the social scourge of irregulars, however, was secondary to charging AMA-affiliated physicians with hypocrisy for their willingness to perform abortions. Published when Chicago was a center of medical training, journalists' exposés took great pains to identify hypocritical practitioners. For example, the *Chicago Times* juxtaposed pencil sketches of "reputable physicians" to "abortionists" and portrayed abortion providers as fur-clad and greedy. In this context, the investigative reports damaged physicians as they "threatened the profession's identity as morally pure and trustworthy."[66] The *Journal of the American Medical Association* engaged anti-Black appeals in its accusations that abortion providers were "blackening the good name of our noble profession."[67] Repeated associations of abortion providers with blackness were no accidental turns of phrase—they reflected a systematic attempt at suturing racial hierarchy and controlling the boundaries of legitimate medicine.

The exposé's attack on the morality of AMA physicians encouraged members to dissociate themselves from physician abortion providers and channel their ire toward women who procured the procedure. Although they had once urged prosecution of abortion providers, the AMA "switched to recommending the prosecution of women" and challenged the quickening doctrine.[68] This shift, which Reagan in part attributes to the status slight brought on by the exposé, was supported by the newspaper's rhetorical association of abortion with infanticide. Cartoons collapsing differences between pre-quickening abortions and the murder of children became a public pedagogy that "taught others a new way to think about abortion."[69] This rhetorical collapse delegitimated quickening by framing even early abortion as the murder of a moral being and minimizing views of abortion as a mechanical way of restoring menstruation.

The greater use of nonmedical instruments to self-manage abortions helped to associate blame with pregnant people themselves. While herbal remedies dominated early nineteenth-century methods for ending pregnancies, by the end of the nineteenth century, rapid urbanization aligned with the shift from home remedies to medical instruments, particularly "true after the invention of the curette in the late nineteenth century."[70] Although the wire coat hanger today visually signifies unsafe, self-induced abortion, it was not invented until 1903 by Albert J. Parkhouse. Instead, "women employed a wide array of instruments found within their homes to induce miscarriages, including knitting needles, crochet hooks, hairpins, scissors, and button hooks."[71] While these instruments amplified infection risk, patients were often just as vulnerable visiting an obstetrician. It is crucial to remember that "puerperal fever was the scourge of nineteenth-century obstetrics, and abortion, like childbirth, makes women vulnerable to puerperal fever by creating sites for infection within the uterus."[72] For most of the century, European and US doctors rejected the idea that they could be the source of puerperal fever. Ironically, as back-alley abortion rhetoric would come to leverage spatial appeals to infection control, obstetrical textbooks did not recommend antiseptic techniques for delivery until about 1880.[73]

Abortion in the Twentieth-Century United States

As the twentieth century dawned, American Medical Association members and obstetrical specialists pushed a second anti-abortion campaign during the Progressive Era. People continued to seek the procedure, and physicians looked toward "therapeutic abortion" loopholes for cases of impending maternal harm to circumvent the law.[74] The AMA offered a three-pronged strategy for shifting the tide of public opinion: reeducating the public with moral "reminders" of the procedure's danger, amplifying anti-midwife campaigns to dissociate abortion providers from the boundaries of professionalized medicine, and assisting law enforcement at the local level.[75] In 1906, the AMA created an investigative organization to "collect information on quackery and patent medicines.[76] As "vice commissions" targeted midwives, hospitals collaborated with law enforcement to gather inquests into presumed abortion deaths: "By 1917, if not earlier, state authorities had persuaded Chicago hospitals to pledge their cooperation in the investigation of abortion cases."[77] Bedside dying declarations that led to the prosecution of abortion providers were common until the end of the 1930s, demonstrating the lengths to which the state would go to regulate sexual behavior and punish patients in their most vulnerable moments. Reagan ultimately describes the complex relationship between the law and medicine: "While some physicians actively sought an alliance with the state in enforcing the criminal abortion laws, most physicians who cooperated with the state did so out of their fear of being arrested as a suspect in an abortion case."[78] Whether an active alliance or fear of their own criminalization, the AMA built extensive regulatory reach in its long-standing efforts to suture professional standing.

In the 1930s, the second period of the illegal abortion epoch, a structural transformation in medicine intensified the visibility of criminalized abortions in hospitals.[79] The Great Depression led to skyrocketing rates of abortions, accompanied by horrific septic infections. While physicians in hospitals performed "therapeutic abortions" for a myriad of physical ailments, hospitals segregated septic abortions from other obstetrical cases because of "the danger of spreading infection and dedicating entire wards to caring for emergency abortion cases."[80] Antibiotics were relatively new and in limited circulation. Although penicillin was discovered in 1928, it would not become widely available until the 1950s.[81] As pseudonymous abortion provider "Dr. Ted" recalled in Patricia Miller's *Worst of Times*: "In 1942, I first saw women with septic abortions . . . antibiotics existed, but they were very scarce. Penicillin was around, but most of it was going to the war effort."[82]

Because of the devastating consequences of septic abortion cases, there were efforts to expand the scope of what would warrant a legal, therapeutic abortion. Dr. Frederick Taussig's notably conservative law proposal expanded therapeutic exceptions to include economic disparity and the threat to the pregnant person's life. The 1930s also saw an expansion of nonhospital abortion providers; specialists provided thousands of procedures in this legal gray area. As such, between the 1930s and 1940s, the definitions of criminal abortion mutated. As Johanna Schoen notes, "Increasingly, it was not the reason for the abortion but rather certain markers of the procedure itself—who had performed it, where had it been performed, how successful it had been" that made the difference. Although police raided providers, they were often willing to look the other way "when abortions were performed in safe environments by skilled practitioners."[83]

Beginning around 1940, what Reagan marks as the third period of the illegal abortion epoch, police involvement and journalistic coverage shifted. Whereas law enforcement had once targeted providers whose outcomes gravely harmed patients, trusted providers and living patients were now caught in the crosshairs. These raids disrupted an established, functional system of referral relied upon by physicians and pregnant people alike.[84] Moreover, pregnant people were more explicitly criminalized. No longer did police simply learn about abortion providers through deathbed confessions from septic patients; surviving patients were now brought to court to testify against providers.[85] Two journalistic trends emerged. First, the press frequently covered police raids, which built larger perceptions of widespread criminality and bolstered the state's justification for engaging in these raids.[86] Second, wartime women's magazines—edited by women—began to discuss abortions more openly, specifically the devastating human consequences of legal repression: "During and immediately after the war, these popular magazines criticized a society too hard at war and too little concerned with the wives and children left behind."[87] This trend should not be read as feminist; rather, it was aligned with a percolation of pronatalism and traditional gender roles among women of color and white women alike.[88] Reagan describes this period as one in which these narratives coincided with stories of women meeting intermediaries and being blindfolded to maintain the provider's anonymity.[89] While some of these stories were the product of first-person journalistic accounts, others were recalled through oral histories conducted decades later.

Between 1950 and 1970, a new fracture in medical authority resulted in fewer abortions being performed in hospitals. Even after state laws criminalized abortions pre-quickening, laws often deferred to physician authority to perform therapeutic abortions when the pregnant person's life was at risk. Although a panoply of physical conditions would previously warrant a "therapeutic" abortion, by the end of the 1940s, the medical community began to debate legitimate warrants for termination. Medicine experienced a newly emergent "professional crisis" that pushed physicians with perceived high ratios of therapeutic abortions to live births into a "defensive" position.[90] Harking back to nineteenth-century AMA anxieties over professional boundaries, physicians caught in this contemporary "bitter" debate "felt that the new disunity over the abortion issue hurt the standing of physicians as expert, objective practitioners of science."[91] The solution became a twenty-year "offensive." Hospitals crafted large committees that required almost unanimous approval, which diffused legal liability from any one provider but had the effect of "legal-izing medicine and medical-izing the law, at once."[92] The fallout of these repressive tactics was devastating. As therapeutic standards tightened, it was predominantly white women with private insurance who could still access the procedure in hospitals; in New York City between 1943 and 1962, white women accounted for 91 percent of the therapeutic hospital abortions.[93] By contrast, Black and Puerto Rican women not only received fewer therapeutic hospital abortions; when they did, they were often coerced into sterilization.[94] At this time, four times as many women of color died from abortions than did white women.[95]

In the mid-1950s, the fourth period of the illegal abortion epoch, reform efforts emerged from several disparate medical and legal sources. Reform rhetorics ranged from sensational visual displays of harm to more affectively muted and professionally enclaved technical deliberations in medicine and public health. In both cases, those suffering from the outcomes of bad abortions were mediated through photographs of tools and aggregated into anonymized statistics. On the one hand, the circulation of crime scene photography created "a visual language of secrecy, criminality, and emotional affect which reflected and reinforced contemporary medical debates on abortion."[96] On the other hand, the Planned Parenthood Federation of America (PPFA) shifted its view on abortion. While Planned Parenthood once argued for the morality of birth control by denigrating abortion, a 1955 conference gathered physicians to share data regarding women who were aborting, whether for therapeutic reasons or not.[97] The statistical aggregation enabled PPFA to position itself in "opposition to the journalistic exposés of abortion that had been a defining feature of U.S. public discourse" since the 1840s.[98] Four years after this conference in 1959, the American Law Institute created a draft of a model penal code that would allow abortions in limited cases, such as physical or mental harm to a pregnant person, fetal abnormalities, and rape and incest. Amid these changes, police raids of abortion providers were still common, frequently targeting Black practitioners.[99]

The 1960s proved to be a transformative decade for public representations of abortion. As mortality and morbidity rates skyrocketed, the connection between abortion law and disability became acute. A rubella outbreak that caused infected pregnant people to deliver disabled children was used to warrant liberalizing abortion exceptions in hospital committees.[100] The 1962 case of Sherri Finkbine, host of the children's show *Romper Room*, was an important moment of public visibility for abortion, routed through themes of ableism and the morality of white motherhood. Finkbine had ingested thalidomide, a sleeping aid subsequently discovered to cause fetal development issues. While Finkbine tried to pursue a therapeutic abortion in the United States, delays and setbacks required her to travel to Sweden. Appealing to her identity as a moral mother of five, the media coverage surrounding Finkbine's story supported reform efforts but simultaneously warranted regulatory practices that restrict abortion today.[101]

The 1960s also witnessed a proliferation of grassroots movements that circumvented restrictive abortion statutes. In 1962, Patricia Maginnis developed the Citizens' Committee for Humane Abortion Laws in San Francisco. By 1965, Maginnis was joined by Rowena Gurner and Lana Clarke Phelan. Together they ran two organizations, the Society for Humane Abortion (SHA, formerly the Citizens' Committee for Humane Abortion Laws) and the Association to Repeal Abortion Laws (ARAL), to normalize abortion and advocate "for a reversal in the power of physicians and patients."[102] SHA was a nonprofit organization that pursued educational and political advocacy, whereas ARAL connected people to quality abortion providers in Mexico, creating referral sheets and personally visiting clinics. Gurner and Maginnis requested that those they referred provide feedback about the quality of clinics and providers. Indeed, as Murillo notes, "in the borderlands, terminating a pregnancy was very much a binational venture. By no means was the abortion business in Juárez, or any other Mexican border city, simply part of inherent Mexican lawlessness or immorality. Instead, it involved a more complicated reciprocal binational relationship between businesspersons, women, doctors, and clinic staff, lawyers, and activists attempting to address a deficit in reproductive health-care services while making a profit."[103] Several years later, in 1969, the Jane Collective emerged in Chicago. While they initially functioned as a referral service to connect women to clandestine abortion providers like civil rights organizer and surgeon Dr. T. R. M. Howard, Jane members eventually began to perform abortions themselves once they realized that some of their chosen providers were not trained doctors. The group was primarily motivated by feminist values of reproductive autonomy and keeping patients out of septic wards.[104] By the early 1970s, the Young Lords Party, a multiracial Puerto Rican group, sought to bring abortions under community control, given the long-standing history of sterilization abuse in Puerto Rico and New York City municipal hospitals.[105] "Their slogan 'End all genocide. Abortions Under Community Control' encapsulated the notion of truly voluntary fertility control."[106]

Between 1967 and 1973, some clergy also helped pregnant people seek safe abortions. Nationwide, there were clergy consultation services (CCS) that helped to connect women to trusted providers. While the CCS mainly consisted of "white, middle- and upper-class, middle-aged" men from diverse faith practices, their statement of purpose declared, "Believing as clergy that there are higher laws and moral obligations transcending legal codes, we agree that it is our pastoral responsibility and religious duty to give aid and assistance to all women with problem pregnancies."[107] Pastor Howard Moody was part of a group of clergy assembled to assist pregnant people with obtaining safe abortions and organized to support legislation such as New York's 1970 reform of existing legal prohibitions to allow abortions until twenty-four weeks gestation. Much like ARAL, CCS created "Negative Lists" to help people avoid low quality providers. The "Negative List" trafficked in back-alley appeals, describing some providers as "butchers," while describing others' clinical spaces as "filthy," "dirty," or "slum offices."[108] With representation in twenty-five states, they used their status as clergy to provide "reinforcement, encouragement, and comfort" to people seeking to terminate unwanted pregnancies as well as to trusted abortion providers.[109] Once abortion laws were liberalized in New York, the CCS shifted attention to ensuring that doctors could not price gouge for services. Anticipating critiques of abortion as a single-axis issue, Moody also specified that advocates do not get so focused on abortion that they fail to see the larger picture of Black self-determination and anti-war efforts.[110]

Ultimately there is no "smoking gun" origin point to back-alley abortion rhetoric: these seeds were sown across the long history of abortion criminalization through a confluence of journalistic, medical, and legal discourses. Although abortion was not always a crime, reproduction was always a way of suturing the US body politic through pronatalist and moralist ideologies as well as coercive means of fertility limitation. Doctors seeking to leverage political power and maintain racialized professional boundaries diminished practitioners who could challenge that authority. Often sensationalist public discourses were shaped by these legal and medical forces, just as the public discourse reciprocally shaped these technical discourses. With any criminalized economy, opportunistic providers emerged, but enclaved grassroots organizations—some fighting on the axis of gender and others articulating intersecting gender, racial, and moral concerns—sought to staunch the impact of restrictive laws by dismantling the very structural issues that led people to what would become abortion's proverbial "back-alley."

Tracing Back-Alley Abortion's Rhetorical History

Whereas many outstanding histories of criminalized abortion address how back-alley abortion rhetoric did not fully mirror individual experiences attaining criminalized abortion care, this book investigates key sites of back-alley abortion's rhetorical power. This study, therefore, traces what David Zarefsky calls "rhetorical discourse as a *force* in history."[111] As a durable rhetorical force in the history of abortion, I look toward how back-alley abortion appeals (and closely related terms such as back rooms and back streets) affectively crafted expectations of medical encounters, sutured public memory, and served anti-abortion interests along racialized, classed, and gendered axes. By centering the circulation of back-alley abortion rhetoric, I follow Robin E. Jensen in investigating the "formation of arguments, appeals, and narratives" within abortion's larger rhetorical ecology.[112] Tracing back-alley abortion's distributed discursive and affective touch points within this ecology reveals how the appeal sticks, transforms, and spreads, much like a virus. An ecological approach suits back-alley abortion because the phrase accrued new weight and persuasive capacity as it traveled through different points of (de)criminalization. Back-alley abortion rhetoric gathered force from how back-alleys were long deployed in public discourse before they encountered abortion and mutated through repeated appropriation. As a fragmented, constitutive, and world-making rhetoric, back-alley abortion also presents a crucial locus to understand "the way we view counter-rhetorics, issues of cooptation, and strategies of rhetorical production and circulation."[113] Understanding its capacity for co-optation makes the anti-abortion uptake of back-alley abortion that

I discuss in chapter 4 all the more intelligible: the back-alley is a variable, multiple, and affectively saturated rhetoric.

Rather than focus on the agential capacities of any discrete rhetor or organization, I center textual and visual invocations of back-alley rhetoric in order to distill patterns among related discursive fragments, assembling them according to their persuasive function for different audiences and contexts. As a rhetorical critic, I approach texts through a variety of rhetorical methods including close textual, visual, affective, and circulation analyses to toggle between different critical vantage points. Sometimes, I zoom in to investigate the minutiae of an artifact's persuasive compositional features. Other times, I zoom out to track how those features reached differently positioned audiences. Toggling between these scales enables me to understand not only *what* was persuasive about a particular text but also *how* it was persuasive in a given moment. In assembling speeches, documentaries, cartoons, conference proceedings, legal decisions, literature, and news fragments, I ultimately resist a totalizing story of what back-alley abortion meant for different audiences and at different times.[114] At the risk of sounding pedantic, this book's title, *Back-Alley Abortion: A Rhetorical History*, is decidedly not *Back-Alley Abortion: "The" Rhetorical History*. I prefer the indefinite article—"a"—to the definite "the" to emphasize the inherent partiality of uncovering and narrating a series of encounters that present coherence only after my retrospective assembly of textual fragments.[115] This kind of retelling hauntingly mirrors our post-*Dobbs* reality: we will only ever grasp the magnitude of harm that criminalizing abortion enacts on reproductive bodies in retrospect, after the individual stories have been told, and they have been circulated and aggregated—once the rhetoric catches up with the experiences.[116]

Because any telling of history is partial, I strive to foreground the theoretical and political priorities of the reproductive justice (RJ) movement while narrating this rhetorical history. Twelve Black women coined "reproductive justice" at a Chicago pro-choice conference in 1994 by "conjoining reproductive rights and social justice."[117] By no means a US-centric movement, RJ has been shaped by global liberation efforts and operates in a globally interconnected context today. Critical of both choice-based rhetoric and the efficacy of US constitutional rights to fully redress reproductive injustices, RJ is grounded in a human rights framework with three pillars: "the right *not* to have a child; the right to *have* a child; and the right to *parent* children in safe and healthy environments."[118] Although the human rights framework is not without its limitations, Zakiya Luna argues that the reproductive justice movement has harnessed some of the more radical dimensions of human rights to enable the movement to maintain a global sensibility, bring those concerns to a domestic US context, and "retain a level of rhetorical flexibility when confronted with unforeseen reproductive concerns."[119] This rhetorical flexibility makes the RJ framework both a rich resource for guiding activism toward a liberatory telos and an indispensable methodology for delineating whether rhetoric effectuates that telos in any given context.[120]

Although some of my assembled archive predates the emergence of the reproductive justice movement, reproductive justice theory provides crucial analytic priorities as the framework germinated by a long legacy of Black feminist political organizing and theory building. Drawing upon the Combahee River Collective's 1977 assertion that "major systems of oppression are interlocking," several exigencies within 1960s and 1970s abortion activism necessitated this RJ framework far before it was coined in 1994.[121] To be sure, women of color have always been active participants in fighting for a robust suite of reproductive rights and access.[122] Black women like civil rights attorney Florynce Kennedy, for instance, not only spearheaded constitutional challenges to abortion restrictions but also saved relevant activist materials that appear in this book.[123] Black women have also built and operated abortion clinics, like Byllye Avery and colleagues' Gainesville Women's Health Center in Florida.[124] However, the quest for legal abortion often focused on the experiences of middle-class white women, even as Black, Puerto Rican, Latina, Chicana, and Indigenous people were most profoundly harmed by the procedure's criminalization. Recognizing how abortion rights activists were motivated by appeals to back-alley abortion, Angela Davis draws on back-alley topoi to illustrate how alienating advocacy abortion rights as a single issue could be:

> As for the abortion rights campaign itself, how could women of color fail to grasp its urgency? They were far more familiar than their white sisters with the murderously clumsy scalpels of inept abortionists seeking profit in illegality. . . . If the abortion rights campaign of the early 1970s needed to be reminded that women of color wanted desperately to escape the back-room quack abortionists, they should have also realized that these same women were not about to express pro-abortion sentiments. . . . When Black and Latina women resort to abortions in such large numbers, the stories they tell are not so much about their desire to be free of their pregnancy, but rather about the miserable social conditions which dissuade them from bringing new lives into the world.[125]

Sterilization abuse, amplified exposure to environmental toxicities, police brutality, and unaffordable childcare—to name a few examples—made the questions of safely having and rearing children as exigent as the need to terminate.[126] Without being guided by an intersectional perspective that critically examines the interactions of race, class, and gender formations in producing reproductive injustice, this book would certainly reinscribe a narrow and decontextualized focus on choice-based abortion rhetorics steeped in whiteness.[127] Instead, taking seriously that an important telos for RJ theory is to dismantle white supremacy, I interrogate the animating role of whiteness as it manifests in back-alley rhetorics of moral purity, sanitation, and criminality.[128] As one example, I show how practitioners of color—often Black men prone to attributions of criminality—defined their clinical practices in contradistinction to the back-alley because the butcher was a racialized rhetorical constraint they had to overcome in their practices.

Similarly, the RJ framework demands attention to how back-alley rhetorics constituted the gendered contours of people having criminalized abortion encounters. While this book follows scholars such as Shui-yin Sharon Yam and Natalie Fixmer-Oraiz who emphasize the need to decouple binary gender from reproductive care,[129] I will frequently use the term "women" to gesture toward the pregnant people largely *framed* to encounter a back-alley abortion. This is not because only cisgender women had abortions—or unsafe abortions at that. Rather, I deploy "women" when they were framed as victims of back-alley butchers to try to generate social and legal change in sometimes racist and often paternalistic ways. In Condit's words, back-alley rhetoric "told the story of a good, ordinary person faced by social (not natural) circumstances that led *her* into evil scenes and self-destruction, magnified by the gory details and scenes *she* was required to face."[130] Understanding how this "good ordinary person" so often fit the subject position of a vulnerable white cisgender woman showcases the very exigencies the RJ framework has long problematized. Considering both that queer activists have long animated reproductive justice coalitions and the continued stigma surrounding queer family formation, I deploy the term "pregnant people" when I am more generally referring to the impacts of criminalized reproductive care.[131] Taken together, the affordances of reproductive justice theory, including the intersecting rhetorics of race, gender, and class, offer crucial ethical priorities when investigating back-alley abortion's participation in a criminalized abortion rhetorical ecology.

Conceptualizing Back-Alley Abortion Rhetoric

Three conceptual coordinates illuminate how back-alley abortion rhetoric operates within the criminalized abortion rhetorical ecology. First, although individuals might define their back-alley abortion located within a specific place, the back-alley is also a rhetorically constructed *space*, a general constellation of features that mark a dangerous threat. Second, back-alley abortion rhetoric invokes a monstrous *kakoethos*, or a stigmatizing negative character that attributes malintent and a lack of scruples to practitioners, their tools, and substandard locations of practice. Third, back-alley abortion circulates public *feelings* rooted in purity cultures, such as horror, disgust, shame and fear. These features, especially space, *kakoethos*, and feeling, are not only familiar concepts for rhetorical scholars; they feature what is unique about the *rhetorical* history undertaken in this book.

A Dangerous Topos: The Back-Alley as Space and Place

When you hear the phrase "back-alley abortion"—and especially if you would define your own criminalized abortion experience as such—your mind might drift to a particular place *where* your criminalized or unsafe abortion occurred and the ambient surroundings of that medical encounter. This place could have been a nonmedical bedroom or simply unsanitary because of wear and tear on the medical equipment or the presence of residual contaminating bodily fluids. Importantly for this book, the back-alley is also a rhetorical *space*—one that is imagined, discursively constructed, and imbued with affective intensities. According to Danielle Endres and Samantha Senda-Cook, the distinctions between space and place are essential but interrelated. Whereas "place refers to particular locations (e.g., a city, a particular shopping mall, or a park) that are semibounded, a combination of material and symbolic qualities, and embodied," space "refers to a more general notion of how society and social practice are regulated (and sometimes disciplined) by spatial thinking."[132] While we may be encouraged to imagine back-alley abortion exclusively in terms of place, this book accentuates its simultaneous status as a *spatial* organizing logic that limits in advance our imagining of specific places that exist in the world. As Raka Shome aptly puts it, space is "a product of relations that are themselves active and constantly changing material practices through which it comes into being."[133] Shome's insight comports with abortion historians' contention that back-alley abortions were actually a function of the law; abortion's criminalized status organizes bodily movement and funnels people into potentially dangerous places while producing an imagined social space of anticipation that we come to define as a back-alley abortion.

While Endres and Senda-Cook speak to important differences between place and space, back-alley abortion illustrates how these distinctions are not concrete and are rhetorically connected to one another. Back-alley abortion occupies an undecided middle point because it is *both* a space and a place—and *neither.* As a space, its invocation and presumed existence often have been invoked to say that social practice, in this case, abortion—should be regulated so that pregnant people avoid dangerous and dehumanizing reproductive encounters. Abortion's back-alley—and as chapter 1 argues, *any* back-alley—is an imagined spatial repository existing in any city or town in which planning has enabled the construction of buildings in such proximity as to produce the emptiness of an alley that can be figured as dangerous. Likewise, self-defined back-alley abortion narratives clearly delineate that they happened *somewhere,* making the back-alley into a concrete *place* that becomes the site of individual recollections of abortion experiences. Back-alley narratives can be emplaced to describe the experience of a dirty, disgusting, and dangerous pregnancy termination. Yet there is one more instantiation of the back-alley that troubles the place/space distinction; the phrase "back-alley abortion" is implied in slogans like "We will never go back." Go back to where? As I discuss in chapter 3, "We will never go back" offers an enthymeme whose missing premise invokes an imagined return to back-alley abortion yet does not fully imply a concrete *place* where such procedures occurred or a defined regulatory *spatial* network of power and control that once criminalized them. Instead, the phrase introduces the notion of time, implying a policy change and a civic regression to a past era that imagines returning people to a dangerous clinic.

Monstrous *Kakoethos*: Butchers, Clinics, and Techniques

Back-alley rhetoric also gestures to how abortion providers become saturated with stigma. In 1963, Erving Goffman theorized stigma as a function of spoiled identities or an "attribute that is deeply discrediting."[134] Understood as a mark of undesirability, stigma has historically been understood as what separates and renders visible—hence the term "stigmata" that marks deviant bodies for surveillant and exclusionary purposes. As Anuradha Kumar and colleagues argue, "stigma can only be created by over-simplifying complex situations and abortion is no different."[135] Due to long-standing criminalization efforts, abortion stigma is a strong generator of feelings of fear, guilt, and shame and is connected to negative views of providers. Abortion stigma can also contribute to delayed care and clinical complications, creating a stigmatizing feedback loop.[136] As chapter 2 discusses, back-alley abortion transpires as a stigmatizing interplay among three conceptual entities: the provider, their spaces of provision, and the methods (both tools and techniques) they employ to perform abortions. As I discussed in the previous section, this stigmatization was evident in the AMA's practices of isolating, separating, and denigrating "irregular" (often racialized) practitioners. Also called "boundary work" by rhetoricians of science, health, and medicine, this stigmatization allowed the nascent AMA to legitimize itself while constraining the medical ethos of midwives and practitioners of color.[137] Back-alley abortion rhetoric enables this medicalized boundary formation in at least three ways.

First, the durability of the back-alley butcher bears witness to abortion stigma's power to constitute flattened and denigrative public opinions about abortion providers' characters. While the ethos of health care providers can wax and wane based on their skill, trustworthiness, and goodwill, abortion stigma does not diminish a provider's clinical ethos so much as it inscribes a rhetorically debilitating sense of *kakoethos*, or bad character. Attributions of ethos in health care and parenthood are not available to everyone, and are often explicitly denied to Black people.[138] Eliminating the possibility for an abortion provider to have rhetorical capacities of good judgment, skill, and trustworthiness for patient well-being that might be enjoyed by "regular" health care providers, abortion stigma reduces abortion providers to a general sense of "badness." As Jenell Johnson aptly notes, stigma generally "allows slippage between many permutations of badness: worthless, evil, dirty, ugly, weak, cowardly, dangerous."[139] The back-alley butcher amplifies the general stigma foisted on abortion providers and enables anti-abortion advocates to generalize *all* practitioners through a back-alley frame.

Second, the back-alley butcher's *kakoethos* and their spaces of practice are mutually constitutive. The "back-alley" presents abortion clinics as dangerous sites of liminality that fail to meet the standards of moral and sanitary arrangement and thus define the *type* of person that would operate therein. They are disorganized, dirty, and disgusting vectors of access to unsafe abortions and bodily harm. Indeed, the back-alley butcher's bad character is conditioned by how we speak of (in)appropriate spaces of abortion provision. In other words, the back-alley butcher is not just intrinsically repugnant; they leach their lousy character from the stigmatized spaces they are said to inhabit. This has deadly material consequences. The stigma attached to abortion clinics renders them targets of terrorism and communicative violence like sidewalk harassment.[140] As Lori A. Brown asserts, abortion clinics are "an obvious choice" to understand how "spaces are inherently contested and politicized" based upon legal strictures and local building ordinances.[141]

Third, the techniques and tools to end pregnancies mediate the relationship between back-alley butcher characters, their provision spaces, and the pregnant people affected. As discussed in the brief history of criminalized abortion above, the means of ending a pregnancy have varied from organic herbs to inorganic metals. Improperly used tools can introduce infection or perforate parts of the reproductive system that become the understandable site of fear, disgust, and horror. The tools constitute back-alley rhetoric because they traverse corporeal boundaries and concretize the relationship between the space, provider, and patient's body. While *Back-Alley Abortion: A Rhetorical History* is interested in the circulation of the phrase, visuality is a component of how back-alley abortion rhetoric circulated through public discourse. As Cara A. Finnegan writes, "images become inventional resources in the public sphere."[142] Examining the production, reproduction, and circulation of visual images of back-alley abortion rhetoric—such as (but not limited to) coat hangers, disgusting spaces, and pregnant people affected—provides insight into the power of the back-alley as a stand-in for all criminalized abortion.

The tripartite stigma that renders the back-alley butcher hypervisible and reduces their every action to bad character constructs what Cassidy D. Ellis theorizes as the "abortion monster." Arguing that the abortion monster is a product of "anti-abortion rhetoric that dehumanizes abortion patients and providers," I point out that abortion rights advocates also invoked this monster—albeit for reasons of health care access and safety.[143] The back-alley, the butcher, and their tools are easily rendered intelligible by theories of monstrosity. For instance, Jeffrey Jerome Cohen observes that the monster is defined by a "refusal to participate in the classificatory order of things." In the case of the back-alley mythos, this refusal manifests as participation in a criminalized underground that violates imperatives of sanitation and moral purity, embedding the monster as a character in the imagined terrain of criminalized reproduction. Moreover, because "the monster stands at the threshold of becoming," an agent who can interrupt fetal becoming is ripe to be labeled monstrous. Monstrosity is not distributed equally across cultures—indeed, the monster "dwells at the gates of difference."[144] Bernadette Marie Calafell extends this observation: "Cultural anxieties and fears around Otherness, whether they are about race, class, gender, sexuality, body size, or ability, manifest themselves in representations of both literal and symbolic monstrosity."[145] As such, the back-alley amalgamates a monstrous character, location, and technique, enveloping many identities subjected to stigma, otherness, and dehumanization. Regardless of its prevalence in the historical record, the sheer endurance of this monstrous figure generates and circulates public feelings about abortion writ large.

Purity, Pollution, and Public Feelings

Back-alley rhetoric is affected by discourses of purity and pollution that attach a suite of public feelings to abortion providers, clinical spaces, and techniques of practice. As Mary Douglas specifies, dirt "exists in the eye of the beholder."[146] Intimately tethered to several religious doctrines, purity and pollution discourses far exceed concerns about personal or spatial hygiene. Instead, as Douglas elucidates, "eliminating [dirt] is not a negative movement, but a positive effort to organize the environment."[147] By positive, Douglas means *productive*—purity practices create moral classification and order practices. Thus, back-alley rhetoric reveals how stigmatized reproductive care is deeply conditioned by seemingly innocuous appeals to clean clinical space. It might feel counterintuitive to be critical of sanitary clinical spaces, given that uncontrolled infection caused many abortion-related deaths. However, as Alexis Shotwell laments, "A great deal of harm is done based on a metaphysics of purity."[148] Purity cultures imbricate physical sanitary questions with sexualized morality, both of which are inextricably raced, classed, and gendered.[149] By investigating how back-alley rhetoric articulates dynamics of sanitation and sexualized morality, this book takes a stance "against purity," which as Shotwell argues is "not to be for pollution, harm, sickness, or premature death. It is to be against the rhetorical or conceptual attempt to delineate and delimit the world into something separable, disentangled, and homogenous."[150] Orienting "against purity" recognizes a long history of public health practices of quarantine leveraging infection control and sexual morality to police national borders.[151] Purity also greases the wheels for racialized attributions of criminality, as Rima L. Vesely-Flad argues: "In the United States, criminal law and institutions of punishment control and contain Black bodies that threaten to pollute society's moral boundaries."[152] As imbricated into back-alley abortion rhetoric, purity discourses index points of white anxiety—sometimes stemming from self-identifying feminist activists—over the porousness of both corporeal and national borders, implicating contagions figured both as microscopic bacteria and providers of color.

If purity culture—operating through articulated appeals to physical sanitation and sexualized morality—offers an ideological setting for this book, then the seepage, leakage, and stickiness of this ideology's attendant anxieties speak to the affective force of back-alley abortion rhetoric. Consider your own embodied reaction to an abstinence educator that Jessica Valenti invokes in *The Purity Myth*: "Your body is a wrapped lollipop. When you have sex with a man, he unwraps your lollipop and sucks on it. It may feel great at the time, but, unfortunately, when he's done with you, all you have left for your next partner is a poorly wrapped, saliva-fouled sucker."[153] If, like Valenti and me, you orient against purity, you likely appraise that statement as "disgusting" and have a visceral reaction of revulsion; your nose might scrunch and you might even feel nauseated. I offer this aversive vignette not because I intend to consistently evoke those feelings as you read this book but to illustrate that purity discourses and back-alley abortion rhetoric circulate public feelings about criminalized pregnancy termination, which include but often exceed the boundaries of any one person's bodily feelings.

Back-alley abortion rhetoric mediates a relationship between individual embodied experiences and public deliberation. To be sure, oral histories cited in the epigraphs throughout this book painstakingly documented the feelings of fear, anger, disgust, horror, and relief felt by those seeking to terminate pregnancies in criminalized contexts. Moreover, my archival work revealed deeply emotional accounts of those writing letters of "desperation" to doctors. As we read narrative recollections of abortions that people may define as "back-alley," it may be tempting to consider those avowed feelings of fear, desperation, and disgust as confined to the experiences of individual bodies. By investigating mostly public discourses of back-alley abortion, I aim not to diminish those like Representative Lee who have had those experiences and felt that fear or disgust. Instead, as Stephanie R. Larson notes, "feeling acts as a kind of circuitry to any rhetorical situation and belonging."[154] This book aims to understand how back-alley abortion rhetoric circulated reproductive feelings rooted in purity culture to shape discussions about reproductive health care, ultimately nourishing abortion stigma.

When narrating this rhetorical history, I refer to affect when I am gesturing to particular points of collective attachment to back-alley abortion rhetoric, when the general energy and atmosphere is nebulous and unformed.[155] However, despite their affective intensities, many back-alley discourses are textually based. Taking the lead of Sara Ahmed's reading strategy in the *Cultural Politics of Emotion*, I similarly ask, "What sticks" when back-alley abortion texts circulate? Ahmed helps us break free from thinking about named emotions like disgust, fear, shame, pity, or horror as either self-contained individual feelings or solely public emotional formations that individuals absorb. Instead, as defined emotions move through public invocations of back-alley rhetoric, they shape the bodies that encounter the rhetoric by creating expectations of what a "back-alley" abortion would be. Last, I invoke feeling to gesture toward the sensorial texturing that connects a more nebulous affect to a more concretized emotional formation. Appeals to awful sights, bad smells, grimy textures, and disrespectful speech do more than affect an individual body—they help to create a shared, collective sense of urgency. Crucial to these textual descriptors are thick sensory engagements that help to condition the circulation of affect and allow an emotion to be recognizable as disgust, fear, or pity. Debra Hawhee encourages scholars to consider a sensorium as a "bundle of constitutive, participatory tendrils that may help to think about the connective, participatory dimensions of sensing."[156] Back-alley abortion's enduring rhetorical power through time tethers each of these concepts together to condition public understandings of abortion's criminalized ecology.

Overview of Chapters

Back-Alley Abortion: A Rhetorical History unfolds over four main chapters, each oriented around a distinct rhetorically inflected analytic. Although the explicit phrase "back-alley abortion" was not a common way to refer to unsafe abortions before the 1960s, alleys had a long rhetorical life before their association with abortion. Chapter 1 argues that the back-alley rhetorics "before abortion" left what I term an "affective residue" that persisted when the phrase was articulated to abortion care. Surveying fictional and nonfictional textual fragments such as British catalogs of city streets; US sanitary trade publications; Progressive Era legislative and community alley-remediation efforts in Washington, DC; obstetrical literature; newspaper articles; court filings; and nineteenth-century fiction, I uncover consistent discourses of sanitation, morality, and criminality. These discourses left a residue of sensory appeals to olfaction, tactility, and vision, granting back-alley abortion some of its underexplored rhetorical power. *Before abortion*, the phrase was a form of racial classification to define low-income city spaces that lacked sanitation, produced immorality, and evaded legal surveillance. As sanitary, moral and criminal discourses circulated through back-alley appeals, they each left vivid sensory appeals that constitute the residual affects taken up when the back-alley met abortion.

Chapter 2 examines how pre–*Roe v. Wade* appeals to back-alley abortion materialized a *rhetorical medical encounter* that anticipated the worst-case scenario of a criminalized abortion. This chapter addresses two questions: Amid the existing landscape of criminalized abortion, how did back-alley abortion emerge as the common way to refer to unsafe practices, unscrupulous providers, and unsanitary spaces? Once established, how did back-alley abortion warn people against *kakoethotic* providers and unsanitary spaces? The affective residue of back-alleys and visual alley aesthetics met three common metaphors used to describe criminalized abortion: *mills*, *rackets*, and *rings*. Drawing from a confluence of archival material including social movement, journalistic, legal, and medical texts, this chapter addresses how the back-alley rhetorical medical encounter drew boundaries around proper spaces and care providers along racial, classed, and gendered lines. While aimed at patient protection, this rhetoric spoke *for* pregnant people, reinforced medical authority, and included fear appeals to warrant overwrought clinical space requirements.

Whereas chapter 2 situates the back-alley abortion medical encounter in the future tense, chapter 3 speaks to how back-alley abortion organizes the memories of the past. Taking *Roe v. Wade*'s constitutional protections as a point of rupture—but recognizing that rights are insufficient to ensure reproductive justice—I argue that back-alley abortion rhetoric began to function as a form of *visceral public memory*, represented by the unstated premise of the enthymeme "We'll never go back." Extending current frameworks for conceptualizing the public memory of criminalized abortion, the visceral public memory of back-alley abortion holds three distinct features. First, it engages graphic images, descriptions, and iconography that make present a returning past. Second, visceral public memory externalizes for public consumption and political contestation the internal organs of bodies harmed by unsafe abortions. Third, visceral public memory figures the racialized and classed anxieties of national and state borders. The chapter compares two exemplary victims of unsafe abortions. The first is Rosaura "Rosie" Jiménez—the first woman known to have died from an abortion because of the Hyde Amendment, in 1977. The second case examines the 1988 death of Becky Bell, a youth who obtained an illegal abortion instead of submitting to Indiana's parental notification laws. Both cases offer insight into the raced, classed, and nationalistic dynamics of post-*Roe* memories of back-alley abortion rhetoric and the limitations of a choice-based framework in moments of reproductive injustice.

Chapter 4 marks a second transformative moment in back-alley rhetoric to demonstrate how anti-abortion activists hijacked the appeal to warrant clinic closures and provider restrictions. In 2010, a multiagency law enforcement team raided Kermit Gosnell's Philadelphia clinic and found abhorrent conditions, which were painstakingly documented in the grand jury report of his case. I argue that without ever using the phrase "back-alley abortion," the grand jury report engaged the discursive and affective residues of back-alleys. Displaying uncanny echoes of chapter 1, discourses of sanitation, morality, and criminality were replete with vivid sensory appeals to olfaction, tactility, and vision. The report's back-alley rhetoric constituted Gosnell's space, character, and techniques as worthy targets of disgust and outrage. It also constituted the state of Pennsylvania's jurisdictional back-alley as a function of failed state surveillance. The report made these moves while eliding West Philadelphia's long history of structural medical racism, which was deeply relevant to the experiences patients had in this clinic. While the report's introduction touted the case's potential to craft an elusive sense of common ground between abortion rights advocates and adversaries, I demonstrate how the anti-abortion *rhetorical uptake* of the case leveraged the back-alley rhetoric of the grand jury report to advocate for the amplified passage of targeted restriction on abortion providers under the seemingly benign appeal to both "clean clinical space" and "protecting" women from "unscrupulous" clinicians. Anti-abortion activists deftly packaged the case into a horror story for public consumption by generating films, visual rhetoric, and books. The Gosnell grand jury report was invoked in the 2016 US Supreme Court decision *Whole Woman's Health v. Hellerstedt* for posing a then-undue burden on people seeking abortions. I conclude this chapter by considering how back-alley appeals were leveraged to place a crisis pregnancy center in the building Gosnell's clinic once occupied.

Given that in many US jurisdictions abortion is once again a crime, the concluding chapter synthesizes the theoretical and analytical arguments in this book. In the wake of the 2022 *Dobbs v. Jackson Women's Health* decision, I draw on previous chapters' analyses to look to the forward horizon. I examine the post-*Dobbs* circulation of back-alley abortion rhetoric in the art of abortion rights and reproductive justice advocates and the invocation by anti-abortion activists of the long-standing residue of the phrase to warrant criminalizing abortion-inducing medications.

This book argues that ultimately, as a rhetorical medical encounter that sutures public memory but also nourishes stigma, back-alley abortion's rhetorical history is complex and has been used strategically to open and close arguments for abortion access, creating affective investment in many of the publics that have touched this phrase over time.

THE CEMENT ERA

Vol. XV | March, 1917 | No. 3

Alleys—Past and Present

By Charles A. Singler

AN Alley was once a spot where cats were wont to meet,
They much preferred the Alley to the brilliance of the street;
With dissonance they flung their feline toasts upon the night,
And no one ever stopped them, for the Alley was a "sight."

The Alley was the birthplace of the weasel and the rat,
And here in sweet seclusion they increased and took on fat.
The common house-fly breeded, and disease germs multiplied,
And people often wondered why so many people died.

Nor was this all the Alley did to make a Boob of man—
It clutched with sticky hands at wheels; to stop them was its plan.
It gave delivery costs a boost, and dirtied up the floors,
And oftentimes when it was wet it kept some folks indoors.

But muddy Alleys, happily, will soon be memories,
Still rife with putrid odors flung upon the summer breeze.
The spirit of Progression has declared disease must go,
And with it muddy Alleys—sanitation's deadly foe.

All hail Concrete, the master Alley, built for horse and man!
Alike in rain or drought it serves the dogcart or the van!
In cleanliness it stands supreme, in sightliness alone
It lends the Alley dignity it ne'er before had known!

The Concrete Alley real estate a higher value gives,
It puts the ban on dust and dirt, but best of all it lives
To render worthy service, holding back the hands of time,
Resisting shock and friction with a courage quite sublime.

Economy, endurance, sanitation, and relief
From black, ill-smelling, rutty mudways, therefore, are, in brief,
The reasons good and mighty why Concrete and nothing more
Should beautify the pathway to the yard and kitchen door.

Figure 1.1. Charles Singler, "Alleys—Past and Present." *Cement Era* 15, no. 3 (1917): 35

CHAPTER ONE

Before Abortion

The Affective Residue of Back-Alley Rhetoric

The poem that provides this chapter's epigraph, "Alleys—Past and Present" (figure 1.1), hails from a 1917 trade publication titled the *Cement Era: Devoted to Cement, Concrete, and Related Machinery.*[1] In his verse, Charles A. Singler praised concrete's ability to sanitize so-called dangerous, disgusting, immoral, and economically destitute urban spaces—cities' own back-alleys. In the waning twilight of the Progressive Era, Singler positioned alleys as thresholds of history that implicated a "barbaric" and "unproductive" past while gesturing toward a more sanitary, moral, and crime-free future. Deploying vivid sensory descriptors with an upbeat ABAB rhyming pattern, readers learned that alleys were, ironically, "a 'sight,'" despite being unseen, sunlight-deprived places where animals like weasels, rats, and cats "were wont to meet." The poem granted alleys malevolent—even criminal—capacity, imbued with the agential quality of human tactility and the intent to halt commerce: "Nor was this all the Alley did to make a Boob of man [*sic*]— / It clutched with sticky hands at [automobile and carriage] wheels; to stop them was its plan." Threatening the porous boundaries between home and city—and thus the distinction between public and private life—alleys made delivery costs more expensive, tracked in residual dirt, and textured home spaces as they "dirtied up the floors." Olfactory appeals signaled a disgusting space, as alleys were "ill-smelling, rutty mudways" and ubiquitously "rife with putrid odors flung upon the summer breeze." Taken together, Singler's alley rhetoric appealed to the sensorium of home-owning city residents to spatialize sanitary, moral, and criminal concerns.[2]

Concrete heroically conquered fear, restored order, and cleaned the alleys described as "sanitation's deadly foe." The phrase "muddy Alleys, happily, will soon be memories" placed the antiquated, dirty, and dangerous alley in the past tense of US civic life unto which an increasingly "Progressive" public need not return.

The poem therefore constituted alleys as a public health exigency that could be abated with "concrete and nothing more." Indeed, the lines, "the common housefly breeded [*sic*], and disease germs multiplied, / And people often wondered why so many people died," implicated concurrent, racialized public health efforts seeking to eliminate vermin and prevent the spread of infectious diseases.[3] Concrete offered a cleanliness of sanitation and a connection to moral improvement insofar as it "lends the Alley dignity it ne'er before had known!" The poem framed concrete as improving the economic conditions of alley life, a durable focus for public health workers and social reformers since at least the mid-nineteenth century. And yet, "concrete is a political material."[4] While concrete gave the appearance of environmental sanitation and improvement, the reality of its production was—and remains—energy intensive and environmentally destructive, introducing carcinogens into the groundwater and soil.[5] Therefore, while concrete made alleys easier to clean, the material's invisible pollution constituted an environmental injustice that disproportionately impacted resource-deprived communities.

The phrase "back-alley abortion" inherits a viscerally resonant history of how "back-alleys" circulated throughout public discourse before colloquially referring to unsafe abortion care. While ubiquitous today, the phrase "back-alley abortion" was not a regular part of our criminalized abortion lexicon until the 1960s.[6] However, references to back-alleys have long circulated; for example, the adjectival preface "back" can be found in Middle English from 1450 ("Backe strete").[7] Throughout the nineteenth and twentieth centuries, public officials and social reformers consistently problematized alleys as unsanitary and immoral spaces with the potential to harbor unscrupulous "bad characters." Such discourses consisted of journalistic, literary, and technical references to back-alleys. The phrase appeared both in the noun form as a physical, primarily urban place and the adjectival form (for example, back-alley obstetrics, back-alley barber). The potential for these abject, unsurveilled back-alleys to permeate the boundaries of upper-class, white urban residents' homes and bodies firmly situated these spaces as fearful, unseen threats. While generally not addressing abortion, these back-alley references so often *feel* like they do.

With the circulation of long-standing terms like "back-alleys," I agree with Karma R. Chávez that "a well-worn rhetorical path precedes them, which means the work of persuasion or shifting public discourse has already begun upon utterance."[8] This chapter detours down that worn rhetorical path to investigate the back-alley *before abortion* and discern the features of alley rhetoric that have "stuck" around and inflected more contemporary framings of pregnancy termination. I argue that back-alley abortion rhetoric retains an *affective residue* from the rhetorical life of back-alley discourses circulating before abortion. Affective residue refers to durable sensory appeals that form public feelings associated with long-circulating terms like back-alleys. As Stephanie R. Larson notes, "Language leaves felt residue . . . persuasion is never an entirely rational operation that acts outside of the physical body."[9] Excavating the back-alley's affective residue reveals the role of sensory rhetorics to materialize public feelings such as disgust, fear, and pity within the rhetorical ecology of back-alley discourses. As the phrase circulated, it spatialized back-alleys as "dirty," "immoral," and "criminal." Sanitation, morality, and criminality were by no means discrete discourses. Instead, they circulated, percolated, and—as I append to Robin E. Jensen's helpful schema for tracing the history of a rhetorical ecology—*left a sticky residue* that shored up economic relationships and racial classifications of alleys as unsavory social spaces.[10] Back-alley discourses' social and classificatory schemas negotiated raced, classed, and gendered relationships as they produced visceral, sensorially grounded standards of dirtiness and cleanliness that remain operative today in back-alley abortion rhetoric. This chapter proceeds by first outlining the concept of affective residue. Then, I tour the tripartite circulating sensory rhetorics and public feelings operative in the back-alley's interwoven discourses of sanitation, morality, and criminality to contextualize the rhetorical assumptions that would come to permeate back-alley abortion rhetoric .

Affective Residue in the "Lower Depths"

Well before its association with criminalized abortion, physical alleys and adjectival references to back-alleys participated in a dynamic rhetorical imaginary of the *bas-fonds*, otherwise known as the "lower depths."[11] A social repository for "places, individuals, and behaviors" linked to an imagined nineteenth-century city experience, the *bas-fonds* consisted of the unseen streets, fetid marshes, institutional "lower" spaces like prisons, hospices, sewers, and pits—and those residing there.[12] Although these locations certainly existed, the affective associations tethered to the *bas-fonds* mythos materialized through a weave of fictional and nonfictional literary, philanthropic, and sanitary reform discourses. Understanding the rhetorical placement of alleys in the larger *bas-fonds* requires a framework for thinking about rhetorical action beyond a situational occurrence. An ecological perspective envisions the "back-alley" as rhetorically materialized over time through "an ongoing circulation process" of repeated denigration of alley spaces.[13] For instance, as this chapter later demonstrates, rather than think about First Lady Ellen Wilson's 1914 Washington, DC, slum clearance efforts within a discrete spatiotemporally-bounded context, an ecological framework envisions her work as part of a dynamic longitudinal process of constituting the public perception of alleyways.[14] An ecological approach asks how alleys accumulated meaning and sensorially resonant feeling over time by considering histories of sociality that inspired policy, iterations of textual invention that touched several authorial bodies, mediated circulatory systems, and unpredictable uptake. Because rhetorical ecologies prioritize rhetoric's movement and distributed emergence, this framework envisions back-alley rhetoric as the product of public discussions about physical alleys and fictional and nonfictional fragmentary textual encounters with *bas-fonds*-related anxieties in this ongoing circulatory system.

Back-alley abortion rhetorics participate in a fluid rhetorical ecology of the *bas-fonds* where interrelated public health issues such as sanitation, racism, sexism, moralized sexual politics, and poverty "circulate and percolate" with remarkable consistency over time.[15] As back-alley rhetoric circulated through public discourse and percolated into attention in any given moment, it did so with an uncannily familiar feeling-association that sometimes seemed to give the appearance of conceptual ahistoricity. As such, back-alley rhetoric before abortion is perhaps best traced through what Debra Hawhee and Christa Olson term panhistoriography—histories where the temporal scope exceeds the boundaries of individual generations.[16] Panhistoriography suits archives like the back-alley before abortion that persist across periods such as Reconstruction, the Gilded Age, or the Progressive Era. This method illuminates the ecological, rather than situational, nature of rhetorical action because it presumes at least some residual rhetorical continuity between one historical period to another.

Tracing the consistent feeling of back-alley rhetoric *before abortion*—what I term the back-alley's *affective residue*—helps account for the persistently durable public meanings, feelings, and sensations accumulated through the repeated references to the back-alley. This residue is a sense of what sticks around within a rhetorical ecology as the back-alley appears to roll through a linear sense of time. Straddling the false distinction between corporeal embodiment and a larger cultural inflection of the body politic, *residue* is persistent, often unruly, but sometimes offers a hopeful aperture into social change.

On the one hand, residue has inevitable embodied associations. Dominique Kalifa shows how the body fluids of people occupying the *bas-fonds* were invoked to create a textured, vivid space in literature: "It was the universe of grease, dirt, excrement . . . what remains is a sense of the 'residue' of everything that is expelled from the body."[17] In other scholarship, residue also gestures toward remaining ambient feelings of bodies having just exited a space. Krishna Savani and colleagues studied the cross-cultural beliefs in what they term "emotional residue" by asking participants to imagine whether they could sense residual feelings from walking into an empty space where other people dwelled in emotionally challenging experiences.[18] Teresa Brennan echoes this question in the opening of *The Transmission of Affect*: "Is there anyone who has not, at least once, walked into a room and 'felt the atmosphere'?"[19] These cases describe what Deborah Gould would also name the "residue," the remaining, deeply felt persistence from previous social encounters.[20] Grounded in research concerning cross-cultural beliefs in a "law of contagion" where "contaminated" and "uncontaminated" objects collide and "transfer some essence or property from the contaminated object to the uncontaminated one,"[21] residue names an "essence" that continually persists in the "uncontaminated" object even after the two objects are no longer in physical proximity to one another.

On the other hand, residue names larger cultural formations that have been supplanted—though not totally displaced—by dominant hegemonic formations. While emotional residue relies upon the assumption that emotion emanates from a person, leaving the space saturated with a sticky, viscous, or energetic remainder, Raymond Williams identifies the residual as a past formation with firm grounding in the present, "still active in the cultural process."[22] Stuart Hall helps us think about how back-alley abortion draws on the residual forms of alley rhetoric as a present-moment instantiation of "forgotten languages."[23] Whereas this chapter traces the rather regressive residue that accumulated with the "back-alley" signifier, it is important to recognize how, in some contexts, the residual retains the seeds of hope to imagine and create, as Emerson Cram so eloquently puts it, "the conditions of possibility for an elsewhere."[24]

Affective residue presumes that the repeated circulation of sensory appeals in association with terms like "back-alley" can imbue physical places and imagined spaces with residue that cements spatial-power associations. The Western sensorium is "embedded within the colonial and national nexus of power" and has long been intimately concerned with "the desire to tame and conquer distant and unruly places, peoples, and times."[25] The back-alley's affective residue accumulates within a dynamic rhetorical ecology of discourse, feeling, and social interaction when there is an object to stick to over time. The temporal durability of the back-alley's affective residue relies on the concerted repetition of similar alley appeals within that rhetorical ecology. Sara Ahmed argues that "stickiness depends on histories of contact that have already impressed upon the surface of the object."[26] Repeated and intense contact with the back-alley produces rhetorical outcomes that limit its possibility to be thought of in more progressive ways. As Ahmed explains, "when a sign or object becomes sticky, it can function to 'block' the movement (of other things or signs), and it can function to bind (other things or signs) together." Repetition creates a "binding effect" that can prevent new modes of meaning making and emotional patterns from occurring.[27] Although this repetition is certainly iterable—in that each repetition includes even the most imperceptible differences—affective residue prevents the back-alley from wandering too far from its well-worn racialized, classed, and gendered meanings and embodied orientations toward sanitation, morality, and criminality. This affective durability was particularly apparent once the phrase began to refer to abortion in the mid-twentieth century.

The residue left by the back-alley "before abortion" consists of the histories of vivid sensory appeals in embodied social interaction, public political action, and textual circulation. Graphic descriptions of the *bas-fonds* commonly hurt "all the senses," demonstrating the centrality of sensation to this particular social imaginary.[28] The senses were long believed to have a formative role in directing feeling and thought.[29] As the sensory rhetoric circulates, "the accumulation of sense patterns" draws attention to how "sensation and feeling are landscapes entangled within sociality and power."[30] Tracing affective residue calls for critics to "apprehend the political and historical conditions that organize the visceral."[31] These conditions are organized by factors such as race, class, gender, sexual normativities, and ethnicity and are intimately tethered to "the generation and activation of bodily memory."[32] Descriptions of sight, smell, and touch grant back-alleys their resonant rhetorical influence and leave the most recalcitrant residue. Although it is impossible to fully fray the interwoven elements of a sensorium, rhetorical vision, olfaction, and tactility are important sensory features that cement our residual associations with back-alleys.

Rhetorical vision—or *phantasia*—is the capacity to imagine an object in the "mind's eye," enabling an embodied, visceral orientation toward imagined life in alleys.[33] Even when grossly inaccurate, appeals to rhetorical vision allow publics distant from the alley to imagine the conditions. Put otherwise, the capacity for rhetorical vision to "fill in what cannot be perceived" allows sense perception to circulate when physical bodies are distanced from the alley spaces.[34] The residues left by appeals to rhetorical vision have kinetic power and are crucial to understanding the role of rhetoric in the "moving of affections."[35] As an embodied locus where we might find a "residue of sense perception," phantasia influences our deliberative judgments.[36] For instance, rhetorical vision can materialize racialized and classed spaces of concern, like alleys, shaping their relationship to national narratives of "progress," "civilization," and other ideals associated with coloniality and whiteness.[37] Indeed, appeals to rhetorical vision enable narrative perceptions of alleys to remain in the mind's eye.

While theories of phantasia tend to privilege the ocular, olfactory appeals also mold perceptions of racialized and classed spaces like alleys and leave a memorable affective residue. Bringing the world before our noses through twin logics of corporeal immediacy and expansive diffusion, Hsuan L. Hsu declares olfaction an overlooked mode of perceiving environmental risk that is "at once materially embodied and spatially extensive."[38] Rhetorical olfaction is well suited to thinking about affective residue, as bad smells can hold a residual presence even when the offensive object is displaced from proximity. Yi-Fu Tuan furthers the sticky connection between space and smell, noting how odors texture the atmosphere and "lend character to objects and places, making them distinctive, easier to identify and remember."[39] Indeed, the capacity for smell to burrow into collective memories is a large part of what makes olfaction a potent persuader, capable of leaving a residue.[40]

Important to the cultural dimensions of sanitary practices, olfaction is intimately tethered to racializing and colonizing practices that distinguish the pure from the impure. The spatial character that Tuan speaks of has often been filtered through classificatory practices that articulate "bad" smells to health problems characteristic of racial and class difference.[41] Despite the connection between "bad" odor mediating the definition of class, odor can also engender possibilities to mobilize for social change, especially when filtered through the lens of environmental justice.[42] In Darrel Wanzer-Serrano's treatment of the Young Lords' Garbage Offensive, the overwhelming stench of uncollected garbage in New York City's El Barrio neighborhood signified an environmental injustice, constituted a public health emergency, and motivated redressive rhetorical action: "Standing amidst the stench, they realized promptly that the all-pervading garbage indeed was an important, if not the most important, issue that they had to address."[43] Bad smells contributed to the visceral urgency of no longer tolerating unhealthy infrastructure. Unlike Yannis Hamilakis's more totalizing presumption that "bad smells are deeply tethered to bourgeois moral sensibilities," Wanzer-Serrano instead notes how garbage and its accompanying odors "represented both evidence of the state's disrespectful and malicious attitude toward the community and proof of the 'system's' incapability to deal with its own intemperance."[44] Whether the rhetors physically bring bad smells before the nose of the audiences or vivid words do so metaphorically, residual olfactions can cement regressive social patterns on the one hand and illuminate histories of injustice on the other.

Although smell can fill physical and imagined spaces, the sense of touch is often more localized in situ.[45] Back-alley rhetoric textures an aversive and fearful physical proximity to dangerous objects like potentially contaminating body fluids and rusty medical instruments. As Eve Kosofsky Sedgwick puts it, "A particular intimacy seems to subsist between textures and emotions."[46] Regardless of the scale of perception, Sedgwick maintains that apprehending a scene's texture leverages a storytelling process that seeks to explain "how physical properties act and are acted upon over time." Sedgwick's texture, also defined beyond a single sense perception as "an array of perceptual data that involves repetition," is an essential intervention into thinking about back-alleys and their affective residue because texture inevitably includes histories of what Ahmed calls sticky "contact zones" in which histories of encounter are erased.[47] The accumulation of sensory material leaves environmental traces. Steven Feld aptly summarizes, "As a place is sensed, senses are placed; as places make sense, senses make place."[48]

The affective residue from circulating back-alley rhetorics also constitutes the stigmatizing boundaries of publics' (non)belonging. Back-alley rhetoric leaves an affective residue whose physical and moral filth "bleeds into the bodies—shapeless, deformed, monstrous—and into characters."[49] As I will discuss in the next section, back-alleys are porous and physical-material boundaries that demarcate the domestic inside from the "dangerous" urban outside. However, back-alley rhetoric also *produces* hardened borders, isolating and stigmatizing those within. Drawing on the notion of residue, Gloria Anzaldúa observes, "Borders are set up to define the places that are safe and unsafe, to distinguish *us* from *them*. . . . A borderland is a vague and undetermined place created by the emotional residue of an unnatural boundary. . . . The prohibited and forbidden are its inhabitants."[50] While, in an alternative imaginary, alleys could thus be considered empty space, Anzaldúa helps us think about their production as a boundary; the publics constituted by the bordering process of back-alley rhetoric are those whose social participation has been similarly "prohibited and forbidden." That unnecessary and unnatural boundary leaves an indelible residual affect on those marked by back-alley rhetoric. In the words of Jenell Johnson, those constituted by back-alley rhetoric are *visceral* insofar as "they emerge from discourse about boundaries, and they cohere by means of intense feeling."[51] Because back-alley rhetorics draw "dangerous" yet porous borders, they also stigmatize the people constituted by these same messages—even historically referring to them as "residue." Indeed, Liberal member of Parliament John Bright used the widely circulating Victorian term *residuum* in an 1867 Reform Bill to pejoratively classify "the worst criminals and indigents," placing them beyond the boundary of a productive society.[52] Johnson reminds us that "one of stigma's most insidious aspects . . . is to designate its bearer as an object that is frustratingly general—to be stigmatized is to be known, simply, as *bad*."[53] By imbuing the stigmatized with *kakoethos*, back-alley rhetorics rendered the alley itself and those living there visible, immoral, and classified as such. This stigma thus subjected those living within to charitable intervention and—more ominously—state surveillance. The residue of this stigmatized public persists today in the uptake of the back-alley into abortion discourse.

The remainder of this chapter traces the affective residue of the back-alley before abortion in the nineteenth and early twentieth centuries to lay the foundation for the rhetorical power of back-alley abortion in subsequent chapters. From London to New York City to Washington, DC, alleys were a significant anxiety amid amplifying urbanization and migration. Initially part of the infrastructural design to encourage sanitation in dense living conditions, US alleys quickly became racially segregated living spaces. Alleys have long been situated as opaque to state surveillance and as unsanitary, pitiful spaces that could impinge on the moral capacities of children and "vulnerable" white women. If left unabated, alleys were stigmatized as harboring criminals and unskilled, uncaring fraudulent operators. As a significant object of fascination in the United States after the Civil War in particular, journalists, charitable entities, and government officials each worked to make alley spaces intelligible using visceral, sensorially resonant appeals to rhetorical vision, olfaction, and tactility that left residual affective qualities lodged in a collective rhetorical imaginary.

Back Alleys and Sanitary Reform

In nineteenth-century London, back-alleys were locations associated with poor sanitation and evil characters. Alleys were part of the urban infrastructure, often enumerated as such in catalogs of city streets. Alleys quickly became associated with worn-down past relics as overcrowded, unclean physical spaces that needed modernization. Robert Chambers's 1863 *The Book of Days: Miscellany of Popular Antiquities* displays a sketch of part of the city that had survived the Great London Fire (figure 1.2). The caption reads, "The churchyard entrance, with the old edifice, and row of ancient houses looking down upon it, seems not to belong to the present day, but to carry the visitor entirely back to the seventeenth century. There is a back-alley encroaching on the chancel, with tumble-down old houses supported on wooden pillars, which gives so perfect an idea

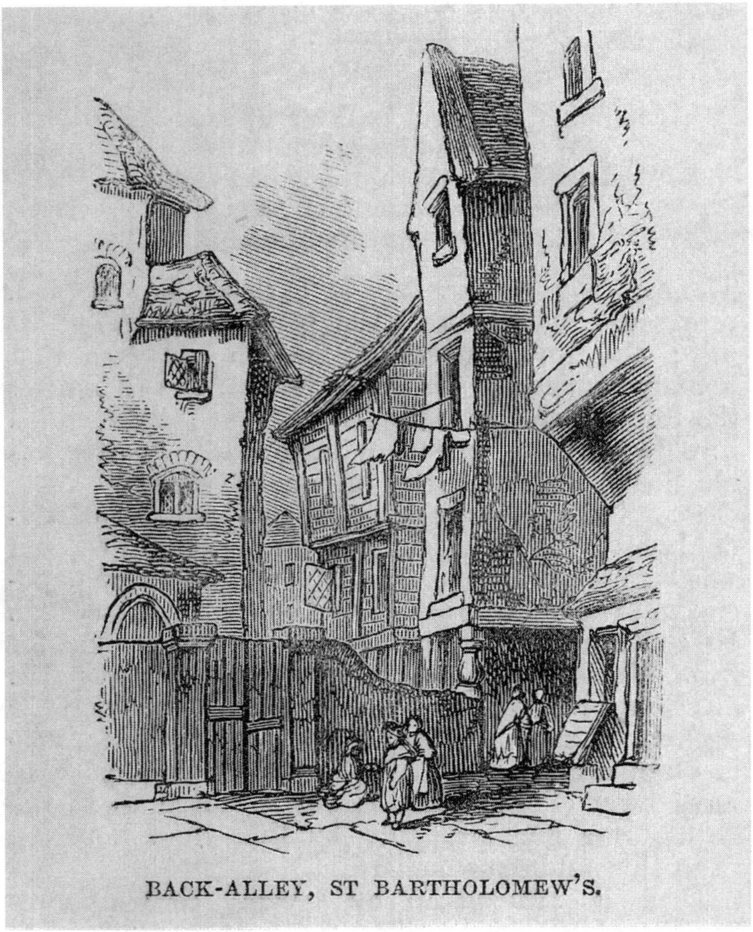

Figure 1.2. A sketch of a back-alley next to a church with wafting laundry. Robert Chamber, ed., *The Book of Days: Miscellany of Popular Antiquities*, vol. 2, 1863

of the crowded and filthy passages, once common in Old London, that we here engrave it."[54] In this case, a fence physically separated the back-alley of St. Bartholomew's church from vulnerable women in dresses waiting outside. The alley's "encroachment" references an unfettered unsanitary intrusion, evoking the agential force of dirt and disease rampant in the centuries before sanitary reform movements emerged in London. The back-alley was also marked by people of bad character. The publication continues, "The Houses are part of those erected by the Lord Rich, one of the most wicked and unscrupulous of the favourites of

Henry VIII." While the church itself was praised, its back-alley was characterized by disorder: wafting laundry, hidden views, and the residual specters of the evil characters therein.

Nineteenth-century British and US sanitary reformers often considered alleys problematic spaces of disrepair and, thus, appropriate objects for state intervention. Sanitary reform emerged in England in the 1830s–1840s and was considered one of the first sustained public health initiatives in nineteenth-century Europe.[55] The Industrial Revolution produced modern commercial agriculture, displacing farm workers and directing them to an increasingly expanding urban environment. With a rapidly growing urban population, it quickly became clear that the capacity of the existing sanitary infrastructure was overwhelmed and outdated. Such was also the case in the United States. By the 1860s, diseases such as cholera and typhoid spread rapidly throughout growing cities as social reformers struggled to make sense of this phenomenon and ameliorate the conditions.[56]

Sanitary reformers were invested in understanding the sensory and spatial connections between filth and disease, which rendered alley spaces some of the more obvious targets of intervention. Before Louis Pasteur's groundbreaking germ theory in the early 1860s, sanitary reformers relied on theories of miasmatism that held that filth, standing water, untended garbage, and human and animal waste produced noxious vapors that autonomously caused disease. British sanitary reformer Edwin Chadwick argued that miasmas could "depress[] the system and render[] it susceptible to the action of other causes" and famously quipped, "All smell is disease."[57] Through this aphorism, miasmatism and sanitary reform functioned as olfactory pedagogies of disgust for those residing near foul environmental smells.[58] In other words, as bad smells became articulated to dangerous diseases, the publicly groomed emotions of fear and disgust each mediated that connection.

For sanitary reformers, environmental fear was also directed toward the people living within "contaminating" alley spaces. With noxious odors seen as the cause of disease before, during, and even after the Pasteurian revolution,[59] race and class differences were medicalized, providing a fearful health-based justification for a social hierarchy that privileged the white and wealthy.[60] Public health discourse often walked in lockstep with this olfactory regime: "Emphasizing the fetidity of the laboring classes, and thus the danger of infection from their mere presence, helped the bourgeois to sustain his [*sic*] self-indulgent, self-induced terror. . . . From these considerations emerged the tactics of public health policy, which symbolically assimilated disinfection and submission."[61] Chadwick fre-

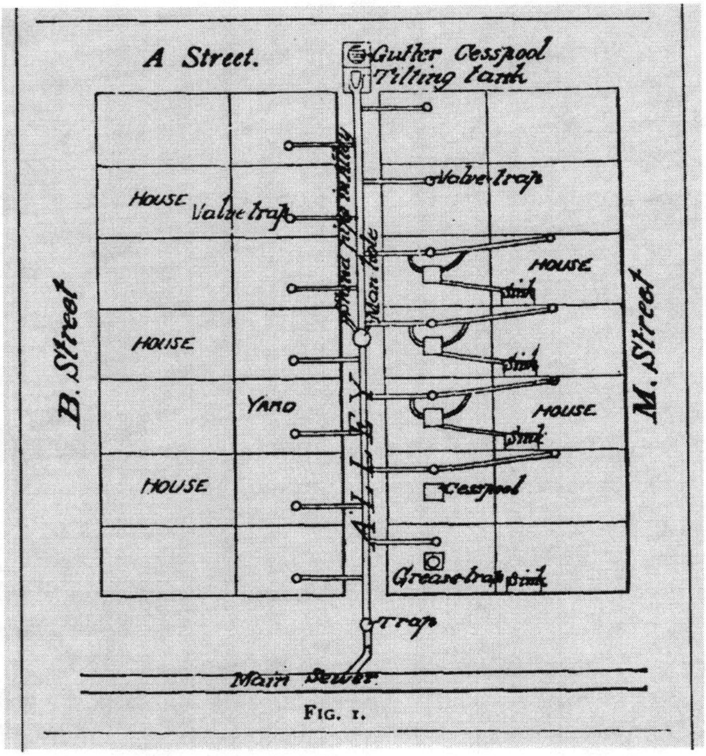

Figure 1.3. Sketch of alley drainage plan. *Sanitary Engineer,* 1883

quently stigmatized those living in poverty, considering the sanitary movement's initiatives an exercise in social control. Importantly, as sanitary movements proliferated across Europe, parts of South America, and the United States, they became part of a settler-colonial logic in countries such as Brazil.[62]

In response to the miasmatic threats, back-alleys were frequently targeted infrastructure, fortifying boundaries between city homes and the waste its inhabitants produced. Operating with a residual miasmatic disease logic, the 1883 *Sanitary Engineer* journal published "Sewer Connections to Private Houses," lamenting the "sewer gases forced out into the alley, thereby contaminating the air in the neighborhood."[63] It instead suggested "an improved plan . . . that all houses be connected to drain in the back alleyway" (figure 1.3).

In this case, back-alleys were designed to control the perceived contaminating gases and therefore enabled sanitary living. Part of these concerns were related to the ability to live a safe distance from waste, problems that modern plumbing and replacing horses with automobiles partially assuaged.[64]

US alley sanitation was an acute public health concern throughout the postbellum nineteenth century, particularly as industrialization took root and migration expanded urban populations. Medical practice considered disease a product of the environment's influence on humans, although physicians still worked to further nuance its role in the process.[65] Alleys were an environment of such concern that implications for their improvement could be situated within various other sanitary contexts. For instance, in 1863, Northern physicians met at a conference to discuss the implications of the Civil War on medicine. At this point, Dr. J. Foster Jenkins, the leader of the organization, anticipated how the lessons of sanitation learned at the soldiers' camp would be beneficial for future alley remediation efforts:

> The private soldier who learns that fever is bred of uncleanliness, and the absence of ventilation to his overcrowded tent, is likely to infer that the same conditions will induce similar diseases in his untidy home up *the populous back alley*. To intelligent soldiers . . . army life demonstrates the truths that personal uncleanliness and foul air, and dampness, and bad cooking, and mental depression, and badly policed camping grounds, and inadequate clothing, and intemperance regarding food or drink, all invite disease, and when they return to the more congenial pursuits of peace, they will from thousands of centers propagate these hygienic truths.[66]

In comparing the wartime encampment conditions with soldiers' back-alley homes, Jenkins hoped that war would prove to be a point of clarity, leading the "intelligent" soldiers to remediate the "miasmatic diseases" back home.[67] Perhaps most notable was his argument that articulated morality with physical cleanliness: environmental sanitary factors such as overcrowding and foul-smelling air combined with personal behaviors such as poor cooking would invite disease. Each of these factors appealed to dimensions of the sensorium: tactile proximity in close conditions, odor of bad air, and taste of bad food. Given the context of this conference, the solution to these exigencies rested in the hands of heroic physicians whose patients were marked by pity, having "hitherto been the unfortunate victims of ignorance."[68] Ultimately, obsolete urban infrastructure often could not keep pace with the hygienic demands of an exploding population. These "hopeful" lessons of the Civil War—that army medicine would translate into improving back-alleys—would not be realized.

As germ theory accumulated more scientific currency in the late nineteenth century, the back-alley began to describe unsanitary and infectious home-based medical care outside the control of reputable physicians. In 1894, physician Ellis P. Townsend, who practiced for thirty years throughout central New Jersey, published "Back Alley Obstetrics." Lamenting the homes he would enter when attending to childbirth, Townsend appealed to what he believed were other physicians' common experiences: "Every physician has had his [*sic*] own experience with what may be termed back alley obstetrics. You have had no previous knowledge of the case, its character or its surroundings."[69] Biographer Sandra W. Moss affirms that "by 'back alley,' Townsend meant poor homes with little or no hygiene, rather than the more ominous modern reference to illegal abortion."[70] Yet if back-alley abortion gains its rhetorical force from the affective residue of social relationships and emotional orientations left behind by work such as this, it is crucial to interrogate the abject rhetorical vision that Townsend set for his peers: "As you enter the door you instinctively feel like holding up your pants to keep them from getting soiled. You find no place clean enough to place your hat; no place to hang your coat. Around you all is confusion and filth, a half dozen children with dirty hands and faces, and unkempt hair and filthy clothing, are rolling around the floor."[71] Under the larger heading of back-alley obstetrics, Townsend's sensory rhetoric created a crucial articulation between sanitary and moral concerns by connecting the "filthy surroundings" with too many "poorly reared" children and with obstetrical disease. A tactile disgust levied at the "filthy surroundings" blended seamlessly into the disorganized "confusion" of too many children living with poor sanitation in a cramped space. The description crafted an aversive social boundary between the physician, the patient, and their family by affirming that rolling up pant legs would be an acceptable embodied response to the "filthy" spaces they encountered. Of course, the physician's efforts to protect his garment neither sanitized the space nor improved patients' health outcomes. Instead, Townsend formed a hierarchical, class-based distance between those existing in unsanitary "back-alley" conditions and those who provide them with medical care.

Much like the poem that opened this chapter, the presence of pests left a sticky tactile residue that concretized the vision of vermin as existing in close relational proximity to low-income communities. Townsend described the insects that joined an already crowded birthing space: "You find your patient in a filthy bed, dressed in filthy clothing, and are lucky if it does not contain more living things than the patient."[72] Townsend's attention to bedbugs, fleas, and other pests situated the space as dangerous to the health and well-being of attending physicians as he castigated families for their unhygienic behavior. To be sure, sanitary reformers often denigrated migrants and people of color for practicing poor hygiene that encouraged pests rather than viewing vermin as symptomatic of structural housing inequities. As Dawn Day Biehler notes, vermin "carry in their bodies the legacy of our past relationships with them."[73] As embodied, visceral anxieties about clean birthing spaces rubbed against a waning birth rate among the white Anglo-Saxon population, the obstetrical back-alley—with its accompanying vermin—similarly carried the legacy of race and class-based fears under the signifier of sanitation.[74] Drawing attention to residual textures, smells, confusion, bugs, and fear allowed Townsend to situate home-based obstetrical care as carrying the qualities of a "back-alley," excoriating the humans in its ecology.

On a much larger scale, alleys were a point of material and symbolic condensation for collective urban racism. Alleys were used to justify segregation because they physically suited larger racial ideologies that environment played a determining role in the formation of race. As Linda Nash notes, nineteenth-century Americans of European descent conceptualized racialized bodies as porous: "Until the late nineteenth century, most Euro-Americans believed that it was the very permeability of the body that created its race and that a person's race was liable to change in a new location."[75] In other words, race was considered materially affected by environmental features such as temperature and humidity. These views fueled segregationist practices that consigned newly freed African Americans to substandard housing on the heels of Reconstruction's failure.

Between 1860 and 1870, thousands of formerly enslaved African Americans migrated to Washington, DC, to escape racial violence and seek economic opportunity, increasing the alley population from 60,000 to 110,000 people. The Great Migration transformed the composition of alley inhabitants, who were of a white majority when tracked in 1858.[76] By 1897, Black Washingtonians constituted 93 percent of alley homes.[77] Racism was constant: "Each wave of black migration to the city was greeted by increased white hostilities. While these influxes did not immediately lead to the massive ghettos of the twentieth century, segregation did take place within the technological, spatial, and mental constraints of the nineteenth."[78] At least one important constraint included a lack of transportation infrastructure in Washington, DC, where many could not travel to work without living in the close physical proximity that alley homes afforded. Segregation also had far-reaching impacts on the health of alley inhabitants: "A long history of residential and employment segregation meant that non-whites were far more likely to live in badly polluted communities and to have more hazardous jobs."[79] These dilapidated alley homes primarily resulted from a lack of consistent building and inspection protocols that allowed opportunistic real estate developers to enrich themselves by exploiting the burgeoning housing demand.[80]

Despite the structural roots of dilapidated alley housing, eugenic rhetoric racialized alley conditions as individual sanitary failings. In 1910, Ellen H. Richards penned *Euthenics: The Science of Controllable Environment—a Plea for Better Living Conditions as a First Step toward Higher Human Efficiency*.[81] While praising the eugenic impulse of "race improvement through heredity," she lamented how its trajectory was future oriented and exceeded the boundary of the current generation.[82] She thus theorized *euthenics* as that which "precedes eugenics, developing better men [*sic*] now, and thus inevitably creating a better race of men [*sic*] in the future."[83] Richards framed inadequate housing conditions as resulting from individual ignorance and moral failing, declaring that homeowners (notably *not* those living in alleys) were explicitly authorized to surveil and intervene: "Unsanitary alleys exist because the abutters do not complain loudly enough to the right authorities."[84] Indeed, as the alley population grew and appeared to threaten the health of mostly white and upper-class people living in homes on the main streets, it inspired different levels of government action.

Between 1895 and 1910, when Richard's book was published, reformers generated abundant social data about the unsanitary conditions of alley life and vividly described the conditions in their arguments for remediation .[85] The body of this work that has enjoyed the most robust uptake was crafted from the perspective of white Progressive reformers. During this time, back-alley concerns appeared as voyeuristic exposés of the decrepit conditions, inviting street property-owning readers to see, hear, touch, and, importantly, *smell* the "invisible" conditions in their back-alleys. These repeated attempts to "unveil" the secrets kept by the alleys amplified public sentiment toward reform efforts. Police journalist Jacob Riis was neither the first nor the last to provide a type of "back-alley" exposé, but his published work *How the Other Half Lives: Studies among the Tenements of New York* is perhaps the most widely recognized today, ascending to a canonical literary status in the United States.[86] Chapter 4 of his widely read text was titled "The Down Town Back-Alleys."[87] Riis's photojournalism was designed to bring the situation before readers' eyes and display the reality that so many more privileged city residents refused to see. Riis wrote of several alleys, labeling one as "a dark and nameless alley, shut in by high brick walls, cheerless as the lives of those they shelter."[88] The entire chapter lamented sanitary issues by personifying the alley, rhetorically texturing the space by declaring, "dirt and desolation reign," and "could their grimy walls speak, the big canals might tell many a startling tale. But they are silent enough so are most of those whose secrets they might betray."[89] Riis's work was not oriented toward social justice but instead appealed to "the propertied classes to destir themselves lest the crime engendered in the slums and the diseases bred there invade the comfortable quarters where ladies and gentlemen resided."[90] Thus, racial and class-based anxieties surrounding the porous boundaries of city life were condensed into the figure of the back-alley—a space that bred social and physical contamination.

Reformers' surveillance of back-alleys amplified the visibility of alley denizens and racialized public feeling of disgust at alleys by appealing to sight, smell, and touch. As New York City police commissioner, Theodore Roosevelt soon became Riis's ardent supporter, carrying that esteem forward during his presidential tenure.[91] Once president, Roosevelt also supported other reformers, like Associated Charities president Charles Frederick Weller and his wife, Eugenia Weller, who used similar surveillance tactics to expose the so-called secrets of alley life. Roosevelt even graced the introduction to the Wellers' 1909 *Neglected Neighbors: Stories of Life in the Alleys, Tenements, and Shanties of the National Capital*, demonstrating his commitment to this expository genre. Roosevelt valued the Wellers' prose and accompanying photographs because they could appeal to the emotional capacities of readers in a way that technical documents could not: "I think that your stories of specific families and typical incidents will be more effective with general readers than the statistics and formal statements which usually characterize reports as to housing conditions. . . . It will afford to any one who reads it a larger and more sympathetic understanding of the problems and difficulties which beset those who live in 'the alleys, tenements, and shanties' of the National Capital."[92] Roosevelt deemed the Wellers' work valuable for its affective capacity for mobilization, in other words, the ability of the vivid descriptions and images to *affect* the bodies of its readership and thus *move* them to reparative, "Progressive" action.[93] Vivid descriptions and appeals to readers' sensory capacities are powerful for lay and vernacular publics because they allow the acquisition of sensory information to serve as embodied evidence to support their view of their surroundings.[94] Generating widespread support for Washington, DC, alley cleanup required that reformers make rhetorical efforts to alert governing bodies and white homeowners to the conditions that lay beyond the boundaries of their homes.

By touring and mapping the alley layouts, Riis and the Wellers became the eyes of distanced white homeowners, as they could see in their minds' eyes the hidden unsanitary conditions in their proximity. While many DC alleys remained nameless, reformers offered others ableist nicknames such as "blind alley" to indicate that white homeowners did not have access or that visually impaired people resided within. The Wellers and other reformers' efforts focused on rendering the alleys visible to the upper-class inhabitants of the city, narrating the embodied process that they took to unveil the alley: "It is with some misgiving that one leaves the well-lighted outer streets with their impressive residences and turns into a narrow passageway where he must walk by faith, not sight. Noises . . . grow louder as the explorer approaches the wider inside alleys. A group of people are seen playing together roughly. A cheap phonograph nearby rasps out a mere ditty."[95] Texture and sound are amplified because one could not use their visual capacities to navigate the area. The "misgiving" of leaving the well-lit and visible streets is perhaps better framed as an anticipated fearful and disgusting orientation to whom (or *what*, in the case of vermin) precisely occupied the occluded alley space.

Appeals to noxious olfaction encouraged homeowners to believe that health-related dangers were lurking in the back-alley. Early on in *Neglected Neighbors*, the Wellers illustrated the features of an "average alley" by offering an olfactory "civic conundrum": " 'hollow like an egg; rotten like a bad egg; what is it?' Answer, 'Average Alley.' "[96] This crude riddle framed the back-alley olfactory threat, as did the Wellers' field note description of the space: "filthy dirty; smells bad."[97] In their explication of the "Average Alley," the Wellers noted that the winding and narrow passages to the homes were "littered with rubbish and malodorous from a toilet often clogged up and overflowing with filth. This dirty toilet stands only 9 feet from the rear of the house and contributes to the constant foul odors which pervade the building."[98] Connecting to the difficult visibility of the alleys with proximal odor circulating therein, the Wellers remarked that with Bassett's Alley, there was "no water supply but many odors . . . [and] one does not need his [*sic*] eyes to find them out." Although many alley homes did not have toilet hookups to the sewer, even those that did, like Bassett's Alley, could be cleaned only by manually flushing with water from the street hydrants. These visceral appeals to noxious olfaction signaled the contaminating and unsanitary conditions of the alleys. Despite these evocative sensory descriptions of this public health concern, reformers were distanced from the alley community and often ignored members of the residents affected.

It was not lost on many politically active African American members of the Washington, DC, community that alley remediation remained in the hands of white Progressive reformers. In 1908, one year before the Wellers published *Neglected Neighbors*, a group of African American interdenominational ministers established the Alley Improvement Association (AIA) in response to white Progressive reformers' failure to seek input from various leaders of the Black community. AIA president J. Milton Waldron spoke of the housing injustice of alley conditions. He deplored the large-scale profits that alley landlords were procuring by ignoring the deadly sanitary conditions: "Of the 19,000 persons living in the alleys, courts, and back-streets, 17,000 are colored [*sic*]. It is not to be wondered that the death-rate . . . is more than twice that of the white inhabitants."[99] Forming a broad coalition with other African American organizations and white political influencers, the AIA improved alley conditions by registering tuberculosis cases, establishing a public hospital, providing free home disinfection, and crafting educational campaigns with visiting nurses.[100] In 1913, Waldron spoke in front of Congress shortly after Woodrow Wilson's inauguration. The AIA joined forces with First Lady Ellen Wilson to support the Slum Clearance Bill, which successfully passed before her death in 1914.[101] This alliance, however, was fraught. According to Constance McLaughlin Green, in a practice similar to that of Riis and the Wellers, Ellen Wilson took "frequent excursions" into the alleys. Despite the First Lady's support of the bill, these efforts had only lukewarm effects in ameliorating more entrenched racial relations with Washington, DC, African American communities. Indeed, "neither her death nor the passage of the Alley Dwelling Act in 1914 modified their feelings."[102]

Through repeated invocation and circulation, the back-alleys of cities such as Washington, DC, and New York were molded by their abjection. Framed as both pitiful and disgusting, alley life was considered dangerous because it could *affect* the viscera of those who resided there and those with whom they might come into contact. While sanitation was undoubtedly a central thread to the affective residue of the back-alley, these appeals to cleanliness also worked to denounce the morality of those living there.

Back-Alley Morality

A second layer of affective residue considers the back-alley as a raced, classed, and gendered (im)moral space mobilized by appeals to discourses of virtue and vice. These categories were tightly braided, so the moralizing appeals often traveled in tandem with sanitation. For example, AIA president Waldron explicitly fused the two, stating, "The alleys of Washington are the moral and physical plague spots of the nation's capital."[103] While Waldron certainly painted the unsanitary alley conditions as a moral failing of the city's resource deprivation of African Americans, he also gestured toward personal moral limitations of those living in alleys. In addition to the AIA's sanitary intervention, the association also held summer school and temperance meetings to allow sanitary education to shape the moral behaviors of those residing in alleys.[104] Alison Bashford similarly affirms that "Sanitary Reform always involved some form of moral reform, which rested upon theories of disease which conflated physical and moral cleanliness and health and perhaps more pertinently, physical and moral dirtiness and ill-health."[105] Indeed, the Wellers' description of the alley space dubbed "Rotten Row" echoed Waldron: "Here the sight and odors of an open bucket of skinned rabbits, a pan of pigs' feet and piles of filth, all black with flies, which were found in the yard one hot day this summer, seemed quite appropriate to the whole effect outside and in of a 'rotten row.' Its constant effect must be to depress and vitiate the manners, morals and general standards of life of all its numerous denizens and neighbors."[106] The filth, flies, and animal carcasses would "depress" the moral capacity of alley residents, rendering their bodies susceptible to disease and their characters susceptible to cultural denigration.[107] Alleys were initially considered amoral, rather than immoral, spaces: "The alley standard represents an undeveloped, and a developing, moral code."[108] In crafting white, upper-class standards of morality, reformers circulated public emotions of pity and fear, materializing raced and gendered standards of vice in the process.

The physical layouts of unsanitary alleys were framed as morally agential because of their ability to *affect* humans and nonhumans contained therein. Because the physical alley layout held agency, those living therein were often deprived of agency, with their so-called immorality met with pity. While alleys were considered dangerous to the health of those living there, dangers were attributed to the capacity for the community to stay out of sight, "which bred conditions of vice, crime, and immorality."[109] The bodies and moral characters of those living in alleys were portrayed as pitiable; "only moral standards which *are impressed upon them*" were considered effective in altering residents' dispositions.[110] Thus, in official documents that held persuasive currency for lawmakers, reformers systematically denied agency to those living in alleys. This deagentification occurred primarily through the Wellers' explicit circulation of pity, a form of empathy whose relational patterning contains a hierarchical relationship between the person who pities and the person who is pitied:[111] "Not only do alley conditions, *because of the moral and physical isolation*, foster a life of license . . . but the narrowness of alley streets and the 'shut-inness' of the place make all that happens common property, so that no one, try as he [*sic*] may, can close his [*sic*] eyes and ears to those vices which it so easy to 'endure,' 'pity,' and 'embrace.' "[112]

And yet, these moments of pity quickly morphed into judgment and contempt for those living in alleys, who could afford to live elsewhere *if only* they could take personal responsibility to prioritize working over "loafing" and "vice." In this sense, alley residents were caught in a paradox of attributed agency. Weller attributed to these "alley loafers" a preference to drink alcohol rather than work to afford a more dignified home. One example is the Wellers' investigation of "Average Alley." There, they established a basis for comparing the dozens of alleys that constituted Washington, DC, and introduced readers to the Keefe family, who, although initially impressing Weller with the unexpected "physical excellence" of their personal space, ultimately embodied "the genius of the alley," having been morally influenced by the larger alley surroundings:[113] "In the wholesome Keefe family even, unwelcome signs appeared. Idleness was the first. Henry, the likeable young gent was found to be loafing every day and it developed that he had been unemployed throughout July, a busy month. . . . In her indignation, Laura [his spouse] explained that Henry could make two-fifty and three dollars daily in cement work but his frequent spells of drunkenness and idling had disgusted his successive employers and finally reduced him to odd jobs, which he is not alert in seeking."[114] Because the alley population at the time of Weller's writing comprised 93 percent African American citizens, "loafing" was a racist and classist indictment of inhabitants' moral conduct. James Borchert confirms that "when Charles Weller referred to 'the usual midday loafers' in the caption to a photograph of Ball's Alley, he did so not to demonstrate neighborly interaction, but for clearly moralistic reasons."[115] Concerned about the idling of potentially productive bodies, alleys—not systemic resource deprivation—were spaces that extinguished an entrepreneurial spirit with immorality and vice. Daniel Makagon notes that age, race, and class influence the distinction between loitering and "legitimate" social interaction, which is deeply tethered to values of capitalist participation: "Loiterers challenge the virtues of production, consumption, and mobility."[116] The "loafing" that the Wellers articulated to moral debasement crafted the expectation that those who were living in alleys were not working.

The Wellers also leveraged sexualized purity appeals to frame alleys as pitiful places that would affect the next generation's civic capacities. Children's immorality was a process of moral transmission from their parents: "The irresponsibility of the alley man and the immorality of both men and women suggest the importance of considering the children. . . . Into what molds of citizenship are alley children being pressed?"[117] Children ostensibly began "pure" but would porously absorb the environment surrounding them: "There is the greatest pity of it all. That the new generation should receive on virgin, fertile soil all the vices of the old, should listen with eager ears and wide open eyes to the evil sights and sounds that in a place so cramped and shut-in must all be common property. Now it is a fight, an arrest, that calls their eager attention . . . where the men at work shout obscene messages to the women across the alley."[118] According to the Wellers, children, the "virgin soil" whose sexual morality was in danger, were affected with an immoral character through their sensory capacities, having been immersed in "evil sights and sounds." The Wellers frequently questioned parental aptitude by printing images of forlorn children with captions indicating they were being left alone for more than fourteen hours with strangers.[119]

It is crucial to note that despite racist indictments of the morality of those who accessed their homes via alleyway, the Wellers' observations were an overwhelmingly inaccurate and decontextualized representation of the African American kinship networks in the Washington, DC, alleys.[120] Elizabeth Clark-Lewis's interview data of African American women and girls who fled southern "violence, intimidation, and suppression" for work opportunities in Washington, DC, showed how expansive kinship ties were crucial for the survival of those who came to work in a strange city to support family back home in the South.[121] Dwight Conquergood maintains that alleys, contrary to the Wellers' characterization, should be considered a shared community space, especially in areas where state neglect materialized as crumbling infrastructure: "Indeed, the chaotic State of disrepair, breakdowns, and emergencies requires for survival a neighborly interdependence unheard of in efficiently managed middle-class properties. Crises create community, but this is particularly true when the crisis relates to physical space that people share over time."[122] Even within "forbidding structures," alleys were also generative, energetic spaces that served as a reminder of the mutual interdependence of social life under segregated conditions.

In addition to providing caring support systems, these extended networks could leverage white fear to protect their communities from racialized violence and police intrusion. The Wellers' travel into the alleys pejoratively proclaimed, "Pandemonium reigns. One sees no immediate cause for fear but feels intuitively a suggestion of evil possibilities and latent danger."[123] Marking the alley's potential danger by what could neither be seen nor surveilled, such intuitions of evil produced a fear-based pedagogy for the predominantly white policymakers who acted on urgent alley conditions. However, Borchert challenges the argument that alley families were immoral or dysfunctional. Ironically, the fear that the Wellers felt in their alley tours was likely a performance choreographed by the alley community: "Perhaps the most striking and interesting aspect of the alley dwellers' methods of defending their 'turf' can be seen in their effective manipulation of white fear. Certainly, some police and non-residents were attacked in alleys; yet these instances were clearly and vastly exaggerated."[124] Members of the alley communities had their own mechanisms for quickly alerting one another to the "outsiders" who found themselves in the alley space.[125]

Fictional Back-Alley Morality

Kalifa reminds us that the *bas-fonds* tethers "a thousand literary references, social inquiries, studies of public hygiene, news snips, the moral and political sciences, songs, and films."[126] As one spatial instantiation of the *bas-fonds*, fictional alley representations featured threats to the virtues of white womanhood, indexing fears of immoral mischief that could occur. In 1849, Edward Z. C. Judson crafted the novel *Mysteries and Miseries of New York: A Story of Real Life* under the pen name Ned Buntline.[127] This story is significant because it is a fictionalized representation of Mary Rogers's abortion-related death, described in the introduction.[128] Although scholars have treated the novel's place as materializing the sensationalism of criminalized abortion, the role of alley references in framing the (im)moral scenes invites further examination.

Readers meet Mr. Precise and his assistant Frank. Mr. Precise wishes to uncover the "truth" of the New York City vice dens and slums, and Frank indulges his desires by immediately hailing a stagecoach. Arriving at a soup-house, "where a good many of these people get all they ever eat!" Mr. Precise's olfactory capacities are saturated: "I feel sick—I shall vomit if I stay here, Oh, *such a smell!*"[129] Wondering what the disgusting-smelling soup was made of, Frank replies, "Out of the offals that are thrown from the market, and the scraps of meat and leaves of cabbage and all that which is thrown out from the kitchens in the back-alleys, sir."[130] Back-alleys here refer to places of refuse, implying an underlying shadow economy wherein children and adults mine the alleys for scraps. The people living in the back-alleys are repeatedly dehumanized as pitiable "creatures."

The back-alley connected virtue, vice, and gendered sexual morality in its assumed, but unlabeled, mention of abortion. Encountering a beautiful three-story brick house with green window blinds, Buntline narrated, that "for some reason or other are never thrown open."[131] Inside, a man named Albert "but a moment before had come into the house by the back alley." Albert is melancholy because although he is married to another woman he nonetheless sent for his pregnant lover, Mary Sheffield—the fictionalized Mary Rogers. While readers already know Albert has no intention of marrying Mary, she believes he merely delayed publicly proclaiming their relationship. Panicked, Mary responds, "In a few short weeks my situation will be but too apparent. . . . [M]y name and shame will be bruited everywhere!" Albert encourages Mary that the kind Mrs. Sitstill—

a fictional representation of Madame Restell (Ann Lohman)—could assuage her pregnancy "situation." A week later, back "in that singular house, with the back-alley entrance, stood Mary Sheffield."[132] Although I do not consider this to be back-alley abortion rhetoric in a contemporary sense, it reflects Mary *accessing* an abortion through a clandestine back-alley entrance—a theme that will emerge in the next chapter. While in the story Mrs. Sitstill is a kindly woman, this was a larger warning tale in the context of the "true stories" of New York City's "urban decay." Sanitation and vice comingled as back alleys became the gateways to modulate Christian men's public feeling about urban vice in the mid-nineteenth century.

Fictional back-alley representation was persistently tethered to the vulnerability of white womanhood, holding considerable literary durability into the early twentieth century. In August 1911, writer George Sinclair published "Actress' Read-Press-Agent," a satirical "series of 'form announcements' that actresses might well enjoy."[133] Sinclair penned ten brief vignettes that could have served as theatrical promotional material—had the play been real. In each case, the "beautiful, young Southern actress, "Miss ———" is preparing to reprise the famed role of Euphronia Smellingsalts in the "forthcoming drama of realistic life: 'The Back Alley.' " Each fictional vignette follows Miss ——— narrowly escaping a dangerous situation such as an automobile accident, a jewelry robbery, and a near drowning—then collapsing from overwhelm onto a fainting couch. While Buntline's *Mysteries and Miseries* was ultimately adapted for stage production, this play, "The Back Alley," never existed. However, its fictional form left an affective residue that the folklore of back-alleys carried into abortion rhetoric. Sinclair's piece is a commentary on early twentieth-century publicity stunts that often had as their focus "vulnerable, yet erotically prone actresses dependent on male assistance," indexing "deep anxieties about modern city life and women's place within it."[134]

These anxieties about the gendered order were simultaneously anxieties about maintaining a white racial order. In one vignette featuring a jewelry theft, Miss ——— defends her housekeeper, Celeste, from police scrutiny by declaring that her trustworthiness stems from Celeste's mother historically having been enslaved on her family's Louisiana plantation.[135] It is also significant that Miss ———'s role is based on the olfactory rhetoric of "smelling salts." Even in fiction, back-alley olfaction persisted—especially when the morality of vulnerable white women was at stake. Reading the emergence of this "play" alongside voyeuristic racialized exposures to alley life situated white women as vulnerable to the agential force of back-alley influence.

As the revelatory documentary exposé intermingled with fictional accounts of virtue and vice, the back-alley held cultural anxieties surrounding the morality of white womanhood. Alleys were places to avoid precisely because their sanitary deficiencies would produce the moral decay of white women and children. Even so-called Progressive reformers distanced themselves through appeals to pity, granting the alley considerable affective agency to mold the manners, morals, productivity, and sexual behaviors of those living therein. Until now, we have been examining back-alleys' sanitary capacities to affect the morality of its residents. Found throughout journalistic textual fragments, back-alleys often became sites of criminality where unskilled "bad characters" with an explicit lack of care intentionally extracted resources to take advantage of those framed as most vulnerable.

The "Bad Characters" of Back-Alley Criminality

As social reformers specified the relationship between the unsanitary spaces of alley life and articulated those conditions to the moral characters of those residing therein, many were careful not to equate so-called alley immorality to criminality. Rather, criminality remained a downstream threat that could result from immoral behavior in unsanitary alley spaces. A confluence of legal restrictions and press circulation stigmatized alleys as criminal spaces that produced the *kakoethos* of those operating in them.[136] Back-alley rhetoric diminished the character of those within it, indicated a malicious intent, and admonished them for lacking quality and expertise. Invoking the back-alley framed these spaces as productive of dangerous criminality, leaving behind the affective residue of both a white, middle-, and upper-class fear and contempt.

On many fronts, back-alleys emerged as locations of crime. Although the affective residue of back-alleys appeared remarkably consistent, the object that mobilized this consistent affect remained contextually contingent. Prohibition of alcohol and pornography emerged in several instances, with back-alleys being places where crime occurred. In 1923, the *New York Times* reported on a ship, the *Manhattan*, that was described as having "a general back-alley appearance," because its aesthetic integrity was challenged: "The paint was falling from her sides in great blistering patches."[137] The dilapidation, or perhaps the residual sanitary discourse, was here, however, tethered to prohibition insofar as this article referenced a decommissioned yacht that had been transformed for smuggling liquor, as its "main street" sales were illegal. A remarkable June 1967 issue of *Playboy* magazine drew on back-alleys as sites of crime, lamenting how prohibition on pornographic material sales harmed youth. While *Playboy* consistently reported on criminalized abortion and advocated for repeal of laws before *Roe* in almost every issue between 1965 and 1973, the phrase "back-alley" in reference to a "quack" provider was not uttered in relation to abortion until 1970. However, a 1967 printed dialogue titled "The Playboy Panel: Religion and the New Morality" featured liberal clergy, notably including Reverend Howard Moody of the abortion Clergy Consultation Service. In this dialogue, Dr. James Luther Adams, professor of divinity at Harvard University, described his preference to keep the government out of vice censorship because it was functioning as a tool of a church "not willing to rely upon its power of persuasion with its own members."[138] He exhorted readers to recognize that "pornographic books and pictures are sold to youth in the back alleys, at exorbitant, exploitative prices."[139] Calling this practice a "very lucrative racket" that gestures to my description of criminalized abortion framing in the next chapter, back-alleys here were not descriptors but rather concrete places of criminal exchange that denigrated youth morality.

Back-alleys emerged as sites of notorious crimes that held the residual memories of criminal events. The November 28, 1926, *New York Times* article "Sale Stirs Ghost of Wilkes Booth" vividly tethered the back-alley to the memory of Abraham Lincoln's assassination. Featuring an enlarged image of Wilkes Booth, the article opened by reanimating his death: "The shade of John Wilkes Booth might have been seen lately stalking about a back alley of Washington, near the site of his crime, if the shades of murderers as they say do not rest."[140] It was a simple report that the US Department of War had decommissioned the barn near the Ford's Theatre, putting it to public auction, where it sold for $4,950.00. Neither a monumental tribute to Lincoln nor Booth, the back-alley played a central role in how Lincoln's death and Booth's escape were remembered. The back-alley separated the space between the Ford's Theatre and the barn where Booth stabled his horse before assassinating Lincoln. The article specifies that Booth "went into the stage door" through the back-alley and left it ajar to escape. The back-alley itself was an object in the narrative, worthy of memory based upon its proximity to Lincoln's death: "This event [the sale], if it did not actually stir Booth's ghost, has been sufficient to stir afresh the memories of that tragic April 14, 1865." Back-alleys recur when memories of "tragedies" lodged in the social imaginary have residual influence in shaping exigencies in the national landscape.

Referencing crimes or surprise attacks in the back-alley as dishonorable tactics were ways to imbue those framed as "other" with malicious intent, crafting a residual fear that easily attached to the mobilities of non-Western people. These durable practices persisted well into the twentieth century. A 1959 *New York*

Times article titled, "Both Sides Sight a 'Dirty War' in Algeria," tethered dirt to criminality. Amid the Algerian War of Independence and its massive resistance to the long-standing French colonization, the article's title borrowed the residue of sanitation. What made the tactics so ostensibly "dirty"? "You see a soldier's face grow taught with weariness and perhaps fear, as a Moslem [*sic*] gets too close to him in the bustle of traffic. Side streets are blocked off by wire netting reaching up to the fourth floor to protect the crowds on the principal streets from a bomb thrower who may be lurking in the shadow of a back alley."[141] The "shadowed" back-alley reference mobilized Western imperialist affects to generate a fearful orientation to Algerian people fighting for their independence. The anti-Islamic sentiment, with an extensive historical articulation to a fearful exoticism, constituted revolutionaries as criminals. Extending four floors into the air, wire netting anticipated that violence would occur from back-alley vantage points where—much like the Wellers' admonition—threats could be hidden from the eyes of controlling military surveillance. The "principal streets"—spaces where privileged citizens would otherwise feel comfortable walking freely—were framed as dangerous in proximity to the alley, as crowds required protection from the "bomb thrower." The secretive lurk of the malicious agent constituted the threat of a "dirty war" where those fighting refuse to play by the colonizer's so-called clean rules.

While back-alleys defined unseen places of criminal activity, they also articulated racial, gender, and economic differences when defining criminalized identity. In Progressive Era Minneapolis and St. Paul, Minnesota, leaders dismantled designated red-light districts in 1910. When the "problem" of prostitution persisted a year later, city officials called for increased police surveillance to combat the effects of the 1910 eviction: "The once segregated sex trade was now dispersed throughout the city—into alleys, residential areas, hotels, and saloons."[142] While sex workers of many races and ethnicities were criminalized, between 1915 and 1919, Black women sex workers were almost exclusively defined as "alley workers" and "alley walkers" in the Bertillon system of criminal identification, one part of a larger policing process of "cataloging and controlling difference" in the urban environment.[143] As Freda L. Fair makes clear, "The codification of alley work within the Bertillon ledger occurred within the context of Black women's labor in the state of Minnesota . . . [as] Black women's work in general is largely undocumented in the state of Minnesota prior to 1920."[144] Alleys were not only sites of crime but, through the Bertillon system, came to materialize the surveillance of racial and gender identity in a devalued sexual labor market.

While back-alleys received uptake as sites of crime requiring surveillance, back-alley characters emerged as unskilled, unqualified, harmful, and thus worthy of stigma and ostracization. Back-alley characters were not who they said they were, and that intentional deception ultimately produced harm within the larger collective. Mark Twain's book *Pudd'nhead Wilson* provides one such textual fragment that, by associating its targets with back-alleys, imbued them with *kakoethos*, that diminished an audience's perception of their rhetorical capacity.[145] Chapter 17, titled "The Judge Utters Dire Prophecy," opens in the summer months as a political campaign is picking up between "the twins," Judge Driscoll, and Pudd'nhead Wilson. Driscoll and Wilson were trailing the twins in popularity and are working in the closing days to save their chances in the local election. With everything coming down to a final appeal, Judge Driscoll makes a speech that, as Twain remarked, is "against both of the foreigners." In this "disastrously effective" speech, Driscoll "poured out rivers of ridicule upon them: He said they were back-alley barbers disguised as nobilities, peanut-peddlers masquerading as gentlemen, organ-grinders bereft of their brother monkey."[146] Common to these character assassinations is Driscoll's description of the twins as "disguised" and "masquerading." They are not gentlemen but peanut peddlers, organ grinders without that which is central to their act. The phrase "back-alley barbers" also tethers a more extended history of the boundaries of medical expertise.[147] As Twain concluded the short chapter, "The twins were defeated—crushed, in fact, and left forlorn and substantially friendless. . . . The brothers withdrew entirely from society, and nursed their humiliation in privacy."[148] The social withdrawal and ostracization here are essential features of stigma insofar as it separates and delegitimates their community standing. Moreover, framing the twins as "back-alley barbers *disguised as nobilities*"—who intentionally hid a weapon to be used at will—allows readers to orient themselves against the twins in terms of their deliberate harm in misleading the public. The disguise alerts the audience that the twins were intentionally effacing, hiding their true selves for political gain.

The perception of unskilled, unqualified, and potentially harmful back-alley dealings could redraw the boundaries of political affiliation while throwing racism and voter suppression into full relief. During the Iowa gubernatorial election of 1891, there was panic among Republican campaign managers after many esteemed members actively repudiated the party. One article discussed the prominent Judge Bishop, who "will give his reasons for opposing the Republican ticket in Iowa in forceful language." Candidate Wheeler was largely missing in action, which was disconcerting to several party members: "It must be very embarrassing to the managers of the Republican campaign to see him continue in his silent ways. There never was a campaign before in the history of this State when Republicans were unable to find out where their candidate for Governor was." The article described the Iowa gubernatorial campaign marveling at the shifting political allegiances: "A horse barn and back alley campaign is the last thing we should expect of a candidate for Governor on the Republican ticket in Iowa. This is one reason why so many Republicans are leaving their party in utter disgust and joining the Democracy."[149] The Republican defection had become so potentially harmful to Wheeler's campaign ethos that the candidate's staff dispersed to several surrounding hotels to recruit the African American service staff to the event. As the *Times* noted, "This putting aside of social bars occurs only at occasional intervals—when the colored [*sic*] vote is wanted. . . . The situation is becoming interesting in Iowa when such cold-blooded aristocrats as Clarkson are compelled to open their parlors to the colored [*sic*] leaders to hold their votes for the once great party." Back-alley campaigning required the presence of hitherto excluded African American men voting, whose participation was described as tantamount to corruption.

Beyond politics, deliberately fraudulent business conduct and poor-quality products were labeled as a back-alley variety—enabling vendors to differentiate higher and lower quality wares while simultaneously hardening the affective residue of sexual purity. A 1919 advertisement for the Rogers Peet Company displayed the image of a cat with the phrase "In the night All Cats are Gray" (figure 1.4). Although this idiom itself has no precise origin, it is frequently attributed to Benjamin Franklin's "Old Mistresses Apologue," a 1745 letter in which he commented on the "benefits" of young men having extramarital affairs with older women: "And as in the dark all Cats are grey, the Pleasure of corporal Enjoyment with an old Woman is at least equal. . . . Because the Sin is less. The debauching a Virgin may be her Ruin and make her for Life unhappy."[150] The Rogers Peet advertisement clarified: "The 'gray cats' in the clothing business include all those back-alley fabrics which, because they're so stylishly gotten up, are hard to tell from all the wool kind such as ours. Know your dealer!"[151] Rogers Peet's association of back-alley fabrics with Franklin's crude gray cat idiom hardens the affective association between the back-alley, sexual impurity, and untrustworthy business practices. The low-quality "back-alley" fabrics may well be inappropriately dressed up and masqueraded as authentic, or pure, wool. Masquerading "in the night" under the moonlight implied difficulty discerning the true qualities of the fabrics. The Rogers Peet Company was not unlike the Pro-

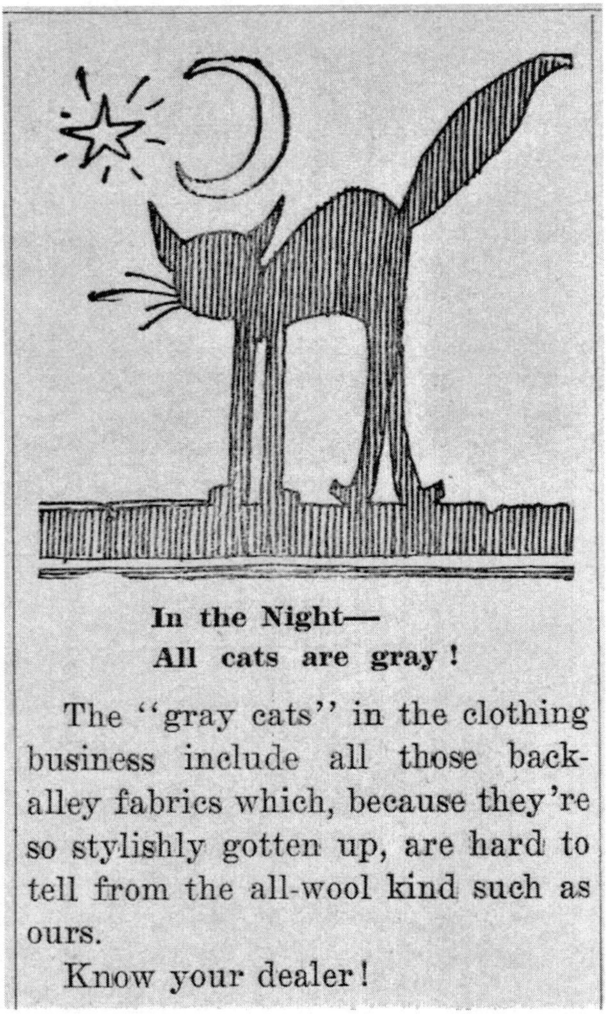

Figure 1.4. Advertisement for fabric made by Rogers Peet Company. *Lehigh Brown and White,* January 16, 1920, p. 2. Special Collections, Lehigh University Libraries, Bethlehem, Pennsylvania

gressive reformers who took considerable pride in themselves for shining the light of day on the alley spaces of the cities. Last, this advertisement brings us full circle to Singler's poem that opened this chapter, as the back-alley of fabrics remained precisely the spot where "cats are wont to meet."

Concluding the Detour

We can gather considerable insight into back-alley abortion by tracing the back-alley *before abortion*. Back-alleys as both physical places and imagined spaces have long occupied public attention. Fictional and nonfictional representations of the back-alley demonstrate its durability as a public rhetorical appeal. Discussions of back-alleys appeared in technical trade journals, antebellum US moral reform literature, Civil War medicine, and Progressive Era urban reform. The back-alley extended through concerns about alcohol and political campaigns. Notably, a robust search of "back-alleys" indicates considerable journalistic engagement. The phrase's durable presence in journalistic outlets, a publication space where the constraints of length prohibit full, nuanced explication of exigencies, also speaks to the power of this phrase to oversimplify complex problems. By examining more than one hundred years of back-alley rhetoric, themes of sanitation, morality, and criminality endure alongside affective orientations of disgust, pity, and fear. As the object of the back-alley changes to address abortion, these affective orientations persist.

Although the back-alley long referred to sanitary concerns, its articulation to morality and criminality complicated attempts at abatement. Between the circulating miasmas of war encampments, the Wellers' descriptions of the nonfunctional, dirty toilets; poor air circulation; and moldy conditions, and Townsend's concerns about vermin and infection in birthing spaces, it is difficult to argue with the harms that unsanitary conditions produce. However, even if some of these back-alley appeals were well intended, this rhetorical work was significantly stigmatizing for actual alley residents. As this chapter has demonstrated, there hardly seems to be a moment when alley space simply referred to sanitation, without a moralizing overlay. The argument that Singler made in this chapter's opening poem was that the weasels, rats, and cats congregated in the alley space, becoming strange bedfellows with humans who, in the case of Washington, DC, were escaping white supremacist violence of the South after the Civil War ended and Reconstruction failed.

This chapter's findings contribute to rhetorical histories of health and medicine by encouraging attention to what remains durable in an ever-moving rhetorical ecology. The affective ecology of back-alley rhetoric here includes a suite of public emotions ranging from disgust, white fear, and pity. Intertwined with durable themes of sanitation, morality, and criminality, these emotions produce a distinct affective residue that travels panhistorically even before the back-alley met abortion discourse. Affective residue refers to a visceral remainder, the remnants of the back-alley that get lodged in the social imaginary. Tracing the discursive strands that left this residue shows that the back alley sedimented a set of social relationships, sensory regimes, and visceral relationships to physical and imagined spaces. Whether it be the Wellers' voyeuristic fieldwork in the African American communities of Washington, DC, or Mr. Precise's tours through alleys in Buntline's *Mysteries and Miseries of New York,* alley abatement was often driven by appeals to the distancing emotion of disgust and the hierarchical emotion of pity for those who were of a marked underclass. This demonstrates that the alleys' visceral associations have long been an influential figure that could mediate hierarchical relationships between race and class.

Gender anxieties about protecting the health and well-being of white womanhood in an urban environment also flourished in the back-alley. This finding was perhaps most acute in fictional representations that placed white women in danger in their alley interactions. Buntline's *Mysteries and Miseries* situated Mary Sheffield's pregnancy and alley entrance as a pitiable and shameful occurrence, the unfortunate effects of an urban life of vice. Similarly, in Sinclair's satirical set of press releases that pointed to the fictitious play, "The Back Alley," we find the "weary" actress, Miss ———, falling into urban dangers such as an automobile accident, a jewelry robbery, a near-drowning, and a deposition where she testified to animal cruelty. The back-alley invited the public assessment that white women needed protection from dangerous, "criminal," and immoral influences. The immoral influences were not only harmful substances and environments but malicious actors—or what we will later learn in this book recurs as the "back-alley butcher." The back-alley organized a relationship between disgusting or fearful surroundings and bad characters worthy of condemnation because they were specifically unskilled, untrained, and *purposefully* deceitful in their business and political dealings. While fragments of this chapter discussed abortion, the next chapter more fully identifies how the back-alley began to slowly emerge in abortion discourse, implicating spaces, providers, and their modes of performing abortion care in the years before *Roe v. Wade.*

CHAPTER TWO

*The Pre-*Roe *Back-Alley Rhetorical Medical Encounter*

All of these abortionists fit the same mold. It didn't matter whether they worked out of houses or the back seats of cars. It was the same dirty routine. The house was usually run down. The room was dirty. The abortion was usually done on a kitchen table, sometimes on the floor. The instruments were wrapped in newspaper. They weren't sterilized. They weren't even washed from one client to another. It was just filth. The abortionists were black and white, men and women, what drew them to it was money. It was terrible.[1] —*Detective Stan*

Contrary to what the police said, my bedroom was neat and clean. So was the rest of my house. . . . I felt so horrible when I was arrested, and my name was in the paper. It wasn't doing abortions that I was ashamed of, it was being arrested. In my mind, the only people arrested are criminals, and suddenly overnight, instead of being a nurse, mother, and productive member of society, I had become a criminal.[2] —*Fay*

Fay functioned in our community for about twenty years, and there were a lot of Fays in other communities all over Pittsburgh. I have no doubt that there were back-alley abortionists—people with little training and little experience—but the Fays I knew weren't like that at all.[3] —*Dr. Clay*

A Landmark Speech

On October 4, 1971, Dr. Edgar B. Keemer Jr. stood in front of a packed press room for the annual gathering of the National Association for the Repeal of Abortion Laws (NARAL). As the vice president of NARAL's central district, Keemer, a Black physician practicing in Detroit, Michigan, surrounded himself with supportive lawyers, clergy, and physicians. He made a startling public admission: "I hereby assert that I have terminated unwanted pregnancies when I professionally assessed them to be a threat to the physical or mental health and, therefore, to the life-prospect of the impregnated females."[4] Although Keemer had been previously arrested, convicted, and jailed for an abortion he performed in 1956,[5] he resumed the practice in 1970.

His justification for doing so drew upon his memorable encounter with Mrs. X, a forty-year-old mother of seven children, who was "frantic for relief." Keemer lamented, "Besides the seven children, she had had two back-alley abortions with serious complications on both occasions."[6] After she "repeatedly expelled the intrauterine device," Mrs. X sought a tubal ligation in a Detroit hospital. During the procedure, Mrs. X's surgeon identified an early-stage pregnancy. Instead of performing an abortion, the surgeon closed her abdomen, informing Mrs. X she could travel to New York, where abortions were legally available as of July 1, 1970. According to Keemer, Mrs. X found this advice "ridiculous." He contextualized the compounding economic and familial factors that she considered in making such a "choice" and pondered aloud, How could she leave her children? Who would care for them? How would she pay for the procedure with only fifty dollars to her name? Considering how these travels would prevent her from raising her children in a safe, healthy environment, Keemer used his best judgment and performed her abortion. His speech closed by exhorting "other midwest physicians to reevaluate their commitment to the patient—be she poor or wealthy."[7] For, while Mrs. X was now "healthy," "happy," and "looking forward to a full life as a devoted mother," Keemer questioned the thousands of others being deprived of the "health, life, and liberty" available to the affluent.

In addition to describing Mrs. X's dehumanizing "back-alley" and hospital experiences, Keemer's speech also managed exigencies experienced within the Black medical community by carefully documenting his educational and professional credentials. Situating himself amid his family's lineage of esteemed medical educators, he explicitly noted that he "graduated from Meharry Medical College in Nashville, Tennessee, in 1936 and interned here at Freedmens Hospital."[8] Holding active staff positions at two Detroit hospitals and memberships in the

Wayne County Medical Society and National Medical Association, Keemer was a thought leader on abortion technique, having published in national medical journals.[9] More than just technically proficient, Keemer was a community *fixture*, serving NARAL, the Black Detroit Medical Society, and the Detroit Civil Liberties Union. Copiously listing these credentials responded to a twofold exigency beyond illegal abortion: the systematic educational segregation and delegitimation of Black physicians and the long-standing propensity for circulating discourses of criminality to denigrate Black people.[10]

Keemer's speech illuminates back-alley abortion's rhetorical power to establish mutually affecting relationships among spatial, provider, and procedural forms of legitimacy before *Roe v. Wade*. By leveraging his credentials to warrant treating Mrs. X following her two previous "back-alley abortions," Keemer resisted being labeled as a butcher by emphasizing the dehumanizing reproductive medical encounters that regularly occurred in hospitals—especially for Black women. Indeed, Keemer sidestepped the delegitimizing *kakoethos* of abortion stigma by maintaining his professional stature and moral character as a function of *where* and *how* abortions could safely be performed.[11] By dissociating himself from the inadequate care Mrs. X previously received, Keemer distinguished his performance of illegal abortions from "back-alley butchery" and positioned his practice, NARAL, and abortion itself as profoundly moral alternatives to existing legal strictures.[12] Importantly, Keemer's address brought the intersection of race, class, and gender to bear on the conditions under which women like Mrs. X would encounter back-alley abortions in the first place.

In light of Keemer's landmark speech, this chapter addresses two questions: How did back-alley abortion emerge as the common way to refer to a criminalized medical encounter with unsafe practices, unscrupulous providers, and unsanitary spaces? Once established, how did back-alley abortion function as a rhetorical appeal intended to prevent patients from having these encounters? To those ends, this chapter examines how pre–*Roe v. Wade* back-alley rhetoric crafted public expectations of a criminalized abortion encounter as the antithesis of legitimate medical care. This chapter frequently places "back-alley" in scare quotes or otherwise uses the phrase "pre-back-alley abortion rhetoric" to account for abortion spaces, providers, and procedures prior to their association with this phrase. Instead, what would become back-alley abortion rhetoric was articulated to rhetorically adjacent locations, characterizations, and techniques. As Nathan Stormer aptly puts it, "when contemplating illegal abortion's history, we tend to think of the 'back alley butcher,' but a therapeutic evacuation was not a fundamentally different procedure from an illicit one. . . . The practical difference between criminal and therapeutic procedures was the raft of untrained, self-taught, or unskilled abortionists in the underground, who undoubtedly accounted for much of the trauma coincident with abortion, but this was a wholly *contingent* difference."[13] This chapter extends Stormer's insight, arguing that the "contingent difference" between illegal and unsafe abortions emerged, in part, from how "back-alley" rhetoric materialized racialized clinical spaces in relationship to providers' technique, bedside manner, and sanitary practice. Before *Roe*, back-alley abortion rhetoric operated in an anticipatory register, sensitizing publics to the unseen potential for dehumanizing and dangerous medical encounters by triangulating provider *kakoethos* with unsanitary clinical spaces and unsanctioned techniques. Although pregnant people were a "dynamic part" of shaping the reproductive landscape during the pre-*Roe* criminalized era, they were rarely centered as deliberative agents in the back-alley rhetorical encounter.[14] By elevating the authority of even trusted medical providers, back-alley abortion also laid the *rhetorical* foundations for the US Supreme Court justice Harry Blackmun's majority opinion in *Roe v. Wade*. As Katie L. Gibson argues, "A central theme of *Roe v. Wade* is the apotheosis of medicine."[15] Although certainly not causal, back-alley rhetoric shaped the larger ecology of criminalized abortion, which percolated in Justice Blackmun's deference to the medical authority of esteemed physicians. Considering that bestowing reproductive *rights* is insufficient to realizing reproductive *justice*, this chapter situates back-alley abortion medical encounters as a constraining racializing health rhetoric and an inventional rhetorical resource for medical and legal discourse.

This chapter proceeds by theorizing the *rhetorical medical encounter*, wherein rhetorics of space, provider, and technique shape public expectations of medical care. I then contextualize the contemporary emergence of back-alley abortion rhetoric by tracing three metaphors that framed criminalized abortion practices before the "back-alley" came to dominate. Overlapping metaphors of mills, rackets, and rings negotiated spatial, provider, and technical legitimacy and mutated into back-alley abortion in the mid-1960s when juxtaposed to appeals to alley aesthetics. As abortion began to experience rolling legalization nationwide, back-alley abortion appeared more explicitly in advocacy, medicine, and the law, cautioning publics about criminalized medical encounters and drawing professional racialized, classed, and gendered boundaries around care guidelines.

Back-Alley Abortion and the Rhetorical Medical Encounter

In August 1941, Jane Ward authored "Don't Have an Abortion," for the *American Mercury* magazine, which was reprinted in *Reader's Digest* and later circulated by Planned Parenthood.[16] Ward's published her article during the wartime period when women's own narratives briefly circulated.[17] Oscillating between her own personal experiences as a pregnant widow seeking an abortion and experts from the New York Academy of Medicine, Ward warned women against navigating a very particular type of medical encounter: a criminalized abortion. To be sure, pregnant people certainly experienced morbidity and mortality following unsanitary clinical encounters with cruel and unskilled providers, aligning with Ward's experience. Simultaneously, testimonials across multiple archival sites and oral histories consistently indicated surprise and relief when an abortion experience did not fit those expectations and was instead marked by provider care, compassion, and competence. Gaps between expectations and outcomes gesture to how rhetoric anticipated what one might experience in a criminalized abortion encounter—such that relief could be a response to a dignified experience.

Narratives such as Ward's shaped a larger genre I term the "rhetorical medical encounter." Especially in the context of stigmatized procedures, "stories, particularly about embodied conditions, provide templates for understanding our own bodies and experiences. . . . When we've heard others' stories, we can use them to frame our own health and medical encounters."[18] Ward's story illuminates the contours of the rhetorical medical encounter for two reasons. Her article invokes proto-back-alley language, such as when she opened the piece by addressing "abortion" as an "ugly 'backstairs' word."[19] By also invoking the tripartite framework of space, provider, and technique, Ward's piece serves as a representative anecdote for pre-back-alley abortion rhetoric specifically and the rhetorical medical encounter more generally.[20]

Contemporary interdisciplinary medical encounter literature concurs: the quality of patient encounters with health care providers profoundly impacts their health outcomes and general well-being.[21] Medical encounter literature was initially provider-centric, detailing a "sequence of ritualized phases" that guided the physician-provider through the process of ascertaining symptoms, rendering a diagnosis, and prescribing treatment.[22] While these interpersonal dynamics certainly present an important aperture into the medical encounter, larger ideological, political, legal, economic, historical, cultural, and institutional dynamics texture the inequitable distribution of poor outcomes by emphasizing the mutually affecting relationship between interpersonal medical consultations and the larger contexts that shaped them.[23]

Criminalized reproductive care demands we center how medical encounters operate within concretized power inequities, including gendered stigma, histories and contemporary manifestations of medical racism, and how these dynamics translate into demoralizing and dangerous patient experiences. While any encounter is mediated through structural forces,[24] a medical encounter is "a product of its encompassing political-economic framework, in which struggle and inequality are central features."[25] As Dána-Ain Davis demonstrates, obstetric racism structures what might otherwise appear to be a communication breakdown in interpersonal medical encounters.[26] In fertility medical encounters, Loretta J. Ross explains how Black women often cannot get gynecological referrals to reproductive endocrinologists and are more likely to be recommended surgical solutions for uterine fibroids that remove the entire uterus.[27] Leandra H. Hernández and Marleah Dean explain how dehumanizing language in medical encounters devalues experiential knowledge and results in patients "feeling discounted and disempowered in vulnerable moments."[28] As individual stories of dehumanizing medical encounters recur, they contextualize expectations for subsequent encounters. Kirt H. Wilson contends, "There is no text without context and no context without text, because both are necessary for the hermeneutic process of understanding."[29] By extension, there is no individual medical encounter without the larger historical context of medical racism and patriarchy, and the structure of medical racism comprises innumerable interpersonal encounters.[30] Sara Ahmed similarly clarifies that a "particular encounter both informs and is informed by the general: encounters between embodied subjects always hesitate between the domain of the particular—the face to face of this encounter—and the general—the framing of the encounter by broader relationships of power and antagonism. The particular encounter hence carries *traces* of those broader relationships."[31] Patients' knowledge systems about the type of medical encounter to expect shapes their behaviors and interpretation of what occurs therein.[32] Back-alley abortion presents a rich site to interrogate the rhetorical-affective dimensions of medical encounters that manage the contingency of procuring criminalized health care within a larger context of structural health inequity.

Given that primary providers often turned pregnant people away (especially after law enforcement raids on abortion providers after World War II), there was often considerable uncertainty about the type of care that a person would receive.[33] *What kind of provider would they meet? Where would the procedure occur? What techniques would the provider use?* In Ward's case, her husband died while she was pregnant and already parenting three children. She visited "the best gynecologist in town" who turned her away: "I'm sorry," he said, "but I can't help you. An abortion is illegal, whether you're a wife or a widow."[34] Stories like Ward's, which would eventually crystallize into explicit back-alley abortion appeals, articulated a worst-case scenario by triangulating a profit-driven provider with bad character (*the who*), an unsanitary clinical space (*the where*), and improper *technē*—the unwieldy use of dangerous, non-sanctioned tools and techniques (*the what/how*).

First, the back-alley butcher or "quack" presents as a monstrous, *kakoethotic* stranger one might encounter when seeking criminalized medical care. As "panic-stricken" Ward sought a different provider, she described encountering "a medical pariah plying his trade in an upstairs office on a back street."[35] Those who fit the "butcher" character were not the trusted neighborhood physician or midwife. Abortion's criminalized status drove even otherwise sympathetic providers to turn away their usual patients, lest they become ostracized from membership in their medical communities, lose their license, or experience legal penalties. Ward described her provider as more concerned with his own legal protection than any complications she might experience: "The doctor had instructed me to not call him or any other physician, so I suffered alone, pulled through."[36] This self-interested callousness affectively illuminates "how the stranger is an effect of processes of inclusion and exclusion, or incorporation and expulsion, that constitute the boundaries of bodies and communities, including communities of living (dwelling and travel), as well as epistemic communities."[37] An exemplary stranger, the back-alley butcher is an exclusionary rhetorical effect of medicine's boundary work; they are practitioners who not only privilege the self at the expense of the other but also operate at the margins of medicine.[38] In Ward's article, Dr. Robert L. Dickinson, chair of the maternal health committee at the New York Academy of Medicine, described how most illegal abortions "are performed by *borderline M.D.'s* [*sic*] *uninstructed* in expert technique."[39] The qualifier "borderline" was no coincidence: as this book's introduction specified, criminalizing abortion has long been a practice of racializing boundary work, as the American Medical Association systematically delegitimated midwives, Black and Brown physicians, and other "irregulars."[40] Ward's article featured frequent pull-out quotations from well-established physicians to reinforce that hierarchy.

Pre-back-alley rhetoric's boundary work delimited not only *who* counted as a bad practitioner but *where* suboptimal procedures would occur. While rhetorician Judy Z. Segal's pathmaking work considers the "physician-patient encounter, a central encounter in medical practice," these interactions are necessarily situated in time and space.[41] I argue that not only does the clinic itself influence these encounters, but public *discussions* of (im)proper clinical spaces set the expectation. For instance, Ward reflected on the waiting room of a clinic she visited: "There were at least 20 people. . . . The atmosphere was tense, heavy with foreboding."[42] Even this rhetorical medical encounter far exceeded the doctor-patient relationship, with Ward describing the place as akin to an overpopulated beauty parlor. As Michel Foucault famously argued, "Medical space can coincide with social space, or rather, traverse it and wholly penetrate it."[43] Whereas chapter 1 demonstrated how back-alley rhetoric racialized imagined space and physical locations, pre-back-alley abortion rhetorics materialized medical encounters in clinical spaces like beauty parlors and Ward's "backstairs."

The pre-"back-alley" medical encounter also implicated *how* practitioners operated, with improper medical tools and unsanctioned techniques. The rhetorical concept of *technē* illustrates improper medical practice occurring in "back-alley" procedures. Jennifer Edwell, Sarah Ann Singer, and Jordynn Jack specify that *medical technē* signifies "knowledge that is pragmatic and bound to exigencies and situations that shape its use."[44] Ward, for instance, described her abortion provider's technique as an "excruciatingly painful scraping of the curette" with "clumsy hands."[45] The *technē* of having clumsy hands, in particular, is intimately connected to provider *kakoethos* and improper clinical space. *Technē* implicates the connection between training and practice: "Thus, medical *technē* denoted a realm of knowledge that was contingent upon the specific context, patient, and symptoms, which a physician would consider in relation to their prior experiences to determine the most appropriate healing practice for each case."[46] Techniques and tools that introduce infection or perforate the uterus braid attributions of improper tools (like coat hangers or knitting needles) alongside improper sanitary practices (unsanitized catheters). With a better understanding of the rhetorical genre of the medical encounter, the remainder of this chapter attends to the gradual emergence of what we today would clearly define as back-alley abortion rhetoric. By tracing the public messages that molded the expectations of *who* would provide care, *where* the encounter would take place, and *how* a procedure would be carried out, I demonstrate how back-alley abortion slowly began to enter US public discourse with regularity.

Before the Back-Alley: Metaphors of Criminalized Abortion Encounters

Before the back-alley became a dominant rhetorical frame for abortion in the late 1960s, criminalized abortion encounters were more commonly represented through metaphors of *mills, rackets,* and *rings*. These three metaphoric vehicles pervaded public discourse from the late nineteenth to the mid-twentieth century and were sometimes used interchangeably.[47] Although these vehicles sometimes overlapped, each generated slightly different rhetorical visions of the criminalized abortion encounter depending upon how (un)sanitary spaces articulated to the provider's motivation and skill.[48] The following cases illustrate how mill, racket, and ring metaphors anticipated the emergence of the more contemporary appeal to back-alley abortion.

The Mill

Dedicated to political commentary, satire, and exposure of the social ills contributing to the waning morals of society, *Jim Jam Jems* was a monthly magazine issued out of Bismarck, North Dakota. Written by Sam H. Clark, but published under the pen name Jim Jam Junior, Clark's investigative reporting titled "A Minneapolis Abortion Mill" led to the resignation and prosecution of University of Minnesota medical school professor Dr. Charles H. Hunter.[49] Ironically enough, the exposé also led to Clark's prosecution. Although Clark obviously derided abortion and aligned with Comstock's morality crusade, *Jim Jam Jems'* denunciation of abortion's so-called moral injuries circulated through the US Postal Service in 1912 and violated the Comstock Act. Dr. Hunter's abortion "mill" was especially significant because of its emplacement in Minneapolis, Minnesota, nicknamed "the mill city" for its prolific—and dangerous—grain mill system on the Mississippi River.[50] Between 1880 and 1930, Minneapolis was the "Flour Milling Capital of the World," kept alive by a steady influx of immigrants who worked in hazardous conditions.[51] Metaphors must resonate with a community to continue circulating as socially meaningful.[52] In the US Upper Midwest, milling metaphors were tangible to the working-class readers who purchased Clark's monthly newspaper.

While the mill was a potent vehicle for *Jim Jam Jems'* readership to imagine criminalized abortion as a means of processing pregnant bodies, it emphasized the sanitary spatial practices necessary to ensure patient safety. Much as nineteenth- and twentieth-century grain mills had a process to turn raw wheat into usable flour, *Jim Jam Jems* walked readers through the process patients encountered in Hunter's abortion mill: "The girl was first taken to the home of Mrs. Pickett, who resides at No. 622 East 17th Street. Mrs. Pickett's is known as 'the first place.' Here, patients are 'conditions.' They are treated for a day or two, and their physical condition brought to a point where the system will best withstand the ordeal of the operation."[53] Although *Jim Jam Jems* did not explicitly reference sanitation by invoking grimy, textured clinic surfaces, regional community knowledge of the physical milling process would assist readers in connecting this stage of the abortion encounter to sanitary practice. The first step of mill processing required that raw wheat be properly prepared to prevent contamination and avoid a system-wide breakdown. The patients who encountered "the first place" were likewise sequestered to avoid deadly infection complications on the operating table, which could alert law enforcement and jeopardize the entire practice.

Clark's mill metaphors encouraged readers to envision the abortion encounter as automated, foregrounding the procedure's process while minimizing attributions of patient agency. Following the preparatory phase, patients were ushered into the actual milling: "She was then removed to the home of Mrs. Susan Northfield at 2100 Garfield, 4th Flat, which is known as 'the second place.' Here the operation was performed by Dr. Hunter, and here the patient remained under the personal care of Mrs. Northfield until the doctor thought her sufficiently strong to make the journey back to her North Dakota home."[54] The passive voice ("She was then removed") limited the agency of the patient while elevating the agency of the milling process itself. Readers familiar with milling would know that wheat is fed through breaker rolls after being cleaned, which "open up the grain by separating the outer layer from the inner components."[55] Abortion perfectly fit the milling metaphor, as the "inner components" of pregnancy tissue were separated from women's bodies. Although the language of "operation" was sanitized and ambiguous, those working in the mills along the Mississippi River would likely find these metaphors vivid and resonant. The patients' final portion of the encounter would be with the "personal care of Mrs. Northfield," until they were well enough to return home.

Although Clark frequently equated pregnant women with the mill's raw wheat, his logic of contamination applied to his floral metaphors that lamented the delicate, lost purity of the women and girls "processed" by encountering Dr. Hunter's "abortion mill." The anonymous subject of Clark's exposé irrevocably ruined her sexual purity through her encounter with a morally contaminating "cesspool of crime."[56] As Reagan reminds us, "The image of the victimized single woman spoke to fears of the city and the changing roles of women."[57] Clark channeled these fears through floral metaphors whose potential could not be recuperated: "The rose does not shut 'to be a bud again' so as far as this child is concerned the cup of life is tarnished and she must face eternity as a broken reed."[58] Within a purity logic, contamination is irreversible. Whether as roses, reeds, or grain, the metaphors of plants circulated lament, pity, and paternalistic grief for a "pure" girlhood that the unfettered processing in the abortion mill would forever damage. When profiling upper-class married "society" women, Clark eschewed sexual purity logics and instead rebuked them for shirking duties of moral motherhood by "prefer[ing] to spend their time and dress and pleasure in bridge and wine."[59] Even without explicit racializing signifiers, these women and girls were likely to be imagined as white. Kimberly C. Harper reminds us that Black women, specifically, "could not claim piety and purity as virtues because they supposedly welcomed all sexual encounters."[60] In this case, even the possibility of *rejecting* moral motherhood was an unavailable subject position for anyone but white women.

In addition to lamenting the lost morality of patients, Clark's mill metaphor connected Dr. Hunter's own immorality with the efficiency of his technique. Hunter's bad character did not emerge because of poor *technē*; instead, as a University of Minnesota medical school faculty member, he was expected to be a moral bastion of the state's medical education program. While Clark certainly excoriated Hunter and his nursing team for their immorality, he did so only insofar as it harmed institutional and patient morals. Indeed, Hunter was perhaps *too skilled* at the operation. Clark's sensational exposure of Hunter's mill claimed to reveal something more significant than an individual case of abortion: an automated and prolific production system that irreparably damaged the moral reputation of Minnesota's major educational institutions and otherwise esteemed physicians.

As a relevant aside to the case's milling metaphors, an alley appeared in the tale of the Minneapolis abortion mill. Like the alleys of *Mysteries and Miseries of New York* explored in chapter 1, the alley functioned as a site of criminalized evasion in *Jim Jam Jems*. When friends made one of Hunter's nurses aware of the publicity that *Jim Jam Jems* had generated, she made a "sensational escape" to Canada: "The woman arose from her bed, where she had been confined for weeks with rheumatism, *and called a taxi cab to her alley door*."[61] While impossible to equate with the more contemporary phrasing of "back-alley abortion," the "sensational" end to the abortion mill exposé connected abortion, alleys, and the evasion of criminal exposure, rhetorically grounding a linguistic connection that enabled mills to later concretize into more explicit back-alley abortion rhetoric.

The Racket

As a journalist writing for *Forum and Century* in 1935, B. B. Tolnai offered something of a grounded theory of the abortion *bas-fonds* using the metaphor of racketeering, which the *Oxford English Dictionary* defines as "a dishonest or fraudulent line of business."[62] In his article "The Abortion Racket," Tolnai's rackets were framed similarly to Hunter's mill as distributing the abortion encounter through the entire city. However, the racket metaphor differed from the mill construct by downplaying the process itself and amplifying the improper spaces and monstrous ineptitude of providers. Encounters with abortion rackets were understood by their conspired protection *from* exposure: "Shielded by an impenetrable veil of secrecy," Tolnai wrote, "criminal abortion thus becomes one of the safest, best protected, as well as one of the most vicious rackets in the city."[63] This "protection" or "safety" did not apply to *patients*. Rather, Tolnai situated the malevolence of criminalized abortion as a more extensive and diffuse illicit network supported by law enforcement.

While the Minneapolis abortion mill required women's bodies to experience lengthy sequestration before their "operation," an encounter with the racket was saturated with disgust at the hurried speed of preparing the clinical space between patients. Unlike Hunter's automated but carefully sanitized abortion mill, racketeers could not see patients fast enough. Tolnai intimated that the flourishing economy of the abortion racket promoted careless septic practices between patients, negatively impacting the clinical space. Tolnai narrated one woman's encounter with the racket's grimy clinic, as she "walks into the abortionist's reception room, to wait her turn on the hastily wiped operating table."[64] As Ahmed argues, revulsion is "fascinated with the texture and qualities of what is felt to be disgusting."[65] "Hasty" antiseptic practices therefore implied that the racket's lack of care for patients manifested in a lack of attention to the space's cleanliness, enabling readers to imagine precisely the contamination that had been left behind: residual bodily fluids capable of introducing infection. With the provider's high velocity patient turnover, the two elements of the rhetorical medical encounter converged: *technē* and space. In the interest of seeing as many patients as possible, ineffective sanitary practices conditioned the type of revulsive space patients would have to encounter.

The racket's hasty sanitary practices also allowed disgust to stick to the abortion provider's character, rendering them both worthy of revulsion and instilling collective fear at the porousness of professional boundaries. Since the American Medical Association's mid-nineteenth-century anti-abortion crusade, maintaining the bounded ethos of the professional organization was an utmost priority, one that frequently referenced quackery or butchery as directly opposed to sound providers. Disgust was central to these practices, manifesting in how "the extent and evil of irregulars was treated almost as a pestilence."[66] However, Tolnai wrote, "Allowing for the fact that a considerable number of abortions are induced by midwives and quacks, the element of secretiveness, lack of proper care, improper sanitation, and very frequently lack of skill still obtains to a high degree in the case of full-fledged physicians."[67] Nevertheless, Tolnai conceded that the possibility of encountering a "full-fledged physician" in a racket should scare the entire community, as even credentialed physicians could hide their greed in plain sight. Toggling between the physical sanitary disgust and the loathsome characters of even "regular" or "full-fledged physicians" created a fearful distrust that warranted a surveillant eye and willingness to fortify professional boundaries against even seemingly trusted providers. Tolnai thus attributed a greedy motive to the quack and full-fledged physician alike, quoting an anonymous provider who referred to the fee-splitting that made referrals so lucrative: " 'I get my part, and I get out,' said a physician who boasts of having been the middleman in over 2,000 abortions in the past four years: 'He can kill her for all I care after that.' "[68] These statements produced the racket as a criminalized abortion encounter marked by bad characters who should instill fear and revulsion in readers. This fear was generalizable insofar as the provider's callousness filled in the underlying thought process of any provider who participated in the "racket," which was tantamount to an underground criminal syndicate.

In January 1951, ten years after Ward's article was published, *Ebony* magazine published a landmark article titled "The Abortion Menace," which used racketeering metaphors in strikingly similar ways to Tolnai's framework. While this article made frequent mention of Black doctors who were convicted of performing sometimes deadly abortions, the article was no encomium to rescue their characters. Rather, *Ebony* excoriated these practitioners, accusing several of being motivated by greed while graphically connecting them to patients' deaths. During the postwar period and through the early 1950s, the magazine largely centered on aspirational middle-class conformity, displaying "the 'happier side' of black life in America" with celebrities and sports stars.[69] While *Ebony* featured articles that combated sexual stigma,[70] "The Abortion Menace" diverged from this trend.

As a picture magazine, *Ebony* staged four captioned images to represent what it called a "typical example" of women's criminalized encounters with the racket: (1) "Meeting 'contact man,'" (2) "Typical abortionist's room," (3) "Abortion operation," and (4) "Tragic death." In the first, viewers witnessed a "contact man," or "go-between," and an "unfortunate woman" standing under a streetlight with their backs turned to the camera to avoid recognition. The second image engaged pre-back-alley language, describing an "unsanitary, *back-room* layout where sometimes as many as 10 such cases are handled a day. Infections usually result from unsterile equipment." Medical instruments were laid on a towel next to an examination table and sink. The third image, "Abortion Operation," featured two medics clothed in surgical scrubs, caps, gloves, and masks. As one performed the abortion, the other cradled the patient's head. The final image, "Tragic death," featured three police officers covering up a deceased corpse with a leg sticking out of the sheet. The "unhappy ending for the woman who risks an abortion" was here attributed to poor aftercare resulting in "hemorrhage, gangrene, or even inflammation of the brain."[71] Taken together, this series of four images walked readers through the entire abortion encounter with the "racket," from the initial meeting, to the clinical space, procedure, and conclusion of the medical encounter.

There are remarkable consistencies between Tolnai's abortion racket and *Ebony*'s. Verbally and visually, clinical inadequacy imputed *kakoethos* to providers while implying a larger network of (mostly unqualified) providers beyond the depicted scenes. Given that *Ebony*'s third image clothed the providers in proper surgical garb, which should signify an aseptic procedure, readers could ascertain that this "minor operation" was performed by an "unqualified practitioner" only because it occurred in "improper surroundings."[72] Similar to Tolnai's "hastily wiped operating table," *Ebony* provided the following context for what distinguished true medical care from the medical racket: "Under the best *conditions* a patient should be given an anesthetic and provided a week of aftercare, but most abortion racketeers seldom provide either. Working out of *cheap hotels and backroom 'offices,'* they are only interested in fat fees and *getting the patient off their hands as quickly as possible* for they well know that when the operation is a failure and the victim dies on the premises, a prison sentence is inevitable."[73] In other words, a criminal conviction was contingent on how quickly the provider could usher the patient *from* their space. *Ebony* also described abortion's social location and shadowy figures in terms strikingly similar to Tolnai's characterization of the racket: "Operating outside the law, shady practitioners include in their ranks a melange of questionable so-called medical men as well as racketeers ranging from frustrated medical students and sexual psychotics to barbers and midwives."[74] Although the article profiled three physicians convicted of performing abortions, *Ebony* indicated that the abstracted descriptions of providers could also include failed medical students, midwives, and barbers.

"The Abortion Menace" also figured clinical space as agential in its capacity to testify against the character of Nashville "racketeer" Dr. Reuben Bartholomew Jackson: "Convicted recently on manslaughter charges in the abortion death of a 25-year-old white secretary, the 50-year-old practitioner told police the woman was brought to his office by an unidentified white man, following an attempted abortion in a neighboring town. He said she collapsed in his office, and unable to revive her, he promptly telephoned fire department officials."[75] Jackson was initially framed as having exercised good judgment by calling emergency services, especially because the woman's autopsy substantiated his claims. However, the article quickly marked Jackson with a spatialized *kakoethos* "when authorities found a four-months-old fetus in his office—in a stove where it had been *hastily* thrown." Jackson's "hasty" disposal of the fetus not only recalled Tolnai's "hastily wiped table"; it also enabled an attribution of bad character that extended to the doctor, his judgment, and his clinic. To be sure, *Ebony* clearly took an anti-abortion stance that figured patients as desperate and unfortunate, such that even well-intentioned abortion providers could be sucked into the criminalized underworld by profit-seeking racketeers.

The Ring

Between 1935 and 1936, entrepreneur Reginald Rankin operated the Pacific Coast Abortion Ring (PCAR), which ran from Seattle to the Mexico-US border in Southern California.[76] In her history of the organization, Alicia Gutierrez-Romine notes that, certainly classified as criminal, the "ring" was remarkable in that none of its patients died, although some experienced profound morbidity and were threatened when they tried to seek hospital care. Rankin recruited skilled provider Dr. George E. Watts and envisioned recruiting "interchangeable" practitioners to move among any of their thirty offices.[77] In addition to recruiting Watts's highly capable but nonmedical apprentice Ruth Barnett, Rankin also pressured independent abortion providers to participate in PCAR to limit competition and insisted that the ring incorporate standardized clinical spaces.[78] Outfitting each space with similar cabinetry and room layouts, PCAR shuffled providers without significant interruption to the speed of abortion procedures and, by extension, the ring's profits.[79] Perhaps most importantly, Rankin organized this standardized space to hide in plain sight. Even though PCAR paid off surveilling authorities, they still wished to remain "unassuming so that every clinic appeared to be a legitimate doctor's office."[80] By taking these steps to blend in, providers became imbued with the bad characteristics of evading professional responsibility.

Ring metaphors remained resonant for decades after PCAR was prosecuted. In a 1954 article in the *Journal of Criminal Law*, Jerome E. Bates defined the contours of the abortion *mill* and dissociated it from the abortion *ring* to better understand the different types of encounters patients would have and how each met "some persistent need or want" within a societal structure.[81] These distinctions nevertheless contained the same categories that have come to define the contours of back-alley abortion encounters: the space, the practitioner, and the methods.

> The records of trial testimony at the New York Court of General Sessions and the files of Kings County, New York, Grand Jury reveal the existence of two fairly complex social structures known as abortion "mills" and "rings." A mill might be defined as an abortionist or several abortionists working steadily in a fairly permanent location and aborting a dozen or so women daily. A ring may be viewed as a number of interacting abortionists or mills working intermittently at several occasionally changing locations and aborting an even more considerable number of women daily. The actors in the ring are totally or largely known to each other, and clients are accommodated at the various locations depending on the pressure of referrals, the availability of operators at the moment of need, and the ability of the client to pay a sliding scale of prices.[82]

Whereas the mill existed in one or more stable locations, the ring produced a wider regional spatiality providing mobility the mill could not offer. The provider of the ring, still needing to "run his [*sic*] establishment with the greatest possible efficiency and safety," required business managers, secretaries, runners, and nursing staff to manage city space and ensure that demand was met.[83] Bates's characterization of mills and rings implied a twofold sense of safety: criminal and sanitary. The ring's provider required safety from possible raids and police surveillance. The labor of maintaining the secrecy of the operation fell to support staff. Secretaries would "judge people and evaluate their social roles" to ensure that they could "raise as high a fee as possible" and protect against "government investigators."[84] Nurses were paid better by the clinic than a hospital and were responsible for enacting necessary sanitary and disinfectant practices between patients.

The metaphors of the mill, the racket, and the ring certainly overlapped, sometimes in the same article. For instance, even as *Ebony*'s "Abortion Menace" featured the subheading "Racket Thrived On," its very first paragraph blended the other two metaphors:

> Ten years ago, reform movements and law enforcement drove practically all the competent abortionists out of business. But sprung up overnight in their stead were hundreds of abortion *mills*, headed mainly by quacks and borderline MD's who carried their lucrative practice underground with the aid of grafting politi-

> cians. In Chicago, one *ring* operated so openly at one time that it was common gossip that they did a booming, *assembly-line* business in a downtown State Street office, handling as many as 50 to 60 cases a day.[85]

Clearly, these metaphors worked together. Although mixing these vehicles might seem to make them unspecific, each shaped a unique vision of criminalized abortion's spatial imaginary, enabling the capaciousness that Rickie Solinger observes in the "back-alley butcher" figure. By representing what Leslie Reagan characterizes as the interpersonal "open secret" of abortion, these metaphors each helped to materialize the spaces where it occurred as a rhetorical secret: a known but unseen underworld.[86]

Consistent across these metaphors was the connection between providers' bad characters, techniques, and (un)sanitary spaces. Whereas mills provided a sense of isolated production and rackets alluded to questionable businesses, rings frequently amplified abortion's geographical spread. When used in tandem, each metaphor laid the discursive and affective groundwork for the emergence of the more contemporary "back-alley abortion" still in use today. By the mid-1960s, alleys became more connected to criminalized abortion in the mainstream, enabling the phrase "back-alley abortion" to emerge with consistency.

The Back-Alley Encounters Abortion: Alley Aesthetics and Biomedical Ethos

Since Lois Weber's 1916 silent film *Where Are My Children?*, television and film frequently represented fictional criminal abortion encounters.[87] However, 1965 marked a momentous year for prime-time US television audiences' visual sensitization to nonfictional criminalized abortion encounters through dedicated alley aesthetics. Aired just weeks before *Life* magazine would publish photographer Lennart Nilsson's iconic fetal images, *CBS Reports* first showcased "Abortion and the Law" to a national audience from 10:00 to 11:00 p.m. Eastern Standard Time on April 5, 1965, with an encore presentation on May 17, 1965.[88] "Abortion and the Law" displayed alley imagery while extending still-circulating spatial metaphors of mills, rackets, and rings. It also exposed a national television audience to the criminalized abortion *bas-fonds*, including physicians challenging archaic laws and statutes in individual states, whether by legal avenue or direct action. Hosted by Walter Cronkite, this documentary surveyed five women, a physician convicted for providing abortions, physicians who supported abortion but would not perform the procedure, lawyers, and clergy—some of whom held "diametrically opposing" positions regarding the moral status of the procedure.[89] However, as Cronkite noted, in what has become a problem of "epidemic proportions in this country . . . a dialogue [has] begun among doctors, lawyers, and clergymen." Cronkite's framing thus excluded pregnant people from deliberation. While women did share their experiences with criminalized abortion in the documentary, they appeared anonymously to provide illustrative testimony and were framed as part of the scenes where abortions occurred rather than as change agents in their own right.

A rhetorical template for mid-twentieth-century criminalized abortion spaces, "Abortion and the Law" articulated alley aesthetics to the public vocabulary of criminal rackets and rings to anticipate a dangerous medical encounter.[90] *CBS Reports* staged investigative real-time moments in alleys as women accessed their abortions, surveyed their surroundings, and met their providers. Reminiscent of the "first" and "second place" of Dr. Hunter's abortion mill, Cronkite described a "twenty-four-year old single girl [*sic*] whom our cameras filmed on her way to have an abortion in a Midwestern city."[91] As the cameras followed the woman waiting in a supermarket parking lot, she met someone, provided a "code name," and got into the "pick-up car which will take her to the abortionist."[92] Cronkite noted, "One hour later, the same car drops her off in an alley on the far side of the parking lot, and she walks back to the car." With the woman's face shielded, she provided testimony to the awaiting interviewers, revealing how her expectations of the encounter did not completely match the reality: "The drive took about seven to ten minutes, no more than that. The driver was very cautious, very alert. He pulled into an alleyway, he pointed out the entranceway. . . . He had keys, he opened the door, and we went into this apartment. And it was dark. It wasn't dingy. It just looked dingy."[93] Between the camera work, Cronkite's narration, and this anonymous woman's vignette, alleys bookended the criminalized abortion encounter, shaping expectations of the sanitary space she would find inside. The lacuna she narrated between the space *looking* dingy and not actually *being* dingy is notable. Although viewers did not receive more context about the surroundings in which she received her actual abortion procedure or the professional comportment of the provider, the woman anticipating the space's "dinginess" reflected the spatial expectations of what people would encounter in the abortion process. The long shot of the woman walking to the car and back from the alley further anchored the experience of travel, mobility, and fearful anticipation. Echoing Ned Buntline's character Mary Sheffield from *Mysteries and Miseries of New York* discussed in the previous chapter, this woman arrived for care through an alley and was returned to the supermarket through another alley to avoid visibility and public recognition. In the liminal moments the woman spent in the alley, viewers vicariously experienced a sense of the fearful contingency of criminalized abortion, witnessing her anticipation of an unsafe encounter and the relief when everything was ultimately okay.

Following these alley scenes, "Abortion and the Law" enacted a reciprocal relationship between unsanitary, disgusting clinical spaces and the *kakoethotic* provider one might encounter in the underworld. Cronkite returned on-screen to connect the dramatic scene with the public problem of illegal abortion, gravely narrating, "Criminal abortions, like the one just described, are big business—big enough to become the third-largest *racket* in the United States. Approximately $350 million are spent for such operations each year. Prices range from $25, charged by the amateur abortionist, to $2,500, charged by the professional. One abortion *ring* in the East, consisting of four doctors, averages four hundred criminal abortions a week."[94] Cronkite's vignette connected alley images to *rackets* and *rings*—combining and mutating extant metaphors with foreboding music. Sanitary revulsion and moral indignation permeated a range of scenes featuring unclean encounters, dangerous techniques, and callous practitioners throughout the program. Although most of the patients represented appeared to be white women, the criminalized abortion encounters displayed a class differential, from seemingly sterile office buildings with the "professional" to seedy motel spaces with the "amateur." One woman testified that the provider took financial advantage of her most vulnerable moment in the medical encounter: "About halfway through, he turned to my husband and said, 'Don't you have some savings that you could utilize and pay me more money?' " The husband testified to *CBS Reports* that "it wasn't clear that he would go ahead and finish the operation if I didn't pay him the extra money."[95] The exchange was set in the motel kitchen where the woman received her abortion "using some of the kitchen equipment, a telephone book, and chairs and so forth."[96] Although kitchen table procedures occurred throughout the history of medicine because of how doctors often provided home care, the kitchen in 1965 suggested substandard clinical conditions compared to the readily available alternative of the hospital.[97] The unexpected request for more money in the dilapidated space connected the physical disgust of the surroundings—something was happening *inside* a space that belonged *outside* of it—to the avarice of the practitioner. The kitchen also signified an arcane moment of the past by its juxtaposition to images of the sterile top-tier hospitals where the program's physician interviewees practiced medicine.

The motel encounter was followed by a long line of licensed physicians who dissociated their moral characters from the provider described in the previous scene. As Solinger confirms, the back-alley butcher "enraged" many physicians and "became a useful marker against which doctors of probity could distinguish themselves."[98] Physician interviewees included those who were convicted of performing criminal abortions for moral or "humanitarian" reasons, like Dr. George Lotrell Timanus of Baltimore. Also featured were white providers Dr. Robert Hall of New York City, who would later join *Abramowicz v. Lefkowitz*, a significant class-action lawsuit fighting New York's restrictive abortion statutes, and Dr. Alan Guttmacher of Planned Parenthood, among several others.

Beyond anger, each of these physicians distanced themselves from anonymized anecdotes of cruel and greedy providers by invoking their guilty feelings at turning "desperate" patients away, establishing their own moral guidelines and walking audiences through unsafe abortion methods whose fallout they had encountered in clinical settings. Dr. Edwin Gold, a white provider, reflected upon his guilt: "I passed on a sentence to this patient . . . which means that she's going to an abortionist. And under these circumstances, she's going to an individual who's usually not qualified, where the termination of pregnancy is going to be carried out under very poor medical conditions. . . . It will not be surrounded with all the safeguards of good anesthesia, blood availability, prevention of infection."[99] Dr. Gold's "guilt"—communicated in his admission that a woman would have to encounter an *abortionist* ("not qualified" and decidedly *not* a doctor) in "very poor medical conditions"—shaped a larger moral display that served to critique the laws and establish a medicalized superiority that could anticipate the sanitary needs of a procedure.

Much like Dr. Keemer's speech that opened this chapter, even physicians who were known providers of criminalized abortion care dissociated themselves from the "butcher's" avarice. Dr. Timanus, another Black provider whose clinic had been raided and who stood trial for providing abortion, described his refusal to participate in providing financial incentives for other doctors, pharmacists, or taxi drivers "because of the criticism that might accrue against the work."[100] Charging a sliding scale between fifty and one hundred dollars and often performing abortion procedures for free, he remarked, "Rather than subject people to quacks, [law enforcement] would allow me to continue."[101] Even as Timanus described his own "criminal" practice, "Abortion and the Law" elevated his expertise to draw boundaries between (un)acceptable spaces, (il)legitimate techniques, and (im)proper bedside manner when delineating the expectations of a criminalized abortion encounter.

After its 1965 broadcast, *CBS Reports*' "Abortion and the Law" circulated widely through activist spaces, serving as a touchstone for abortion rights groups to generate discussion topics. The documentary was a shared text that enabled groups to facilitate dialogues about the problem of criminalized abortion and to drum up support for repealing restrictions. The New York City–based Association for the Study of Abortion (ASA) referenced the CBS documentary, declaring that "it seems essential that the problem be opened for the public." The ASA generated a tool kit guide to "initiate discussion" regarding awareness of the "abortion problem" at local, national, and international levels. Discussion leaders were reminded that "a prime objective of the Association for the Study of Abortion is to ascertain and evaluate attitudes of lay and professional groups toward existing abortion practice."[102] Leaders were encouraged to involve viewers by asking them to reflect on the existing legal exceptions that authorized abortion as an acceptable practice.

For these focus groups, back-alley rhetoric crafted the illegal abortion's scenic ambiance. It served as the implied premise of the following enthymeme: women cannot legally access abortions; watching the video instructs you that illegality means access through the alley to the kitchen table; therefore, shifting the laws will prevent alley-based abortions. The sanitary, moral, and criminal discourses were points of affective stickiness, generating emotional commonplaces for the participants to return. For instance, the discussion guide prompted participants to provide their "reactions" to Dr. Timanus's conviction for performing abortions. Questions about the guilt Dr. Gold felt for turning pregnant women away from hospital abortions prompted shared dread: the alternative to the hospital was the alley. Participants were, finally, exhorted to react to Dr. Guttmacher's belief that "this 160-year-old law is puritanical punishment," lending viewing audiences the opportunity to express their moral outrage.[103] When coupled with exposure to the alley imagery from the film, these prompts leveraged the anticipatory fear of a dehumanizing abortion encounter to amplify affective investments in the movement to remove criminal abortion statutes.

A second way that activists took up "Abortion and the Law" concerned its circulation by the California-based Society for Humane Abortion (SHA), incorporated in 1965 by activists Patricia Maginnis and Rowena Gurner. Maginnis had previously organized the Citizens' Committee for Humane Abortion Laws in 1962. Between 1962 and 1964, Maginnis gave regular speeches to media and business professionals, organized public debates, and created public opinion polls to generate support for abortion in California. A nonprofit educational organization, SHA would publish newsletters addressing issues such as publicly unreported injuries and deaths of women who had received abortions alongside testimonies of those who were denied abortions by hospital therapeutic abortion committees. In conjunction with the Association to Study Abortion, SHA engaged in conference organizing and public education, including offering numerous public viewings of "Abortion and the Law" in neighborhood gatherings and various college classrooms across California.

Elsewhere, the Society for Humane Abortion represented the criminal abortion encounter by extending alley imagery that reinforced the connection between a greedy practitioner and the "dingy" alley space. Months after "Abortion and the Law" debuted to national audiences, SHA published a newsletter in November 1965 that included women's comments about restrictive abortion laws, reports on skyrocketing statistics of child assault, and the censorship of SHA's advertising in publications like the *National Review* and *Saturday Review*. The newsletter also included a political cartoon drawn by T. Carroll (figure 2.1) that invoked an alley to connect legislative decisions to their natural outcome: the misery of those who could not legally access a safe abortion in the United States.[104] A lawmaker in the upper left-hand corner looks triumphantly down at eight distressed women lined up outside the office of "Dr. Qwak, M.D." The caption reads: "Yessir, our abortion laws REALLY keep women in line." The meaning of keeping women in line was doubled: While it emphasized the control that laws could hold over reproductive bodies, the cartoon's irony emerged from the laws inability to fully control what women would do in response. Indeed, "keeping women in line" also resonated with *Jim Jam Jems*' metaphors of mills. Spatializing a moment of contingency, the cartoon depicted pregnant bodies waiting in an alley space and anticipated the fear of an unpredictable—and presumptively suboptimal—medical encounter.

This cartoon's composition centers alley aesthetics while generating assumptions about who gets abortions, where, with whom, and at what stage in pregnancy. Unlike previous instantiations of back-alley abortion aesthetics in "Abortion and the Law," the women in the cartoon are not quickly traveling through the alley to evade visibility. By treating the alley like a waiting room, the cartoon blurs the boundaries of inside and outside the clinic. Furthermore, the line visually invokes the metaphors of raw wheat that would be fed through a mill system. That cartoon, of course, represented all the patients as white women, lined up deep into the alley waiting to enter the dark office, with faces reflecting distress, anger, and uncertainty concerning what they would encounter inside. Each woman is also represented as heavily pregnant with exaggerated breasts and buttocks, potentially feeding the perception that terminations regularly occur in the later stages of pregnancy.

Representing a dangerous city space, the bottom left-hand corner includes a broken wagon just in front of an open trash can enticing a black cat that, as the

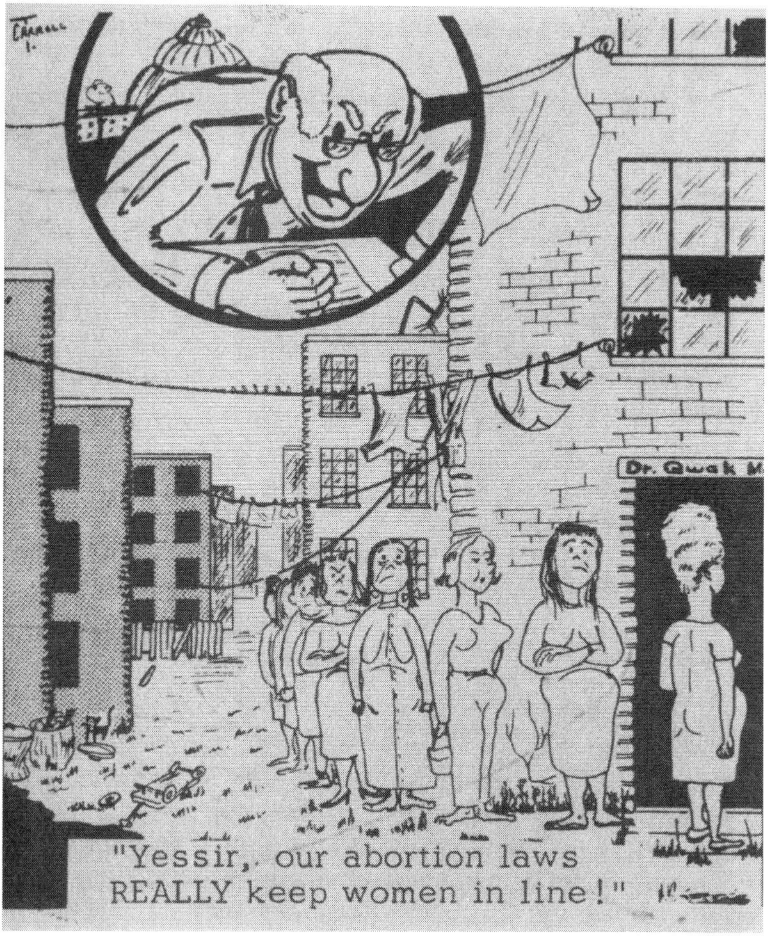

Figure 2.1. T. Carroll cartoon, Society for Humane Abortion. Public domain

poem that opened chapter 1 noted, one "is wont to meet" in the alley. The open trash can, in turn, stimulates a viewer's olfactory imagination to assess the space as a disgusting, dehumanizing way to access medical care because the unsanitary pathogens from the atmosphere could easily breach each patient's corporeal boundary. Broken windows, dilapidated fencing, and laundry strung between buildings paint the area as run-down and unkept, invoking the back-alley's affective residue. These features invite the viewer to imagine the possibility of criminal victimhood without a moment's notice.[105] Although viewers cannot see the clinical conditions inside, the cartoon's broken windows also invite them to anticipate a disordered office inadequate for practicing medicine. Including this cartoon in the SHA newsletter visually solidified a connection between the gleeful cruelty of lawmakers, unsanitary alley conditions, and the unqualified provider with a steady stream of gloomy patients.

The spatial imagery of "Abortion and the Law" was also taken up by future journalists seeking to survey the affective landscape of criminalized abortion. In December 1966, Stanford University student Larry W. Howe submitted a script for a communication studies course titled "Abortion and the Law: A California Report." This script centered alley imagery to capture audience attention while introducing California physicians and social movement organizers seeking to improve the criminalized climate.[106] Although never filmed, this proposed script for a thirty-minute television documentary engaged key advocacy stakeholders in its creation, including physicians affected by abortion laws and grassroots activists such as Patricia Maginnis, who consulted with Howe in his project. The proposed script was split into two columns to indicate how video and voice-over would represent the unseen criminal underworld of illegal abortion in California. For the first minute and a half, viewers would see images of three women: a married forty-five-year-old Woman A; a younger wife of a college student, Woman B; and Woman C, defined only as being "from slum area."[107] Representing the economic stratification that affected one's access to safe abortion, Howe proposed quick cuts between the three women: Woman A, who already has three children, flew to Japan, where she paid $100. Woman B, wishing to wait until her spouse finishes college to have children, crossed the Mexico-US border, pays $600, and reports that her encounter with "the doctor was efficient and clean."[108] Woman C, by contrast, who was not indicated as being in any relationship, reports that she has seven children and used word of mouth to find a practitioner who fled with her money after the procedure ended, leaving her hospitalized for the next two weeks.

The script indicated action shots that would, much like the *CBS Reports* production, follow each woman through her abortion encounter into the spaces where the procedure occurs. Unlike Women A and B, Woman C's life appears to be in disarray: a split shot of her and the others shows her "preparing food for her children, who are running around her."[109] Woman A, on the contrary, is waiting at the airport for her flight to Japan while Woman B is dutifully observing her husband studying next to a large stack of books. A subsequent voice-over rehearses a common class-based access refrain to discussions of criminalized abortion circulating elsewhere: "Those with money travel to Mexico or Japan, where they can secure proper medical treatment. Those less fortunate are forced to risk their lives *in motel rooms, back alleys, filthy apartments*."[110] The back-alley remained a dangerous and clandestine space that generated a sense of anticipatory dread "simply because," as the voice-over warns, "a trained doctor cannot legally give them medical assistance."[111] Stage directions suggested filming a long shot of a motel and then a medium shot of a "dirty alley," zooming in to a door before a focal shot to a "grubby apartment," where the camera was directed to "PAN to messy bed," intimating that these were all potential sites of Woman C's abortion. At this point, the script indicated dramatic orchestral music. The title, "Abortion and the Law: California Report for KPIX," would flash across the screen to demonstrate that the abstraction of national news that Cronkite reported on was also a local reality.

Considering that the program was never brought to fruition, these three women functioned as positional placeholders for the criminalized medical encounter. When considered through the lens of the alley's affective residue, however, Woman C held a critical racialized function in relationship to the alley even as her situation was narrated as solely a function of her class. Although Howe's script did not specify Woman C's race, her juxtaposition to the back-alley materialized it nonetheless. As addressed in chapter 1, beginning with the Great Migration, real estate opportunism allowed alley homes to become sites of racist spectacle and dehumanizing sanitary conditions synonymous with stigmatized anti-Blackness. Dominant city planning discourses such as Ellen Richards's *Euthenics* associated alleys with racialized and individuated moral failings such as criminality, poor sanitation, and greater rates of disease.[112] By invoking the "dirty alley" without further context, "Abortion and the Law: A California Report" elided the structural and economic reasons for inadequate housing conditions.

Without explicitly labeling Woman C's race, her subjectivity was nonetheless constituted by the residue of alley clearance efforts and powerful controlling images about Black mothers' presumed promiscuity.[113] Living in the "slums" with seven unsupervised children as a single mother, Woman C implicitly fails to meet the moral expectations of white motherhood. According to Harper, Woman C's seven children would situate her as a "breeder woman" or "jezebel," feeding into images of the "welfare mother" or "crack addicted mother" who was "not able to provide a moral foundation for her children."[114] Thus, the fate Howe imagined for her criminalized abortion encounter—the dirty bed, motel room, or alley—was conditioned by the larger racialized history of back-alleys in conjunction with controlling images of Black women.

Although Howe recognized his depersonalizing moves and framing limitations, he did not reflect upon his use of controlling images of Black women or on how his alley rhetoric pushed him toward such assumptions: "If the script appears a bit like a magazine or book, I fear this is a result of my distance from the subject, in spite of my inundation with basic research on abortion."[115] While alley clearance surveyors of the past prided themselves on their objectivity, Howe instead considered his distance from abortion experiences a shortcoming of his proposed project. His solution was to redouble his efforts to gather more stories: "To make it a live and persuasive documentary, much more personal detail must be presented, more women, everyday women who are among the 100,000 California women who yearly have abortions. To find these women would be my next task."[116] To be sure, Howe's reflection indicated a desire to nuance his assumptions by elevating the perspectives of those who would be most affected by legal restrictions on abortion. However, his invocation of alley spaces nonetheless defaulted his proposed program to reductive caricatures of racialized and criminalized medical encounters, inviting responses from pity to the moralizing disgust and contempt.

Ultimately, "Abortion and the Law" drew on existing circulating metaphors to make visible criminalized abortion and introduce alley aesthetics to a nationwide prime-time audience and circulated to foster activist engagement. Alleys were prime spaces to receive this articulation to abortion owing to the affective residue that sanitary, moral, and criminal alley discourses left behind. As this program and others like it indicate, back-alley abortion appeals offered rhetorical affordances to physicians who were part of a "splintered group": they could claim the morality of abortion while maintaining their professional ethos.[117] By connecting to skilled physicians who could lament the situation, the documentary drew a boundary around appropriate spaces of provision and the doctors operating therein, demonstrating how the *kakoethos* of abortion stigma was reciprocally constituted by the back-alley space and the bad character of its provider.

Within social movement, journalistic, and legal discourses, back-alley abortion appeals and imagery picked up considerable circulation after *CBS Reports*. Often working together, doctors and activists used the back-alley as one rhetorical strategy in the pre-*Roe* movement to legalize abortion. These appeals ranged from public protests to activist-organized conferences about the proper spaces of abortion care. Even with legal protections emerging, back-alleys continued to anticipate the worst-case scenario: the spatial, technical, and provider expectations of a dehumanizing medical encounter.

Repeal or Reform? Back-Alley Deliberations over Proper Abortion Spaces

In 1969, New York legislators considered repealing the state's abortion laws and brought predominantly male experts—judges, psychiatrists, legislators, and physicians—to testify. As attorneys Diane Schulder and Florynce Kennedy later wrote in their book *Abortion Rap*, only one woman was called upon to testify—a Catholic nun.[118] The Redstockings, a radical feminist group, stormed the hearings demanding to testify. Republican senator Norman Lent dismissed their efforts, arguing that the hearings were designed to gauge expert testimony, not public opinion. Declaring their experiences with criminal abortion a necessary part of this medical encounter, the Redstockings instead organized an abortion speak-out at the Washington Square Methodist Church.[119] While the exact phrase "back-alley abortion" was not recorded, one person described the differences between medicalized clinics and criminalized spaces in terms of *technē*: "It's a very simple procedure. Takes the doctor twelve minutes if it's done in a hospital. If it's done in the *back room* of some hotel, it's not such a simple procedure."[120] In clinical spaces, abortion techniques were assumed to be simple; "back rooms" were ripe for complications. Another speaker similarly exhorted:

> The reason we have the laws that we have now is because men want to make us suffer for their sins because it's a sin to get pregnant. And women are forced to carry an unwanted pregnancy. If you do not want the pregnancy, you are faced with the very clear reality, and that is you are sacrificing your life when you go to a hotel or when you get into a car on 54th St. and Lexington Avenue and you're blindfolded and taken somewhere, you don't know where. You're not given anesthetic. The instruments are not even sterilized. You wind up with an infection. . . . And this is what women have to go through. This is our debt to society.[121]

This speaker set an anticipatory scene much like that depicted in "Abortion and the Law": a patient would be taken *somewhere* and would likely not be able to trust the provider. They might be denied access to sanitary tools, skilled techniques, or adequate pain medication. Not knowing *where* the abortion would take place, *who* would complete the procedure, or *how* it would be done, the blindfolded moments were those of liminal anticipation.

As New York reformed its restrictive abortion statute in 1970 to allow abortions until twenty-four weeks gestation, appeals to back-alley medical encounters gained traction. Newfound legalization produced new regulatory exigencies about where abortions should take place, who was qualified to perform them, and what techniques were appropriate. Considerable debate commenced between those doctors who wished to see abortions still performed in hospitals and movement leaders who, in conjunction with progressive medical professionals, recognized that abortions could be safely performed elsewhere. In fact, they reasoned that financially inaccessible hospital care could lead pregnant people to the same harmful encounters showcased in "Abortion and the Law." One crossover between these contexts was Robert Hall, who appeared in the *CBS Reports* documentary. Hall advocated for hospital-based care, arguing that botched jobs could set the movement *back* at least five years.[122] His argument was visually bolstered by a photograph of a surgeon carefully inspecting sanitized tools. Others, like Lucinda Cisler of New Yorkers for Abortion Law Repeal, argued that limiting abortions to hospitals was barely more than a reform initiative.[123] Back-alley appeals mediated deliberations about spatial propriety, provider stature, and techniques across the country in newly legalized states.

Between New York's legislative decision in March 1970 and July 1, 1970, when the legal changes went into effect, back-alley appeals proliferated in two notable symposia that directly addressed the safety and wisdom of out-of-hospital abortion encounters. The first was the Society for Humane Abortion's Symposium on Office Abortions held in San Francisco on May 16, 1970, following California Supreme Court's 1969 *People v. Belous* decision. The second was NARAL's First Symposium on Hospital Abortions, held in New York City the day after the legal changes went into effect. Under Patricia Maginnis's leadership, the California-based SHA was the first to organize a Symposium on Office Abortions. Maginnis and her associate Rowena Gurner had coordinated a referral program for women traveling to Mexico to obtain safe abortions. The referral service allowed Maginnis to confidently assert that abortions could be safely performed in offices rather than hospitals, presuming proper antiseptic techniques and provider motivation. Throughout the mid-1960s, Maginnis and Gurner's referral program also offered word-of-mouth surveillance, tracking providers and their spaces of practice. To guarantee safe care, they procured post-abortion reviews and kept meticulous records of trusted practitioners. These reviews were overwhelmingly positive, with patients and partners commenting on the kindness and high-quality care they received. Occasionally, reports raised sanitary concerns, and, in these cases, Maginnis and Gurner frequently followed up by allowing practitioners to clarify their aseptic practices. Less frequently, providers demonstrated inappropriate bedside manner and price gouging, resulting in their removal from the referral list.

On the morning of May 16, 1970, a group of seventy-two gathered for the SHA symposium. Introducing Maginnis as the "Florence Nightingale of pregnant women," Dr. David B. Cheeks applauded her work in abortion-related border crossings from the United States to Mexico and post-abortion care facilities in the United States.[124] This comparison was significant, as Nightingale spent her career championing principles of clinical spatial organization to decrease the risk of infection in hospital encounters. Cheeks noted that specialists presented "a great deal of experience" and could share techniques for performing the procedure well in doctors' offices. These techniques would, in turn, allow women to avoid traveling long distances for the privacy and security of a safe abortion.

Maginnis's introductory remarks explicitly connected financial inaccessibility to the likelihood of a back-alley abortion encounter. She situated the realities of New York's reproductive landscape as an exemplar of class discrimination enacted by socioreligious pressures, which had established "arbitrary standards" for practicing reproductive health care consisting of confining abortion to hospital spaces that generated enormous fees. As Maginnis explained, "If doctors fail to abide by these politically motivated health department 'standards,' they will be vulnerable to malpractice suits." She targeted "legislators, health departments, medical associations, and anyone else who will force abortions to be done only in hospitals." She also threw the financial disparity into sharp relief: "A principal reason why we are frantic about the hospital requirement is that in hospitals, abortions now cost from $400–$1000, while in the office, the procedure can be performed safely and profitably for less than $150.00. And I don't think we can tolerate the attitude that says, 'Well, you can get an abortion if you've got the money.' Good medical care only for the affluent is blatant discrimination, totally out of step with democratic and humane ideals." She closed with a powerful appeal that contrasted the back-alley to these ideals: "With only high-priced abortion available, the stage is still set for back alley operations. The basic question of this symposium is whether or not abortions should be restricted to hospitals."[125]

The connection Maginnis made between the exorbitant costs of hospital abortions and women seeking substandard "back-alley" care was not a new appeal. While she had printed T. Carroll's cartoon in her SHA newsletter, Maginnis was herself a prolific cartoonist and illustrator. In 1969, she published a pamphlet titled *The Abortee's Songbook* that included her own illustrations and lyrics that helped provide context for the images. The songbook critiqued medical surveillance and religious control—but one cartoon connected the exorbitant costs of hospital abortions and alley spaces (figure 2.2). The image on the left page of *The Abortee's Songbook* presented a woman collapsing over broken stairs leading out

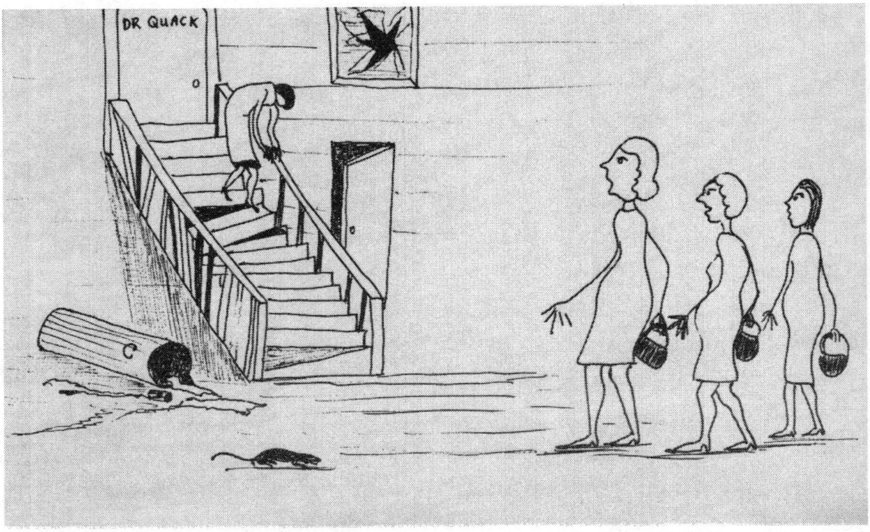

Figure 2.2. Patricia Maginnis, *Abortee's Songbook,* Society for Humane Abortion. With permission from Schlesinger Library

of the office of another Dr. Quack. A broken window and open door promise the same dangers to the pregnant women approaching the entrance from the street. As the other three women approach the clinic, ostensibly readying themselves for their own abortions, they anticipate their own outcome based upon the first woman's clumsy descent down the stairs. Seeing the woman leaving in such an unstable manner primed their shock, fear, and dismay, demonstrated by their mouths agape. Next to the stairs, a tipped-over garbage can attracts a rat to the image's foreground. Recall how the poem that opens chapter 1 also remarked that the alley was the "birthplace of the weasel and the rat." Thus, while the alley imagery was less explicit than in T. Carroll's cartoon, affective residuals remained.

A brief limerick contextualized the image on the right side of the songbook: "You go to the quack up town; Hospitals want four hundred down! Their blatant extortion; of you for abortion; is dressed in a surgery gown!"[126] In no uncertain terms, this two-page spread in *The Abortee's Songbook* constructed the "quack up town" as the necessary choice when high costs and hospital committees gatekept hospital abortions. In juxtaposing Dr. Quack to the hospital doctor's extortion dressed in a seemingly sterile surgery gown, readers were forced to confront an important question: Who was the actual immoral provider in this context?

Returning to SHA's conference, back-alley rhetoric continued in Lana Clarke

Phelan's aspirational luncheon address "Can We Build a Better World?" Lamenting the "wretched profiteering and exploitations of underprivileged women," Phelan echoed Maginnis's point that with modern office-based techniques, "abortion will be decently, safely performed under proper medical circumstances and at modest prices rather than in the vast underground racketeering facilities which have been the lot of American women denied access to normal channels of medical care."[127] She closed her speech by connecting NARAL's advocacy with an alley appeal: "In short, we are bringing a relatively simple medical treatment out of the alleys of America into doctors' offices, clinics, and hospitals, in which care should have been provided for the past century."[128] A notable difference between Maginnis and Phelan was the way each figured the role of the alley in relationship to the hospital. For Maginnis, hospital prices ushered patients toward back-alley practices through inaccessible costs. For Phelan, however, alleys were the criminalized point of origin enabling hospitals to become part of a suite of "normal channel[] of medical care" in contradistinction to still-existing abortion rackets.

The published proceedings also expressed the benefits of physician-office abortions in contrast to the back-alley. Not only would office procedures enhance privacy and lower cost, but a well-sanctioned environment would also mean greater access to the procedure: "Fewer women will seek back alley 'bargains' because there will be many skilled physicians doing office abortions under good conditions at reasonable prices."[129] This availability would ensure that patients procured the procedure earlier in their pregnancy than if they were "obtaining a high-cost hospital abortion or a dangerous back alley abortion." A number of attendees ultimately speculated that office-based procedures could expand abortion access, serving as a point of equilibrium between two nonideal options: the overly expensive hospital procedure on the one hand and the "back-alley bargain" on the other. This statement ultimately demonstrates the flexibility of a back-alley abortion rhetorical appeal within the same symposium. Whereas this symposium participant speculated about the "bargain" of a back-alley procedure, descriptions of back-alley abortion often came with price-gouging narratives resembling the motel room incident in "Abortion and the Law." Either way, back-alley abortion became the foil for advocating for better spatial options.

Despite these deliberations about where abortions should be performed to prevent recourse to "back-alley bargains," arguments against hospitals were largely grounded in patient cost rather than racism. However, hospitals proved to be sites of obstetric racism in abortion care, especially illuminated by the death of Carmen Rodríguez, a thirty-one-year-old Puerto Rican woman, after her abortion at Lincoln Hospital—just eighteen days after New York's law went into effect.[130] Rodríguez was given an asthma medication in anticipation of her abortion that was contraindicated for her heart condition. Her heart stopped, and she experienced irreversible brain damage as the provider tried to revive her. One of the "chief demands" of the New York–based Young Lords Party was dignified health care for low-income people, especially "Third World" people who bore the brunt of racially stratified medical care like medical experimentation and sterilization abuse.[131] Throughout the YLP's newspaper *Palante*, several articles spoke to horrific treatment at New York municipal hospitals. In "Murder at Lincoln," Gloria Cruz equated city municipal hospitals to "butcher shops" as she excoriated the lack of care and technique that Rodríguez experienced at the hands of the inexperienced medical staff: "They never bothered to check her chart. The punk that was treating her was a student."[132] While she did not use the phrase "back-alley," Cruz nevertheless wove the tripartite framework of the back-alley medical encounter, joining the likes of Dr. Edgar Keemer in arguing that hospitals often were dehumanizing and dangerous clinical spaces for women of color. Making a similar argument, connecting inexperienced, unqualified providers (medical students) with inept technique (not checking her chart for existing health issues), the municipal hospital emerged as a site of reproductive injustice—what Cruz called a "butcher shop."[133]

Ultimately, while some activist and more enclaved technical communities situated the back-alley as a speculative horizon justifying improving medical encounters, others like the Young Lords grounded their appeals in frames of medical racism. Although back-alley abortion arguments sought to improve outcomes in their own ways, some individual abortion providers still found the back-alley to be a concrete rhetorical constraint that they had to overcome in their own practices. Indeed, back-alley descriptions of clinical space shaped the attributions of individual providers' legitimacy in terms of care and judgment, demonstrating how medical encounters inevitably implicate space, provider, and *technē*.

Spatializing Providers: The Dissociative Power of Back-Alley Abortion

Back-alley spaces went beyond articulating abstracted arguments for policy reform; they also mediated the rhetorical production of provider character. Back-alley appeals distinguished between worthy practitioners who operated in proper clinical spaces and practitioners whose poor judgment was reflected by their choice to haphazardly operate in an unclean space, as evidenced by the distinct medical practices of Dr. Edgar Keemer, whose testimony opens this chapter, and Dr. Robert Stanley Nixon. Whereas Keemer's anonymous interview was relaxed and publicly circulated in a newspaper, Nixon is instead *spoken for* in a declined criminal appeal that crafted legal precedent.

Although Keemer would not publicly announce having performed illegal abortions until his NARAL speech in 1971, he provided an anonymized 1969 public testimony in which he dissociated himself from back-alley providers.[134] Arguing for the moral necessity of removing restrictive laws in an interview with journalist Helen Fogel of the *Detroit Free Press*, Keemer maintained that he wished to remain anonymous not because he was "cowardly about [his] position" or shirking professional responsibility. Instead, his extensive family practice, membership in medical societies, and affiliate status with large hospitals necessitated that he speak off the record. "You can't imagine the pressures involved in this," he confided to Fogel.[135] As he later elaborated in his 1980 autobiography, these pressures were deeply tied to the racial politics of performing abortion as a Black physician. Adamant that he was "never one of these back-alley men," Keemer refused to equate his anonymity in this interview with a lack of skill or profit motive. Quite unlike the "motel kitchen" abortion extortion discussed in *CBS Reports*' "Abortion and the Law," Keemer "charged an average of $150," often offering the procedure for free. Indeed, the article emphasized his decided lack of financial interest by comparing how "fees for dependable medical abortions, legal and semi-legal, start at $500." Instead, the anonymous doctor was driven by care and the well-being of patients—quite unlike the hospital system Maginnis critiqued.

After establishing his altruistic motivations, the article described Keemer's clinical space to bolster his capacity as a medical practitioner. As Fogel wrote, "The doctor and I stay in his well-appointed office in a Detroit professional building." Far from the "dingy" space anticipated in "Abortion and the Law," Fogel characterized Keemer's "well-appointed" clinic as easily capable of passing sanitary inspection. Within the scene of this office interview, Keemer argued that, with changing laws, abortions could be safely performed in similar nonhospital settings—including the very space of this interview—with techniques that could prevent sepsis and patient harm. Specifically, he recounted the cases of people who sought his care after they self-managed their abortions or went to an unqualified provider: "One went at herself with a straightened coat hanger. The other went to a layman. . . . He stuck a catheter up there. It wasn't sterile. There were no antibiotics. She may have to be hospitalized."[136] He subsequently argued that removing the red-tape requirement for therapeutic abortion committees would enable more rigorous discussions about how to improve nonsurgical techniques to make the procedure more accessible.

Part of Keemer's dissociation from the back-alley occurred through his skilled technique that elevated the type of care one could expect with him. Keemer explicitly mentioned the possibility of incorporating Luenbach paste: "It can be safely done in a doctor's office such as intrauterine infiltration of chemical paste."[137] Keemer would not only publish about Luenbach paste in the *Journal of the National Medical Association* in 1970 but would write in his 1980 autobiography that the paste was an essential way he learned to perform abortion procedures. Together with his father, a pharmacologist and medical school professor at Meharry Medical College, the Keemers would improve the Luenbach method to minimize patient health risks. Keemer described the paste in such a way as to situate it as cutting edge *technē* rather than allow the relative obscurity of the paste in US medical practice to reflect poor clinical judgment: "The method is almost unknown here, but it is preferred by many European specialists."[138] By taking techniques unfamiliar to therapeutic abortion committees in US hospitals and establishing the feasibility of incorporating them into appropriately sanitary medical office spaces, Keemer created a firm medicalized and ethical boundary between abortions performed outside a hospital setting and back-alley abortions.

Moreover, the article's description of the physical space of the doctor's office communicated that illegal abortion did not necessarily mean encountering a cruel, self-motivated, or untrained "back-alley" practitioner. Instead, the piece connected Keemer's practice to a larger sense of community care by comparing how patients felt after receiving abortions from him versus those received from "back-alley" practitioners; his office was "filled with certificates of memberships in professional groups, licenses, and citations from civic organizations for the Doctor's work in community improvement projects."[139] Not only was this physician immensely *qualified* to practice, but the presence of civic organizational work also demonstrated him to be a caring and trusted fixture of his community. Keemer reflected on the moral dimensions of performing criminalized abortions, specifically addressing patient desperation and provider guilt. He declared that fear and desperation were much more common ahead of the procedure than post-abortion guilt: "I've never known anyone to be affected by guilt feelings. Every Christmas—holiday season—I get cards without signatures. 'You saved my life,' they say."[140] Distinguishing himself from a mobile and transient back-alley practitioner, he spoke of how patient economic privilege did not necessarily mitigate against a back-alley encounter: "You know if these girls with education are going to these back-alley people, you can imagine how desperate they are."[141]

Although sustained attention to Keemer's office space could help him dissociate himself from back-alley providers and practices, the inverse occurred in the case of Robert Stanley Nixon—also of Michigan. Specifically, Nixon's case emphasized how an unsuitable clinical space could rhetorically connect a physician with back-alley practices, regardless of whether they were licensed and credentialed. Like most back-alley rhetoric, this association was leveraged through troubling appeals to "protecting women's health," which the conclusion of this chapter will investigate more fully.

In 1971, Robert Stanley Nixon was found guilty by a jury of a felony for providing an abortion in his office in the *People of the State of Michigan v. Robert Stanley Nixon*.[142] Following his conviction, Nixon appealed the ruling in 1972. On August 23 of that year, the court rejected his appeal based on improper clinical space. Although the court upheld his conviction, it simultaneously critiqued what the court saw as outdated dimensions of the law based on appeals to sanitary medical progress. As abortion statutes were being lifted in various states, this Michigan court critiqued the legal framework that warranted Nixon's conviction as antiquated because it reflected a historical moment when a lack of sanitary technologies would produce significant health impacts.

The ruling clarified the nature and intent of the original abortion statute, offering a protective buffer against dangerous medical encounters. Although "an induced abortion of an unquickened fetus did not constitute a crime," an 1846 law maintained that the abortion of a "quickened child" constituted manslaughter.[143] Noting this gap in the criminal jurisdiction, the court reasoned that the statute's purpose was "to protect the pregnant woman," for "when one remembers the passing of the statute predated the advent of antiseptic surgery, the legislature's wisdom in making any invasion of the woman's person, save when necessary to preserve her life is unchallengeable."[144] The decision explained how sanitary exigencies warranted the statute considering that no such prohibition existed for a "pre-quickened fetus." Even the restrictive revision in 1931 "predates the existence of the multitude of broad-spectrum antibiotics which have substantially reduced the dangers arising from infections."[145] By historicizing the sanitary history of the abortion statutes and appealing to medical progress, the court conjoined the "protection" *of* a pregnant person's health with the "protection" *from* infection.

The connection between a licensure requirement and antiseptic space produced a dividing line between the goal of "protecting women's health" and sentencing them to encounter a dangerous "butcher." Preventing a pregnant person from accessing abortion created a disjuncture between rights and health outcomes: "To recognize the woman's right to abort and simultaneously deny her the right to seek proper medical aid, except where necessary to preserve her life, does not encourage and promote the health and safety of the woman; but rather, it encourages the woman to place herself in the hands of those not properly skilled."[146] The possibility of rejecting the antiquated statute was predicated on the skill of the practitioner as recognized by medical licensing boards. Appeals to recent "tremendous" progress in "medical science" also enabled the court to rethink the statute, but only to the extent that a qualified practitioner would have the good sense to ensure that the procedure was performed in a "proper medical setting." Drawing on the 1969 California Supreme Court decision *People v. Belous*, the court in Nixon's case concluded that there was no state interest in prosecuting abortion providers "when performed by a licensed physician in an antiseptic environment."[147]

However, the decision deployed a back-alley appeal to specify a spatial loophole that would still render the Michigan statute valid. A licensed physician would still be considered a back-alley practitioner if they failed to practice in an antiseptic environment. Should a licensed physician practice in an infection-conducive environment, they would still be subject to prosecution: "While we do not believe that the intended aim of the statute is effectuated by the continued prosecution of licensed physicians to perform abortions in the first trimester of pregnancy in an antiseptic clinical environment, *we do not intend to convey the impression that a license to practice medicine leaves a physician free to practice "back-room butchery," any more than his* [*sic*] *unlicensed counterpart*."[148] While a license certainly would signal skill, the space of the medical encounter was of critical importance when considering the relative criminality of the procedure. The decision created the back-alley (and back-room) as a spatial boundary defined by its relative sanitary qualities. The spatial-provider was so crucial to the decision that the court repeated the sentiment: "While a licensed physician may well be more skillful than one not trained in medicine, if the physician practices that skill in the septic environment of the backroom rather than in an antiseptic clinical environment, that physician, like his less skilled brother, will be amenable to prosecution under MCLA 750.14."[149] Because the court argued that Nixon performed the abortion in his office and his colleagues testified that his practices were likely to introduce infection, his appeal was denied: "He may not use his professional status as a shield."[150] In this case, the clinical space superseded the technique and the provider ethos when considering the safety of the medical encounter.

Discussions of clinical space held rhetorical power in constituting the quality of a practitioner and their techniques in the medical encounter. Whereas rhetorical theories of *kakoethos* locate a rhetorically disabling "badness" in an individual, the juxtaposition of Keemer and Nixon show how criticism of space and technique substantially mediated provider legitimacy and stigmatization when considered as part of a larger encounter. Indeed, the back-alley butcher could not be delegitimated without thorough discussions of the "dangerous" clinical spaces.

Conclusion: From Back-Alley to "Lunchtime" Abortion

Months after the *Roe v. Wade* decision—on March 22, 1973—*Jet* magazine editor Robert Edward Johnson published a striking cover image of an abortion being performed at Chicago's Black owned and operated Friendship Medical Center.[151] The cover showed clinic director Dr. Theodore Roosevelt Mason Howard, with the title "Legal Abortion: Is It Genocide or Blessing in Disguise?" Cynthia R. Greenlee astutely observes that this image has been underappreciated for two reasons. First, the striking presence of Howard on the cover of such a widely circulated magazine challenges the idea that abortion activism emerged from "a mainly white mainstream feminism."[152] Second, this image also dampens the anticipatory fear of a back-alley medical encounter: "This is not the makeshift and blood-splattered back-alley room in a shady neighborhood. Howard appears in a sparkling white lab coat, and his helper is decked out in scrubs and a hairnet. They seem the picture of medical efficiency and professionalism, not untrained shysters."[153] Pictures of Howard warmly conversing with patients peppered the deep dive into his practice—and protests surrounding it—as the article described the dignified treatment one would receive at Friendship. Details of the state-of-the-art space and fair fees contextualized these friendly images: "At $125 per operation, the modern, 16,000-square foot medical center was on its way toward becoming one of the largest and best-operated abortion clinics in the country."[154]

The article nonetheless warned readers about proposed statewide legal constraints that Howard and Friendship Medical Center would soon face: "Already, a move is afoot in the Illinois legislature, where a white lawmaker has introduced a bill that abortions must be performed by a specialist in gynecology and obstetrics. Dr. Howard is a general practitioner." Much like Keemer in his NARAL address, Johnson copiously listed Howard's medical credentials that included his prior service as chief of surgery at a hospital in Mound Bayou, Mississippi, a specialization that demands astute knowledge of maintaining an aseptic clinical space. Relatedly, Johnson warned that "effort is also underway to pass a law that would require that abortions be performed in hospitals." Interventions that required a provider to have an obstetrical specialization and operate in a hospital were overwrought to Howard—he believed that in his clean and modern clinic one could feasibly get a "lunch-hour abortion for early pregnancies." Howard believed smaller doctor's offices could be a safe site for abortion: "I don't think abortions have to be performed in hospitals, but I think they should be performed in clean, efficient, well-equipped clinics. . . . I maintain that a working woman doesn't have time to go to a hospital, nor does she have the money they charge. Friendship is as equipped as any hospital in the city and can deal with a woman in a much more peaceful, friendly atmosphere."[155] Dr. Howard's profile in *Jet* imagined a safer medical encounter in a freestanding clinic that could fully meet the needs of Black patients who frequently experienced medical dehumanization in hospitals.

One day later, the Women's Health Consumers Union, a feminist watchdog organization, published a March 23, 1973, report sounding the alarm regarding "sneaky, behind-the-scenes maneuvers" being used to circumvent *Roe v. Wade.*[156] They warned that an Illinois-based company, Mediclinic, "which 'coincidentally' franchises prefabricated surgical clinics," offered model legislation that state legislatures could adopt to "evade the Supreme Court decision."[157] The watchdog group realized that only nine days after the *Roe* decision was handed down, California had "*already* responded to Mediclinic's 'suggestions' by quietly adopting sixteen pages of regulations."[158] Women's Health Consumers Union warned that Mediclinic's success in California was an ominous harbinger of things to come. Mediclinic painted a dystopian vision of a new landscape of legalized but unsurveilled medical encounters, lamenting, "Thousands of abortions will be performed in physicians' offices and ill-equipped clinics, without certification of physicians qualified to perform such surgery, a transfer agreement with a hospital in case of an emergency, an anesthesiologist, skilled nursing care, sterile conditions, and other needed facilities." With a catastrophizing fear appeal, Mediclinic warned that "the result will be infections, deaths and human tragedy on a large scale."[159] Coining the term "Surgiclinics," Mediclinic touted their prefabricated surgical center as a cost-effective alternative to hospital-based abortions, comparing the need for their services to the demand for nursing homes. Given their stated need that abortion spaces accommodate general anesthesia, a trained nursing staff, and a "sterile laboratory facility alongside other diagnostic tools," Mediclinic maintained that these provisions were "neither medically feasible nor economically practical in the physician's office."[160] While appeals to a techno-utopia with medical amenities and economic efficiency initially warranted the introduction of Surgiclinics, the company quickly pivoted its rhetoric, seeking to limit *where* abortions could be performed. Unlike Keemer's office use of Luenbach paste, the Mediclinic presented Surgiclinics as the *sole* spaces that would prevent morbidity and mortality outside of a hospital.

Mediclinic deployed a strikingly similar argument to contemporaneous abortion law reformers like Robert Hall, who advocated for abortions in hospital settings by invoking the back-alley: "The poor, who suffer the bulk of the abortions performed in this country, are least able to pay the cost of an abortion in a hospital, and will resort to back-alley practitioners if no alternate to such cost exists."[161] For Mediclinic, the inevitable alternative to a hospital was the back-alley, obfuscating the extant conversations that grassroots activists and NARAL-associated health care providers had held for at least five years. The legal requirements that Mediclinic hoped to instantiate far exceeded what was necessary to perform a safe abortion and included licensure requirements that limited those who could perform the procedure to a physician. Mediclinic's model laws also proffered overwrought spatial requirements, especially for an abortion within the first twelve weeks of pregnancy. The recommended state statutes would require "a list of routine surgical procedures which may be performed in the outpatient surgical center, including therapeutic abortions under twelve (12) weeks of pregnancy performed by a physician."[162] First-trimester procedures in a Surgiclinic would also require clinics to have *two* operating rooms, a recovery room capable of containing five patients, x-ray capacity (which would require a radiologist on staff), hospital admitting privileges, and an on-site laboratory. By issuing this sample legislation and arguing that anything less would be tantamount to a back-alley practice, Mediclinic produced a false choice for lawmakers under the guise of protecting patient health.

There is much at stake in situating pre–*Roe v. Wade* appeals to back-alley abortion as a *rhetorical medical encounter* that could anticipate a worst-case scenario and advocate for better options within the landscape of criminalized abortion. First, pre-*Roe* back-alley abortion rhetoric demonstrates that the medical encounter is often communicated far in excess of the doctor-patient interaction by introducing the influence of clinical space on provider ethos and *technē*. When brought into conversation with structures of health inequity, segregated licensure, demonization of Black physicians, and a dearth of access to care, these factors mutually affected one another.

Second, understanding back-alley abortion as a rhetorical medical encounter illuminates how rhetorical cultures of medicine embedded in media, entertainment, and deliberative activism can offer aesthetics and emotional touchstones that influence the public vocabularies taken up in landmark Supreme Court decisions, like *Roe v. Wade*.[163] As Gibson reminds us, beyond the well-taken critique of *Roe*'s privacy framework, another of the decision's fundamental issues can be located in Blackmun's deference to medical authority and subordination of the "woman-as-patient."[164] While abortion and medicalization certainly have enjoyed a long history dating back to the American Medical Association's nineteenth and twentieth century campaigns, the proliferation of back-alley abortion rhetoric offers a more recent context to the emergence of *Roe* and its reliance on medicalized framing. Although Gibson identifies the downstream effects of this medicalized framing in decisions like *Maher v. Roe, Harris v. McRae,* and *Gonzalez v. Carhart,* this chapter demonstrates that back-alley abortion rhetoric—with *kakoethotic* providers, unsanitary spaces, and unsanctioned *technai*—was an indelible part of the rhetorical culture that influenced *Roe v. Wade*. Even as "doctors of conscience" admitted to participating in the so-called criminal underworld, many strategically dissociated themselves from "back-alley" practitioners by invoking appeals to sanitary clinical space and a larger sense of moral duty to prevent patient harm from bad providers and self-induction techniques. At the same time, sanitary clinical spaces also served as the legal boundary between legitimate abortion provision and back-alley providers. The next chapter examines how, after *Roe v. Wade,* back-alley abortion coalesced as a more explicit appeal to prevent the "return" of criminalized abortion in the face of heightened anti-abortion pushback.

CHAPTER THREE

*The Post-*Roe *Visceral Public Memory of Back-Alley Abortion*

> The dead women we saw had either bled to death, or they had died from overwhelming infections. Some had tears along the vaginal tract where they had used coat hangers to get up into the uterus and break things up—like rupture the amniotic sac.[1]
>
> —*Coroner Fred*

> The official word at the time, and what I was brought up to believe was that she died of pneumonia. . . . The knitting needle perforated Mother's uterus, and she developed peritonitis and then gangrene. . . . There is a lingering visible trauma, or maybe a sort of emotional fallout that we all still carry around.[2]
>
> —*Marilyn*

In April 1973, just months after the *Roe v. Wade decision, Ms.* magazine published Roberta Brandes Gratz's article titled "Never Again," which featured a graphic front-page coroner's photograph of a white woman's corpse.[3] Nine years prior, the housekeeping staff at the Norwich motel in Connecticut had discovered the deceased woman exactly as she appeared in the grainy black and white photograph: nude, facing away from the coroner's camera, kneeling on the floor with a bloodied towel between her legs, and gripping another towel in her right hand. Centered in the image's frame were the residual textures of the last moments of her life: her bloodstained, fully exposed buttocks narrated the trauma that her body experienced before death. Perhaps the most stomach-churning part about this image was that viewers witnessed a graphic trace of desperation—with no support present, the woman was alone and frozen in a position of fearful vulnerability as she tried to contain the uncontrolled bleeding on the floor.

As journalist Amanda Arnold explained, "People knew of Geraldine 'Gerri' Santoro's cause of death—an air embolism caused by a back-alley abortion—before they ever knew her name."[4] While her identity was unknown, the photograph of her body was a devastating reminder of illegal and unsafe abortion before *Roe*. Rhetorical critic Sara Hayden affirms, "Indeed, precisely *because* this image was meant to stand for all victims of illegal abortion, such details would have been counter-productive."[5] Santoro's image circulated widely after *Roe*, appearing in several feminist publications and adorning protest signs with the phrase "Do You Remember?" as a veritable counterpoint to gory images of fetuses.[6] During this time, her children were unaware of their mother's cause of death, believing she had died in a car accident. By 1995, filmmaker Jane Gilooly lifted Santoro's anonymity by creating the documentary *Leona's Sister Gerri*.[7] Naming Santoro and interviewing her family, the documentary detailed the ripple effects this image had on public discourse and Gerri's own family. Although Gerri Santoro died years before *Roe*, the post-*Roe* circulation of her image was a bone-chilling reminder that unclean instruments, a lack of caring support, and improper care spaces could quickly return pregnant people to the "back-alley."

This chapter argues that after *Roe v. Wade*, back-alley abortion rhetoric took on a unique rhetorical force. Whereas journalists, activists and sympathetic physicians deployed back-alley appeals and aesthetics to argue for law repeal, reform, access, and medical authority, the procedure's constitutional protection under *Roe* generated new exigencies. As the newly legalized procedure invited immediate anti-abortion pushback, back-alley abortion rhetoric mutated into a form of *visceral public memory*: a vivid reminder of the embodied horror of unsafe abortion. Specifically, while pre-*Roe* back-alley abortion rhetoric typically anticipated medical encounters featuring unclean spaces, unskilled practitioners, and unsafe techniques, the previous chapter demonstrated that these appeals were often disembodied, speculative, and mediated through the voices of physicians, journalists, and lawmakers. The visceral public memory of post-*Roe* back-alley abortion was distinct from earlier invocations of the phrase, as it vividly returned publics in both image and graphic description to the embodied corporeality of reproductive bodies harmed by unsafe procedures. While still not narrated by the voices of people directly harmed by unsafe abortions, the public memory of back-alley abortion is a "bone-deep, felt sense of communication that transpires from a position of flesh and wound."[8] The visceral public memory of back-alley abortion situated viewers in relationship to embodied harms done by financial inaccessibility and criminalized reproductive care. Circulating public feelings ranging from disgust, outrage, pity, and shame, exemplars of butchered women fed advocacy for public funding for abortion and against mandatory parental notification while illuminating long-standing critiques by feminists of color who frequently drew attention to the inadequacies of a reproductive rights legal framework.[9] After all, while *Roe* enabled wider abortion availability for affluent and middle-class white pregnant people, root causes of reproductive injustices such as systemic medical racism and poverty were never resolved. Instead, the distribution of reproductive precarity more intensely impacted low-income pregnant people of color.

To illustrate the differential dynamics surrounding the visceral public memory of back-alley abortion rhetoric, this chapter juxtaposes the cases of Rosie Jiménez and Becky Bell. Rosie Jiménez, a twenty-seven-year-old "mestiza Mexican-origin Latina" woman residing in McAllen, Texas, was widely framed as the first victim of the Hyde Amendment, a perennial fiscal appropriations rider prohibiting federal abortion funding.[10] Becky Bell, a seventeen-year-old white youth, sought an unsafe abortion rather than involve her family as mandated by Indiana's parental notification laws. Each case offers a perspective into the raced, classed, and nationalistic dynamics underlying post-*Roe* appeals to back-alley abortion that ranged from an uncritical deployment of border rhetorics to the normative formation of the white nuclear family in crisis. Moreover, Jiménez's and Bell's memories have rhetorically traveled *together* since the 1990s. Despite an almost ten-year gap between their deaths, Rosie Jiménez and Becky Bell would come to be, at times, commemorated alongside one another.

This chapter contributes to understanding the rhetorical relationship between memory and history after *Roe v. Wade*.[11] Post-*Roe* back-alley abortion rhetoric is unique insofar as it is marked by exemplary bodies harmed by unsafe abortions. The bodies of Gerri Santoro, Rosie Jiménez, and Becky Bell each served as public reminders of visceral trauma—or trauma done to the viscera. As Marita Sturken has argued, cultural memory is distinct from but inextricably entangled with history.[12] Thus, "back-alley abortion" produced a notably limited range of memories about the experience of illegal abortion. While this range of experiences was narrow, it was not free of feeling—quite the contrary. True to Celeste Condit's observation that back-alley rhetoric bore strong emotional force in the pre-*Roe* days, these post-*Roe* memories of the "back-alley" are saturated with the residue of the phrase's use before its intersections with abortion.[13] "Back-alley abortion" also reverberated with the contextual reproductive injustices that triggered its repetition and recirculation, such as the Hyde Amendment and parental notification requirements, which disproportionately harmed women of color. Gerri Santoro, Rosie Jiménez, and Becky Bell were not the only people affected by these legal and funding strictures; they simply occupied public memory spaces most enduringly. This chapter proceeds by first explicating *visceral public memory,* drawing on Gerri Santoro's image as an example. Second, I critically examine back-alley rhetorics associated with both Rosie Jiménez and Becky Bell. I conclude by discussing the implications of their convergence into the visceral public memory of unsafe abortions.

Abortion Rhetoric and Memory

The long-standing connection between abortion and memory provides a rich site for understanding the history of criminalized abortion and more contemporary back-alley appeals. Nineteenth-century anti-abortion medical rhetoric frequently framed abortion as a form of "cultural amnesia," insofar as the American Medical Association used the *exposure* of female bodies to remind women about their life's reproductive purpose—knowledge that they had ostensibly forgotten when they ended pregnancies.[14] Demonstrating how abortion rhetoric has always implicated population management and racial hierarchy, the AMA's goal to reanimate women's forgotten knowledge spoke to "native-born, white privileged Americans" as population increases in immigrant communities threatened the waning white population with "race suicide."[15] Anti-abortion medical rhetoric assumed that criminalized abortion reflected a larger sense of "cultural decay" that justified biomedical ethos to remind white privileged Americans of what had been lost.[16]

Public memory scholarship acknowledges that symbolic and material practices capacitate memories for institutions, publics, and individuals.[17] Engaging the Greek term *mnesis,* Nathan Stormer argues that the capacity to remember and forget is a quality of *all* discourse that "enacts the persistent yet changing relationship of the present to the past and future."[18] Rhetoric may spotlight the past less to invoke a historical fact and more as a way to enlist the interpretation of earlier happenings for an exigent, present-day need.[19] For example, memories of back-alley abortion mediated present and future exigencies when Dr. Jane Hodgson—the first licensed physician convicted of performing an illegal abortion in a hospital in 1970—decried the AMA's endorsement of the federal "partial birth abortion ban" in a 1999 issue of *JAMA*: "*Lest we forget*—legal, competent, medical professionals are all that stand between safe health care for women and the dark days of the back-alleys."[20] Hodgson's back-alley invocation drew on the past "dark days of the back-alleys" to argue about the then-present danger

JAMA's regressive editorial endorsement was creating. Lamenting that the "editorial statement further marginalizes abortion providers in the eyes of medical students," Hodgson's allusion to not forget the back-alleys of the past also spoke to a downstream concern: *JAMA*'s present-day endorsement could produce a future knowledge vacuum if the AMA dissuaded medical students from seeking training in this crucial form of health care.

While public memory work can exist in technical medical journals like *JAMA*, it also occurs through a range of cultural objects, practices, and documentation technologies, insofar as "memory emerges from the news, art, stories, celebrations, customs, literature, rituals, monuments, films, photographs, clothing, mementos—and on through the full panoply of signifying forms including social data—that people use to call on the past."[21] Objects of public memory enfold the past, present, and future with the phrase "Never again," which appeared on *Ms.* magazine's 1973 cover with Gerri Santoro and its permutations like, "We won't go back."

The maxims "Never again" and "We won't go back" have graced yard signs, billboards, bumper stickers, websites, and other media in the United States since *Roe* and in the wake of the 2022 *Dobbs* decision, appearing in contemporary protest moments with images of Santoro (figure 3.1).[22] The implication that "we will never go back to the era of back-alley abortion" connects the recollection of this past to the continual formation of a collective "we," which is constituted through circulating back-alley rhetoric and as an unfolding process of identification among its adherents. The phrase positions subjects squarely within a present moment of precarity when safe, sanitary, and empathic abortion care is threatened. This threat has historically included absent state funding apparatuses for pregnant people living in poverty, legislative restrictions demanding spousal or parental notification, and spatial restrictions that segregate abortion procedures from "legitimate" hospital procedures.[23] The refusal to "go back" also recalls the abortion speak-outs of the late 1960s and early 1970s, themselves a form of recollection of previous experiences.[24] Back-alley abortion rhetoric appears across each of these mediated forms—as both fiction and nonfiction—to produce a vivid reminder of the past. The phrase "We'll never go back" presumes that the shared "we" who will "never go back" occupy a present that threatens regression to an earlier, more dangerous time. The formation of this "we" is a crucial function of public memory insofar as back-alley rhetoric at least partially "narrate[s] a common identity, a construction that forwards an at least momentarily definitive articulation of the group."[25] From the standpoint of the precarious present, the collective emphatically rejects a promised future that resembles

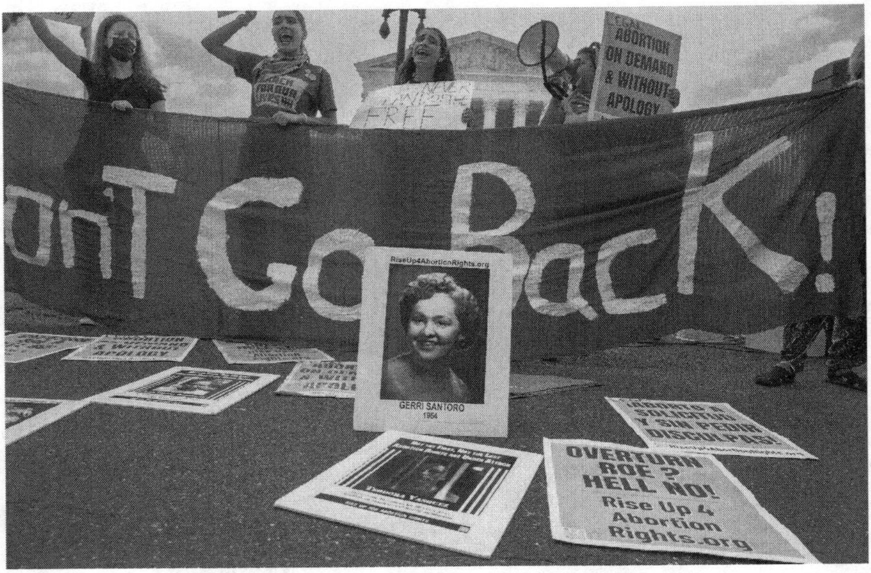
ABORTION ON DEMAND & WITHOUT APOLOGY
onT Go Back!
RiseUp4AbortionRights.org
GERRI SANTORO
1964
OVERTURN ROE ? HELL NO!
Rise Up 4 Abortion Rights.org

Figure 3.1. A group of protesters, holding a banner that reads, "Won't Go Back," stand behind photographs of Gerri Santoro and Teodora Vásquez. Photograph by Mridula Amin

the dangerous past, suturing their motivating values while taking pride in the movement's past accomplishments.[26]

However, the post-*Roe* (but pre-*Dobbs*) memory work implied in the phrase "We'll never go back" erroneously presumed that unsafe abortion was a hermetically sealed past relic and temporally centered subjects most closely related to white cisgender womanhood. As Ersula Ore and Matthew Houdek explain, "White temporal rhetorics reinscribe a linear conception of time that employs closure to achieve ideological and political ends."[27] Even as Black and Puerto Rican low-income pregnant people disproportionately occupied New York City's hospital septic wards, for example, "We'll never go back" most centrally addressed those with the presumed capacity to presently access the procedure—those for whom a legal *right* equated with the closure of an era of reproductive injustice. This rallying cry continues to exist in profound tension with the lived realities of pregnant people of color who continue to navigate structures of medical racism.[28] As this chapter's juxtaposition of Rosie Jiménez and Becky Bell elucidates, the visceral public memory of back-alley abortion is often narrated and understood through experiences of middle-class and affluent white womanhood, even as back-alley rhetoric is residually marked at the intersection of racist and classist discourses. Ultimately, the memory work accomplished through "We'll never go back" often assumes the closure of an era of reproductive injustice without interrogating how racialized and classed stratifications of reproductive health care have yet to improve in the ways the phrase presumes.

Back-alley abortion rhetoric incorporates what rhetorician Kendall Phillips theorizes as two ways of conceptualizing public memory: the memory of a public's past and the publicness of memory. The former addresses "the struggle of publics to assert their memories."[29] One example is Florynce Kennedy and Diane Schulder's 1971 book *Abortion Rap*, which commemorated the illegal abortion stories of women who testified in the 1969 class-action lawsuit *Abramowicz v. Lefkowitz*.[30] While the attorneys made arguments they hoped to shepherd to the Supreme Court, the 1970 New York state law reform rendered the case moot, threatening to bury the narratives of those who worked up the courage to testify. By compiling and publishing them, the authors ensured that the memory of these women's unwanted pregnancies would persist in future public discourse.[31] Another example of the "memory of publics" appears in attorney Sarah Weddington's memoir, *A Question of Choice*. Known for arguing on behalf of the plaintiff Jane Roe (Norma McCorvey), Weddington recalled how "people often tell me where they were when they heard about two events: the death of President John F. Kennedy and the decision in *Roe v. Wade*."[32] These flashbulb memories constituted important moments of emplacement in time and space, enabling people to remember where they were, how they felt, and how their identities were affected by the experience of that moment.

Conversely, the publicness of memory encompasses "a complex set of factors: the subjunctive nature of the loss of presence inherent in appearance, the mutative nature of repetition, and the efforts of cultural forces to combat this inherent instability through hegemonic practices."[33] The circulation and percolation of Gerri Santoro's body exemplifies the "mutative" and hegemonic dimensions of public memory. Although Santoro died in 1964 and her image experienced some circulation in print outlets like the *Village Voice* before *Roe*, the image's post-*Roe* circulation transformed the original coroner's image. Each iteration of the image's circulation held a different power: its famed initial publication in *Ms.* magazine produced public shock. When it was reprinted on the cover of several feminist publications throughout the 1970s, including *Goldflower, Our Bodies Ourselves*, and *Off Our Backs*, it responded to legislation that threatened *Roe*'s underpinnings.[34] In 1974, NARAL encouraged activists to use Santoro's image when debating anti-abortion activists to counter their wide circulation of images of fetal remains. Exhorting budding debaters to "know your audience,"

NARAL prepared advocates with evidence of back-alley abortion's mortal cost, providing supporters with a form to order multiple copies of Santoro's image.[35]

The 1995 documentary *Leona's Sister Gerri* generated a more radical mutation of memory by deanonymizing Santoro and reconnecting her to affiliative networks. Coinciding with the release of this documentary, Brandes Gratz took to a 1995 issue of *Ms.* magazine, writing alongside the image: "She had a name. She had a family. She was Leona's sister Gerri." Brandes Gratz reflected on her complicated feelings in the wake of her 1973 article, admitting "I didn't even think about who the victim actually was." However, demonstrating the tenuous connection between history and memory—and the criminal associations of back-alley abortion rhetoric—Brandes Gratz considered the culture of secrecy surrounding pre-*Roe* abortions: "Revealing the identity of the woman in the photograph would have been viewed as another kind of crime. So I thought then. Today, everything is different."[36] Such contextual differences were on full display when Karyn Sandlos assembled a focus group among abortion activists who viewed Gerri's image and reflected on its collectivizing force in the year 2000. One participant spoke to the mutative role of memory based on a shifting historical context:

> I don't think [Gerri Santoro's image] does work anymore, personally for me. . . . I think that the issues have changed, I think that the focus has changed, I think that the political landscape has changed too much, I think that feminist politics have changed too much. I think that it [the photograph] could play an important role, but not as an all-encompassing symbol anymore, as maybe a reminder of what we have had to avoid, and what we have to, you know, prevent things from going back to.[37]

Even as this participant identified as a reproductive worker involved in the daily banalities of scheduling appointments and caring for patients, their presumption of temporal closure imbued the image with limited political efficacy at the end of the Clinton administration.

Indeed, shifting electoral climates made a difference in the Santoro image's mutative circulation. Following the 2016 election of Donald Trump, *Vice* magazine morphed the image's rhetorical force once more. Instead of reprinting the photograph, *Vice* published an illustration representing the original image. Illustrator Julia Kuo drew Gerri Santoro's body cloaked by a *Ms.* magazine, producing a doubled sense of coverage.[38] Blanketed by *Ms.* magazine, Santoro's body drew an association between press coverage and privacy by symbolizing how the widely circulating periodical had unwittingly covered up her identity. However, contrary to this symbolic depiction, the very creation of this illustration circulated

Santoro's image and identity, making it into yet another iteration of coverage-as-exposure. Even the illustration's more modest depiction of Santoro's body proliferated the original image's visibility. Returning full circle, *Ms.* magazine also reprinted the original image of Santoro's body following Trump's 2016 election, demanding, "We must bring back to life the stories of women like Gerri, who died because they had no choice and the thousands of women like her whose lives were forever altered because they didn't, either."[39] The pre-*Dobbs* circulatory life of Santoro's body exemplifies the iterative mutation of public memory and the ways it has been deployed to signal temporal closure in the "return" of a past threat.

The Visceral Public Memory of Back-Alley Abortion Rhetoric

The *visceral public memory* of back-alley abortion complements current frameworks of abortion memory by showcasing how vivid visual or descriptive representations of internal bodily harm can mobilize public feeling to "never forget" a harrowing past. Jenell Johnson reminds us that visceral publics emerge "from discourse about boundaries, and they cohere by means of intense feeling."[40] Bringing Nathan Stormer's notion of *mnesis* into conversation with Johnson's theory of visceral publicity, visceral public memory externalizes another person's internal viscera to vividly orient a public in relationship to the causes of bodily harm.[41] The visceral public memory of back-alley abortion attunes publics to the damage wrought by unsanitary (and often nonmedical) instruments traversing the bodily envelope, detailing the impact of that boundary-breaking upon the pregnant person's well-being. The visceral public memory of back-alley abortion holds three distinct features. First, it relies on graphic images, vivid descriptions, or visual iconography that appeal to rhetorical vision to generate fearful public feelings that make present a returning past.[42] Second, whether vividly narrated or represented visually, a body's internal viscera are externalized *for* a nontechnical public as a central object of image, narrative, and memory. Finally, visceral public memory figures the racialized and class-based relationships between victim, perpetrator, and activist, situating these actors alongside state and national borders.

Visceral public memory demands that bodies function as evidence of the harm done to them at a physical and an institutional level, forging an affective connection "between bodies and institutions."[43] While somatics generally refer to the skin, muscle, and other soft tissue of bodies, the National Institutes of Health define the viscera as deeper levels of organs "including the lungs, the heart, and the organs of the digestive, excretory, and reproductive systems."[44] Although a seemingly troubling binary opposition between the surfaces and deep interiorities of the body, the body's inherent porousness resembles more of a "Mobius strip-like border between the human body's insides and outsides."[45] Johnson also asserts that the viscera simultaneously imply the presence of "crude or elemental emotions," which accounts for the intense public feeling generated by the memory of back-alley abortion.[46] Indeed, my theory of visceral public memory invokes Sara Ahmed's observation that inner and outer bodily boundaries are a contingent effect of circulating emotions.[47] Appeals to disgust, fear, outrage, pity, and sympathy are the collectivizing "affective supports" that enable visceral public memory to take root.[48]

Human bodies are essential for producing, holding, and transmitting memory. Stormer aptly notes that "the moment a body gains a cultural purpose, it becomes rhetorical."[49] To avoid abstracting harmed bodies into a decontextualized and universalizing form of white cisgender womanhood, Karma R. Chávez argues intersectional analysis is necessary to "attend to actual bodies and bodily difference."[50] As my juxtaposition of Rosie Jiménez and Becky Bell will show, harmed viscera shape memory differently based on how bodies materialize as raced, classed, gendered, and abled subjects. As Sturken argues:

> Like a memorial quilt, or an image, the human body is a vehicle for remembrance—through its surface (the memory that exists on physical scars, for instance), its muscular and skeletal structure (the memory of how to walk, the effects of a physical injury), its genetic tissue (the marking of one's lineage and genetic propensities), and its immune system (the memory of the body's encounters with disease). . . . Bodies are social texts whose meanings change in different contexts; there are distinctions between the gendered and racially marked body of cultural identity, the social body regulated by government institutions, and the biomedical body.[51]

Bodies are indissociable from larger, contextually situated networks of sociality, power, and oppression. Scars are not only the physical trace of skin split apart; in cases of interpersonal and state violence, they communicate past social and institutional encounters for those attuned to read those memories.

If visceral public memory relies on image or narration of graphic harm to flesh, then we must also reckon with the public life of the wire coat hanger, an instrument of public memory that has visually condensed "back-alley abortion," scrubbing bodies from sight. Considering how the pre-*Roe* era of criminalized abortion was marked by the procedure's status as an "open secret,"[52] bodies have not always been available or even the preferred method of enacting abortion activism. Although coat hangers were certainly used as methods of self-inducing abortions, the hanger's visual iconography took on a life of its own as it collapsed the difference between self-induction and encountering an unsanitary space and inept provider. The coat hanger both enables this rhetorical collapse *and* stands in as a part for a larger whole, invoking spatial sanitation and provider *(kako) ethos* while implying the potential for harm to a body's internal organs. Although not itself flesh, the wire coat hanger works by indelibly pressing upon the psyche as it is imagined to be pressing through the cervix.

The contested and hijacked memories surrounding origins of coat hanger iconography have a racialized history of their own. Law student Nina Harding asserted herself as the first person to place a coat hanger on a protest sign in 1969. In a 1992 interview with Barbara Winslow, Harding recalled having "traveled the back-alley route" for her criminalized abortion.[53] As she began to fight for abortion liberalization with Seattle's Radical Women, she crafted a bold poster using a tool from her own criminalized abortion: "I still had the coat hanger and catheter tube hanging from it, and I got an older knitting needle, and old crochet hook and an old rusty nail and I scotch-taped it to the sign that said 'Tools of the Trade.'"[54] As Harding later lamented in 2004, "The clothes hanger that conservative feminists use as a symbol for abortion is in reality ***my*** symbol. . . . What pains me is that we, African American women of color advocating abortion rights . . . were set aside by conservative feminists for not being 'ladylike' and invisible. When we gained the victory of abortion rights in Washington State, the conservatives not only claimed the victory but also took my coat hanger symbol for abortion and claimed it as their symbol."[55] Meanwhile, understanding the importance of combining legal intervention with public spectacle, civil rights attorney Florynce Kennedy co-organized the New York class action lawsuit *Abramowicz v. Lefkowitz* to repeal New York's restrictive abortion laws while encouraging protesters to march the streets with coat hangers in January 1970. Just months later, on March 28, 1970, Kennedy co-organized the Coathanger Farewell protest march to Bellevue Hospital in her capacity as a member of the feminist coalition People to Abolish Abortion Laws. As Sherie M. Randolph aptly summarizes: "The *Abramowicz* case and the various pro-abortion protests during this period helped to make the coat hanger the major symbol of the growing reproductive rights movement because it symbolized the dangerous methods women were forced to use to abort pregnancies on their own."[56] Although they were operating on separate US coasts, Harding and Kennedy—two Black feminist attorneys—demonstrate pivotal moments in the history of abortion advocacy when the coat hanger was used to bring forth harmed viscera in the mind's eye.

Coat hangers proliferated after *Roe* and were, at times, triumphantly claimed as the rhetorical invention of white feminists. One example appears in Merle Hoffman's memoir *Intimate Wars: The Life and Times of the Woman Who Brought Abortion from the Back-Alley to the Boardroom*. Hoffman recalled a moment in 1985 when she believed there needed to be a deep reckoning with circulating fetal images: "I suggested we use the simple image of the wire coat hanger, which represented all of the awful homegrown abortion remedies." Hoffman reasoned that the hanger would provide a counterpoint to potent fetal images "without stooping to graphic shock tactics" of the circulation of the still-anonymous image of Gerri Santoro. Despite pushback from Planned Parenthood, which was worried about upsetting funders and the (un)intelligibility of the hanger for younger generations, Hoffman plowed forward and "used the hanger as a symbol myself. It went on to become a ubiquitous symbol of reproductive rights and a powerful visual cue that reached younger women."[57] *Intimate Wars* features several images of Hoffman holding oversized coat hangers. Indeed, juxtaposing these contested racialized memories of the coat hanger's origins demonstrates the erasure of Black women's contributions to the rhetorical history of abortion.

Visceral public memories iteratively constitute racialized bodies by enacting a more extensive relationship between publics, victims of unsafe abortions, and emerging political exigencies. While publics certainly fight *about* abortion, they also vigorously fight *through* abortion to negotiate larger social and political dimensions of race routed through deliberation about the management of life itself.[58] Visceral public memory involves the traversal of a bodily boundary and national and community borders of belonging. As such, visceral memories lay bare the political, cultural, and historical assumptions that work with our sensory equipment to shape flesh into racialized bodies.[59] Because back-alley rhetoric elevates tactility, vision, and olfaction as considerable persuasive drivers, visceral public memories of back-alley abortions contribute, in Lisa A. Flores's words, to a "rhetorical racialization as [a] public . . . seeing and sensing of race."[60] In other words, visceral public memory mobilizes vivid descriptions and sensory rhetorics to delineate racial difference by evoking a distinction between the inside and outside of bodies, clinical spaces where viscera are exposed to infection, and—importantly—national and state borders where abortion care is more or less available.

The visceral public memory of back-alley abortion shapes the nation, cohering cisgender white nuclear family ideals and othering those outside its often-impermeable boundaries. As Patricia Hill Collins reasons, "If the nation-state is conceptualized as a national family with the traditional family ideal providing ideas about family, then the standards used to assess the contributions of family members in heterosexual married-couple households will become foundational for assessing group contributions to overall national well-being."[61] Within nineteenth-century medical discourses, the memory of abortion was always about reminding female reproductive bodies of their place in reproducing the nation.[62] For anti-abortion advocates, this manifested in an "American heritage tale" to narrate "a selective and coherent account portraying a specific strand of white, Western, Christian history as the authoritative and legitimate American heritage."[63] As the cases of Rosie Jiménez and Becky Bell show, back-alley abortion draws upon some of these nascent ideals of the nation and white cisgender familial ideals. Hayden recognizes how different public formulations of the family will produce "differing priorities for experiential wellbeing."[64] Such normative family formations can produce regressive affiliative boundaries as they circulate profound affective intensity. Shui-yin Sharon Yam observes, "Because political membership, legal recognition, and national identity are filtered through a familial lens, relationships among citizen-subjects and those between citizens and aliens and the nation are rendered much more intimate and visceral."[65] In other words, visceral public memories of back-alley abortion can have much in common with US heritage tales: both frequently draw on deep feelings associated with maintaining normative family structures while also eliding nonnormative family formations.

Considering that images of "certain death" pervade back-alley abortion discourse, this form of memory requires that the deceased be spoken *for*.[66] As a result, visceral public memory often foregrounds the stated feelings of those who narrate the deceased's experiences of back-alley abortion rather than the perspective of those who experienced the procedure themselves. Doing so can make those narrating the visceral public memory of back-alley abortion particularly susceptible to what Mariana Ortega calls "being lovingly, knowingly ignorant," especially when well-meaning white feminists narrate the back-alley abortion deaths of women of color.[67] Grounded in a more-or-less explicit fear of plurality but still holding innocently good intentions, white feminist narrators of back-alley abortion can speak in place of—and perpetuate racist assumptions about—people who endured unsafe procedures and the locations in which they received them. The evocative, emotional narratives of back-alley abortion often are about—but go without—the voices of people unable to obtain safe clinical care. Ultimately, visceral public memory envisions the past and future of abortion care in light of a present threat. The visceral public memory evoked by exemplary bodies and texts registers complex trauma that leaves an imprint on memory, cognition, and affective capacity. It is both "encoded in the viscera"[68] and most often tells a partial story from a white spectator's point of view.

After *Roe v. Wade*, the United States in the 1970s experienced increased legislative, fiscal, and other access restrictions related to abortion. Whether it was proposed amendments to the Constitution seeking to imbue fetuses with human rights, the Hyde Amendment, or parental notification requirements, *Roe* energized anti-abortion groups to circumvent the decision by any means necessary. However, these restrictions had deadly consequences for pregnant people in vulnerable positions. The remainder of this chapter traces the key cases of Rosie Jiménez and Becky Bell, two people whose postabortion deaths were substantially characterized by the visceral public memory of back-alley abortion.

Back-Alley Visceral Public Memory of Rosie Jiménez

In late September 1977, Rosaura "Rosie" Jiménez discovered she was pregnant. Jiménez could not access affordable abortion care in McAllen, Texas, because of the newly imposed Hyde Amendment restrictions on Medicaid. After seeking an abortion in McAllen with an unlicensed practitioner, Jiménez contracted a bacterial infection. After a week of fighting for her life in intensive care, she passed away on October 3, 1977. After her death, loved ones found a $700 scholarship check for her education that she had refused to spend on her abortion. The *New York Times* and Rewire News Group each attest that twenty-seven-year-old Jiménez was "the Hyde Amendment's first victim."[69]

Originally introduced in 1976 rider to the 1977 fiscal appropriations bill for the Department of Labor, Health, Education and Welfare (Labor-HEW), the Hyde Amendment prohibits federal Medicaid funding from being used for an abortion. The perennially reauthorized amendment has been one of the most sustained longitudinal efforts to eliminate or severely restrict federal abortion funding. Condit traces how, from its outset, federal restrictions on abortion funding reflected a moment when appeals to choice that had been primarily the rhetorical domain of abortion rights activists were turned against them: "The anti-funding advocates insisted that if abortion was a matter of individual conscience . . . then the Congress had no business forcing taxpayers whose consciences compelled them to oppose abortion into paying for the abortions of others."[70] In other words: you—the pregnant person—can ostensibly *choose* to have an abortion, but "we"—the mythical subject position of the unimpeded "taxpayer"—can *choose* not to pay for it. Of course, this reasoning has the effect of disenfranchising low-income pregnant people because *choice* ultimately implicated a larger constitutional right recognized by *Roe*. As Michele Goodwin argues, the "Hyde

Amendment is particularly distressing Constitutionally, because it not only excludes indigent pregnant women in dangerous pregnancies from Medicaid benefits, even when recommended by a doctor, but also demands the expenditure of millions of federal dollars in order to impede the exercise of a constitutional right."[71] As outlined in *Roe*, the constitutional right that Goodwin speaks of is *privacy*. Khiara Bridges makes an important connection between poverty and privacy when she argues that rather than being given ineffective privacy rights, "poor mothers have been dispossessed of privacy rights" altogether.[72] Even as constitutional challenges to Hyde made their way through the courts, deadly consequences were left in the amendment's wake.

While Rosie Jiménez may have been the first publicly amplified case of the Hyde Amendment's wrath, around the time she died, regional hospitals around McAllen saw a rapid influx of patients experiencing similar septic abortion-related complications. This cluster of postabortion morbidity rates prompted a McAllen physician to alert the Centers for Disease Control, which triggered the agency's surveillance practices. Jiménez's death illuminated several structural limitations of the reproductive rights movement's rhetorical frameworks. As Rocío García summarizes, "Rosie Jiménez's story is a powerful reminder of the shortcomings of mainstream notions of access that do not acknowledge how settler colonialism, heteropatriarchy, and racial capitalism are designed to work in tandem to grant access and visibility to some at the expense of others."[73] While access to federally funded abortions was *without a doubt* a driving structural reason for her inadequate abortion experience, reducing Jiménez's material constraints to the Hyde Amendment also risks erasing reproductive injustices that lower-income Mexican-origin women experienced when trying to procure reproductive health care in the United States. Indeed, Jiménez navigated life in the context of what Gloria Anzaldúa defines as the Borderlands. As Sarah De Los Santos Upton aptly summarizes, "The Borderlands draw[s] from the Mexico-US borderlands as a geopolitical region and expand[s] this concept to psychological, spiritual, and sexual Borderlands."[74] Jiménez's experience should thus be considered in terms of her physical proximity to both the border and the psychic spaces that influenced ideologies of coercive reproductive control and how Mexican-origin women were stereotyped by mainstream white reproductive rights organizations. One such example was the coerced sterilization of Mexican-origin women at the Los Angeles County Medical Center between 1971 and 1974.[75] Ultimately, Rosie Jiménez had few "choices." She could put her $700 scholarship toward abortion, leading to a less economically stable life, or put it toward her education, leading to fewer affordable options for her abortion procedure. Her decision threw into sharp relief Catalina de Onís's and Jennifer Nelson's respective observations that choice-based frameworks rarely align with the needs and lived experiences of low-income women of color.[76]

Unlike the many others harmed by the Hyde Amendment's restrictions, Rosie Jiménez's memory was granted *profound* visibility through explicit back-alley framing. An important text that generated this visibility was Ellen Frankfort's *Rosie: The Investigation of a Wrongful Death,* which named Rosie Jiménez and viscerally figured the racialized, nationalist, and classed dynamics of her memory in the wake of her death.[77] With an afterword by National Abortion Federation founding president Frances Kissling, this book is the product of Frankfort and Kissling's investigative journalism and subdivided into three parts, "Feeling My Way, Knowing Nothing," "The Government Enters the Investigation (Again)," and "Taking Action." Laudably, the authors rectified many incorrect and downright racist assumptions circulating publicly about the then-anonymous Rosie and her abortion. Because she was previously able to access an abortion with Medicaid funds, they clearly demonstrated how structural constraints like the Hyde Amendment—not individual moral feelings of shame—were responsible for her fatal abortion. By also collaborating with her friends Pauline, Evangelina, Margie, Diane, and Marta, who refused to allow her memory to succumb to reductive and violent stereotypes, the text connected Jiménez to her extended kinship network. Yet, I would be remiss if I did not acknowledge García's reticence toward such humanizing rhetoric insofar as "the discursive politics of Latinx representations tend to reflect a contentious and bifurcated ideological terrain, where harmful misrepresentations of Latinxs are often met with counter-discourses that humanize Latinxs."[78] While keeping García's warning close at hand, I specifically examine how the book's back-alley visceral memory work amplified some racist narratives while it tried to dispel others. Doing so reduced the complex Borderlands contexts impacting Rosie Jiménez's reproductive injustice to funding access, while simultaneously erasing the history of border crossings that many US residents took to procure safe and dignified abortions in Mexico through the Association to Repeal Abortion Laws, Patricia Maginnis and Rowena Gurner's referral service.

Alley spaces mediated the book's spatial investigatory work, crafting the container for memorial possibilities. It foregrounded the "foreboding" city spaces surrounding medical clinics in Reynosa, Mexico, only to contrast this scene with the "modern" medical buildings located on the main streets of McAllen, Texas. Without yet knowing Rosie Jiménez's name, Frankfort arrived in McAllen determined to discover what happened to the anonymous woman who had died from an abortion widely believed to have occurred in Reynosa. Upon her arrival to Reynosa's Calle Dias, "a street dense with medical activity," Frankfort's sensorium was overwhelmed by "exhaust fumes from the oversized iron boxes remain[ing] trapped in the narrow streets."[79] Alley implications gave way to explicit alley tours when Frankfort connected the outdoor urban spaces to the presumed poor clinical conditions that hypothetically *could have been* inside the buildings:

> Between the office of a cardiologist and Universal Radio and Television Store is a narrow alley. It is filled with tanks of gas, old seats from cars, the top of a shopping cart, a rusty coke machine without wheels, boxes of empty bottles, a wooden doorframe, shells for fluorescent lights, car tires without treads, and a water-stiffened mop—an inventory of truncated limbs and dissected parts for an anatomy class in American know-how. A woman comes to the door of a house at the end of the alley. . . . Is this where she went instead? Down this alley to abort?[80]

Disorienting yet anthropomorphized garbage marked the alley's mise-en-scène. The rusted textures of the Coke machine met the smoothness of treadless tires and broken glass—all physical threats to those walking down the alleyway. The mop, stiffened by saturation with dirt and mop water, could no longer effectively clean. Each of these items, importantly, were equated with body parts; the "truncated limbs" and "dissected parts" oriented readers to a graphic sense of bodily harm, even though no bodies were present.

On first blush, Frankfort's thick description of the environment around her merely set a vivid scenic foil that would later be undermined by her own investigation. After all, by the time she wrote the book, Frankfort knew that Rosie's lethal abortion did not occur in or near any alley in Reynosa. However, her description of the trash strewn about the alley drew upon long-standing racial scripts associating Mexican border cities not only with dangerous abortion procedures but unsanitary danger writ large. As Sarah De Los Santos Upton, Carlos A. Tarin, and Leandra H. Hernández affirm, "The US-Mexico border region is a toxic landscape." However, they clarify that such toxicity is due in part to multinational corporate dumping and precarious labor exploitation, which has generated severe health disparities and reproductive injustice.[81] Lina-Maria Murillo further contextualizes that dehumanizing policies ultimately distilled structural inequities into personal moral failings: "Immigration and public health regimes, militarization, de facto segregation, and outright neglect produced the mechanisms through which both the state and nonstate actors racialized generations of people of Mexican descent as uncivilized, dirty, and dangerous to a (presumed) white American body politic."[82] Frankfort invoked these racial scripts when describing Reynosa's offices of dentistry, radiology, and emergency surgery as "primitive" and "outdated," as "their signs jut out like rickety canopies."[83] As Frankfort wandered through Reynosa's alleys, her incredulous narration repeated well-worn tropes of medical primitivism promulgated by the American Medical Association for more than a century. The *bas-fonds* imaginary she narrated presented an abject scene that cast doubt on the quality of abortion a person could receive in Mexico. And yet, as evidenced by pre-*Roe* efforts like that of ARAL's Patricia Maginnis and Rowena Gurner, US residents had long traversed the US-Mexico border to obtain abortions with overwhelmingly positive outcomes.[84]

Frankfort entrenched attributions of fear and danger in Mexico by juxtaposing her excursion through the Reynosa alley system to what she considered to be a more modern clinic and capable provider back in the United States. Returning to McAllen, Frankfort continued her pursuit of the still-anonymous Jiménez by speaking to several physicians who could have treated her. Describing the US clinical surroundings as a "professional" space with "legal" abortion, Frankfort elevated the McAllen clinic by contrasting to the imagined one in the Reynosa alley: "Although the pleasant new professional building resembles all the others clustered around McAllen General Hospital, it differs in one important respect: it is the only place where a woman can go to have a legal abortion."[85] Frankfort described the clinical space in McAllen as new, pleasing, and by implication a safer place to procure care than anywhere one would access via an alley entrance. When Frankfort met a second physician on her quest to identify Jiménez, she connected his clinical space to his professional ethos: "Right across from the street from McAllen General Hospital, on the outside of a new one-story professional building . . . a fancy script spells out the name of Raphael Garza, followed by the letters *M.D.* and the medical symbol."[86] The new medical spaces were framed as sanitary, disarming, and safe—a striking departure from Reynosa's alleys.

As Frankfort spoke with McAllen's physicians, journalists, and reproductive health advocates, she attuned readers to how many of her interviewees affixed discourses of racialized morality to both Rosie and Mexican-origin women writ large. Some of these references were explicit, such as when Lila Burns, the wealthy, well-dressed, and white executive director of the McAllen Planned Parenthood, proclaimed, "There's a very low abortion rate in this area. Our people are very moral."[87] Frankfort's other interviewees coded their racialized moral judgment by elevating white temporal standards of immediacy. As Frankfort visited the local newspaper to triangulate the still anonymous Rosie's death date with a named obituary, the newspaper employee initially struggled to locate the entry. While they knew the date of death, October 3, 1977, they had no idea when an obituary might have been sent. The newspaper employee assumed "Mexican-Americans don't have a sense of time. They could have sent it much later."[88] Ultimately, Frankfort and the journalist discovered that the Jiménez family had provided an obituary just one day after Rosie passed away—October 4, 1977. While this assertion proved to be one of the many racist assumptions channeled through white moralism, it was also part of a larger trend of similar newspaper coverage of illegal abortions. As Murillo notes, borderland newspapers frequently leveraged racist and sexist appeals when addressing criminalized abortions, "vilifying those caught in the crosshairs of unjust laws in both countries while also promoting nationalist narratives of decency, law, and order."[89] Frankfort's exchange with the newspaper revealed how its employee fabricated the false expectation that her family would not care to operate according to white "civilizing" Anglo-American standards of timeliness and care when it came to memorializing her death.

Once Frankfort was finally able to pinpoint Jiménez's identity, the book's memory work entered a more visceral register when physician interviewees vividly centered trauma on Rosie's organ systems. As Dr. Dan Chester recalled Rosie's demise, he provided Frankfort with a graphic overview of the infection that took her life, *Clostridium perfringens*: "It's an organism that is present in dirt, feces, and can come out of the intestinal tract. . . . This particular micro-organism produces a variety of toxins. One breaks down the red blood cells. . . . The debris from the red blood cells had accumulated in the filtering mechanism of her kidney. There were other toxins that are harmful to different systems. The muscle cells of her heart and liver and the immunization systems were all adversely affected."[90] The *Clostridium perfringens* attacked her muscular, organ, and immune systems, collapsing the walls of her red blood cells and damaging them beyond repair. Frankfort printed several similar graphic descriptions, testifying to this book's frequent reliance upon visceral rhetoric to produce this public memory text. By centering her body with thick description, Frankfort oriented readers to Rosie's corporeal interiority, externalizing her viscera for public remembrance and political deployment. Vivid visual and olfactory references to biological decay also appeared on the book jacket, which cited Rosie's friend Pauline at her death bed: "It was hard to look at her. She was a dark greenish-brown, and there was blood coming from her eyes. . . . But that smell. Pauline remembered it. It was the same smell her father gave off as he lay dying." The sensory appeals that materialized the mortal harm done to Rosie Jiménez's viscera were a significant way the book enticed readers to open it.

One consistent assumption across several of Frankfort's interviews was that abortion seekers like Rosie were morally ashamed and that, aligning with the protections of *Roe v. Wade*, desired privacy. According to the interviewed doctors and medical providers, moral shame and privacy were the likeliest motivations for Rosie and other Mexican-origin women to seek abortions in Mexico. Attributions of (im)morality were perhaps strongest when Frankfort interviewed physicians who had encountered Rosie. Dr. Chester rehearsed his statements on *Good Morning America* when discussing the case with Frankfort: "No you could not conclude that Rosaura crossed the border because she couldn't pay for a safe abortion. . . . Mexican American women might go over to Reynosa for a number of reasons. They have a fair amount of shame about sex as well as a need for privacy."[91] Not only did this attribution of shame and a desire for privacy evacuate Rosie's agency; it entrenched individual moralized explanations for the structural difficulties of accessing affordable care. Indeed, Chester's assertion of Rosie's shame-based motivation was patently false. Her friend Pauline declared, "I heard on TV that the reason she went to have an abortion in Mexico was because she was embarrassed. That's a bunch of bull. Just money. All the time it was just money. Rosie was such a unique person. . . . She got me by the hand and took me to school. Like this check that was in her bag for seven hundred dollars. It was her scholarship money. That was sacred."[92] Burns repeated Chester's attribution of shame almost verbatim. When Frankfort asked whether Rosie would have preferred to procure an abortion in Mexico over an assumed safer one in Texas, Burns spoke for Mexican-origin women *in general*: "Yes. They want privacy. And it feels more like home. There is a pharmacy, the Guadalupeña, where they all go for illicit drugs and abortions. That's where the woman who died went."[93] Because readers would later discover that Jiménez procured her fatal abortion in Texas, Burns's testimony elided the sheer number of US women of many ethnicities who traveled *from* "home" to seek care. Burns's speculation ultimately cast aspersions upon people like Rosie by presuming they had criminal motives or were more at ease in an inhospitable and dangerous environment. To the contrary, Rosie had obtained a previous abortion procedure with Chester using Medicaid funds in 1975, demonstrating that Medicaid funding had produced safer abortion conditions. Additionally, Frankfort interviewed Rosie's friends Evangelina and Pauline, who confirmed that the abortion that took Rosie's life occurred in McAllen, Texas, with midwife Maria Pineda. With this knowledge, Frankfort, Rosie's friends, and surveillance team members of the Centers for Disease Control decided to investigate Pineda and ultimately stage a raid.

Reminiscent of her opening tour of Reynosa, Frankfort circulated back-alley residue to describe Pineda's neighborhood landscape to spatialize her medical incompetence. Before participating in the raid, Frankfort and CDC employee Julian Gold visited Pineda's home to see for themselves where Rosie had received her fatal abortion and try to elicit a confession. Driving through Pineda's neighborhood, the "unincorporated areas where the migrants live," Frankfort's descriptions of the "closely bunched bungalows . . . kept in a careless sort of fashion" with "dogs laz[ing] in front . . . trying to rid themselves of fleas" bears a striking resemblance to other alleyway topoi this book traces.[94] As they pulled up to Pineda's home, Frankfort expressed relief at the space's basic sanitary provisions, remarking how "at least [Pineda's house] has electricity and running water."[95] Before leaving the car, Frankfort described Julian's fear of impending criminality in his desire to park the car in close proximity to the house, "so he could look out and see me in case I come running out of the house, behind me a mad Mexican with a butcher knife."[96] Frankfort initially dismissed Julian's racist comment as having "seen one too many American movies," and stressed to readers that *she* was not afraid. Just a few pages later, however, Frankfort described how the environment *did* concern her. She decided to proceed because "the bicycle in front of the house and the sight of small children inside make the setting unconducive to crime."[97] She then offered a decidedly racist justification to quell her fear of violence: "Despite previous fears, I am convinced that Mexican-Americans rarely murder Anglos; in fact, all evidence points to the contrary. And in cultures where *macho* runs amok, a crude chivalry often prevails with white women."[98] Their exchange along with her own narration clearly "relied upon racialist imagery deeply embedded in the American psyche about Mexico and Mexicans as inherently criminal and immoral."[99] Frankfort's engagements with back-alley affective residue rhetorically transposed the earlier narrated dynamics of Reynosa into McAllen's migrant neighborhood.

While it is important to recognize that Maria Pineda provided Rosie Jiménez with unsafe abortion care, Frankfort's narrative molded Pineda into a back-alley practitioner through intersecting sexualized and racialized stereotypes that diminished her capacities to practice medicine and amplified her capacities to spread disease. Keeping in mind that Frankfort showed up to Pineda's home unannounced, Frankfort nonetheless held Pineda up to the expectation that she be clothed for an unexpected aseptic medical procedure. Although irrelevant to Pineda's capacities to practice medicine, Frankfort gave a sexualized description of her appearance: "Her hair is covered with a short scarf tied behind her head, exposing large loop earrings. She is wearing a faded pink ribbed-cotton turtleneck top; it is too tight and pushes her full firm bosom upward where a swell of womanly flesh rises above the outlines of her pointed brassiere, making a sexy cushion for the rhinestone cross resting between her breasts."[100] Isabel Molina-Guzmán and Angharad N. Valdivia argue that a corporeal emphasis on breasts, hips, and buttocks in Latina media representation can signify both "fertility as well as bodily waste and contamination."[101] In Frankfort's narration, Pineda signified both: as a midwife who practiced at the threshold of human fertility, her ill-fitting clothing emphasized her breasts and conveyed the possibility of contaminating abortion practices. Indeed, Pineda's impurity in this description was doubled: her sexual impurity enabled readers to assume that she was also introducing bacterial impurity into Rosie's body.

Touring the house and yard, Frankfort snapped photographs that would later be deployed as a cautionary tale at a medical conference, cementing alleyway aesthetics into public health practices:

> She may do her artwork in the shed, but there is nothing to indicate she does abortions there. She must perform that activity in the house. I try to pass the snarling dog with nonchalance. He pulls on the chain, but I make it to the front, where a wooden pen serves as a makeshift container for two garbage pails, their lids askew. I photograph the pails with their overflowing bags of garbage, a photograph Julian would later use as part of his presentation on family planning at a medical conference in Reynosa.[102]

Specters of journalistic muckraking in Frankfort's tour invoked the residue of alley clearance efforts with dangerous animals and "makeshift containers." Her photographs would serve as decontextualized "proof" of "primitive" medical care spaces. Without losing sight of the unsafe abortion care that Maria Pineda provided Rosie Jiménez, the debunked assumption that the abortions would be completed in the shed generated an additional layer of medical primitivism that aligned with Frankfort's opening alley tour.

At the end of the book, visceral rhetorics mediated the harm done to Rosie through the medical tools that law enforcement removed from Maria Pineda's home. Kissling joined the others at Pineda's home to stage a police raid. Pauline and Frankfort went into Pineda's home asking for an abortion while wearing a surveillance wire. Once the raid was complete, Frankfort situated herself as an objective journalist who could no longer suppress her feelings, admitting, "Whatever distance I had maintained until now dissolved. I was at the house where

Rosie had the abortion that killed her, watching the police carry out filthy instruments in kidney-shaped pans."[103] Harm to Jiménez's body was mediated through the unsanitary tools in a pan resembling human kidneys. Imagining those same tools capable of introducing the *Clostridium perfringens* into Rosie Jiménez's bloodstream, the book closed with their removal by law enforcement, ostensibly signifying a safer reproductive futurity enabled by the criminal justice system. That very same criminal justice system, however, did not seem to appreciate the group's investigative work, and Kissling, Frankfort, and Diana were detained by police under suspicion of colluding with Pineda. As Kelly O'Donnell and Naomi Rogers reflect, "The feminist visitors were shocked to find that their race and status did not protect them from the arm of the law."[104]

"Look at it this way, Pauline. With so many investigations, it's like she's not really dead. Rosie's going national."[105] Margie's comment could not have been more prescient. Rosie Jiménez subsequently experienced profound postmortem coverage, circulation, and commemoration to repeal Hyde and support abortion funds. A memorial fund was crafted in her name, with 5 percent of Frankfort's book proceeds going toward it. Jiménez's memory was kept alive to prevent further harm that would occur with additional funding and legal restrictions.[106] The next section critically examines one such effort to mobilize in her name. Even within an organization dedicated to the tenets of reproductive justice, back-alley abortion appeals limited collective identification across different languages.

Back-Alley Advocacy in Rosie's Name

Activism on behalf of Rosie Jiménez was swift after her death, led by organizations like the Foundation for the Feminist Majority and state chapters of the National Organization for Women. In some cases, "Rosie Jiménez Day"—October 3—became an aperture to bring funding injustices to the foreground. Despite important advocacy and efforts undertaken to fight for Medicaid abortion funding, back-alley rhetoric elided important differences between abortion-seekers' race, ethnicity, and social position. These elisions demonstrated how back-alley abortion rhetoric failed to exceed the boundaries of English-speaking audiences, which, given the ubiquity of such appeals in US abortion rhetoric, further nurtured existing patterns of single-issue advocacy.

Juxtaposing a formally identical advertising flier in English to one in Spanish reveals critical differences in the positioning of the memory specters of back-alley abortion for different language–speaking audiences, even as both were targeted for participation.[107] For example, the Coalition for Reproductive Freedom had a more expansive set of reproductive politics that did not solely focus on abortion rights. As a member of the Reproductive Rights National Network (R2N2) that sought "reproductive freedom for all," the Coalition for Reproductive Freedom committed itself to "safe, legal and accessible abortion; protection from sterilization abuse and an end to population control policies; reliable, safe birth control; an end to racist and lesbian oppression; childcare supports; a safe workplace; incomes sufficient to support a family and accurate sex education." R2N2 was cofounded by the Committee for Abortion Rights and Against Sterilization Abuse (CARASA). Formed in 1977, CARASA separated itself from organizations like NARAL and Planned Parenthood whose predominant focus was on lobbying, legislation, and media education.[108] As a member of a network dedicated to enacting advocacy to address the systemic causes of gendered violence and reproductive oppression, it was unsurprising that the coalition would resist proposed Massachusetts changes to state-sponsored abortion funding.

Indeed, while Jiménez received her fatal care in Texas, her narrative resonated in Jamaica Plain, Massachusetts, several years later. R2N2's posters relied on the alignment of remembering her death on October 3, 1977, mobilizing to build a shared sense of urgency to gather on the Massachusetts State House steps on Monday, October 4, 1982. The poster in English (figure 3.2 left) and the version in Spanish read (right): "**ES URGENTE QUE ACTUEMOS AHORA! / It is urgent that we act now!**" collapsing the years between 1977 and 1982 that saw a state-level version of the Hyde Amendment.

Both posters attended to Rosie Jiménez's affective orientation to her future before seeking her abortion. Even in the condensed space of the advertising flier, viewers learned remarkably intimate details of her life:

> Rosie era una madre de 27 anos que vivia sola con su hija. Rosie tenia la esperanza de que sus estudios universitarios podian ayudarle a ella y a su hija a superar los problemas de la pobreza y del subempleo. Per ella necesitaba un aborto. Su beca de $700 estaba asignada para sus estudios y nada mas, y la Enmienda Hyde [Hyde Amendment] habia eliminado el uso de fondos del Medicaid para los abortos. Ella logro ir a un abortador. Por el use de instrumentos no esterilizados le dio una infeccion que exige su hospitalizacion al dia siguiente. En una semana Rosie se murio.
>
> (Rosie was a 27-year-old single mother who hoped her university studies would be her and her daughter's way out of a cycle of poverty and underemployment. But she needed an abortion. Her $700.00 scholarship check had to go for school, and the Hyde Amendment had cut all Medicaid funds for abortion. She went to an illegal abortionist. Infection caused by unsterilized instruments sent her to the hospital the next day. Within a week she was dead.)

Rosie's raced, gendered, and economic existence was framed as "hopeful" before the Hyde Amendment. Describing a cyclical route through underemployment and poverty, the hope that the poster attributed to Rosie was based on her determination to survive and thrive within racialized capital structures. This attribution of hope also prepared viewers for a rapid descent into a dialectic of desperation—a despair that could easily befall others thousands of miles from McAllen, Texas, under Massachusetts's proposed funding restrictions. The implications became clear: she needed an abortion and could not afford to choose a licensed OB-GYN. She also could not afford a dignified future with her daughter in her current economic position. Having chosen an abortion with the wrong person, her future hope was condensed into the $700 scholarship check that signified taking responsibility for a better future, which ultimately cost her life. Ultimately, Rosie's choice was not a choice at all.

The significant differences in the flyers included the presence and absence of back-alley abortion and appeals to *choice* when referencing the vigil held in Rosie's name. The phrase "back-alley abortion" crafted different boundaries for memory, identification, and relationships to the State. In the top third of the flier, large bolded text aligned with a black-and-white photograph of Jiménez smiling at the camera. While the English version used the wording "On October 3, 1977, Rosie Jiménez died from an illegal back-alley abortion," the Spanish version read, "En el 3 de Octubre, 1977 Rosie Jiménez murió de un aborto ilegal tal como ocurre con la vida de tantas mujeres cada año." While both referred to abortion being illegal, the Spanish version specified that these procedures occurred in the lives of many women every year, but without the added "back-alley" modifier. The English version individuated Rosie's experience, as the title did not have the same collectivizing appeal to others who experienced Jiménez's fate. The narratives below the headings and images were similar in that they both spoke of the check she had in her purse and having her abortion performed with unsterilized instruments. However, only the English version exhorted audiences to specifically remember back-alley abortion nine years after *Roe*'s legalization and six years after Hyde went into effect. Moreover, the Spanish-language version relied on Rosie being one among many impacted by the restrictions. In the English version, readers encountered this relationship between the one and the many only in the middle of the narrative: "Rosie was only the *first of many* victims of the Hyde Amendment cut-off. Untold numbers of women, especially poor and women of color have suffered and died from illegal abortions, because they did not have access to legal ones."

That back-alley abortion was meant to be persuasive to English- but not

On October 3, 1977 Rosie Jimenez died from an illegal, back-alley abortion

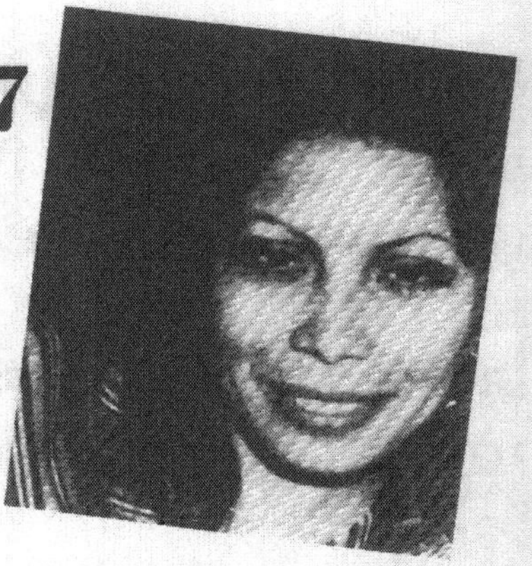

Rosie was a 27 year-old single mother who hoped her university studies would be her and her daughter's way out of a cycle of poverty and underemployment. But, she needed an abortion. Her $700.00 scholarship check had to go for school, and the Hyde Amendment had cut all Medicaid funds for abortion. She went to an illegal abortionist. Infection caused by unsterilized instruments sent her to the hospital the next day. Within a week she was dead.

Rosie was only the *first of many* victims of the Hyde Amendment cut-off. Untold numbers of women, especially poor and women of color have suffered and died from illegal abortions, because they did not have access to legal ones.

Massachusetts is one of the few states where funding is still provided for women who cannot afford abortion. However, proposed changes to the state constitution threaten to end this funding. Our legislature is overwhelmingly anti-choice: what happened to Rosie Jimenez could happen here. We must work to keep abortion a right for all, not a privilege for some.

It is urgent that we act now!

PRO-CHOICE VIGIL

Monday, October 4
4-6 p.m.
State House steps

The Coalition for Reproductive Freedom
P.O. Box 686 Jamaica Plain, MA 02130
For more information, call 524-2542.

Member

The **Reproductive Rights National Network (R2N2)** is an organization of local groups throughout the country committed to reproductive freedom for all. This includes safe, legal and accessible abortion; protection from sterilization abuse and an end to population control policies; reliable, safe birth control; an end to racist and lesbian oppression; child care supports; a safe workplace; incomes sufficient to support a family and accurate sex education.

Figure 3.2 left and right. Flyer with a picture of Rosie Jiménez that advertises a Massachusetts protest against abortion funding restrictions. Courtesy of the Abortion Action Coalition records at Northeastern University Archives and Special Collections

En el 3 de Octubre, 1977 Rosie Jiménez murió de un aborto ilegal tal como ocurre con la vida de tantas mujeres cada año

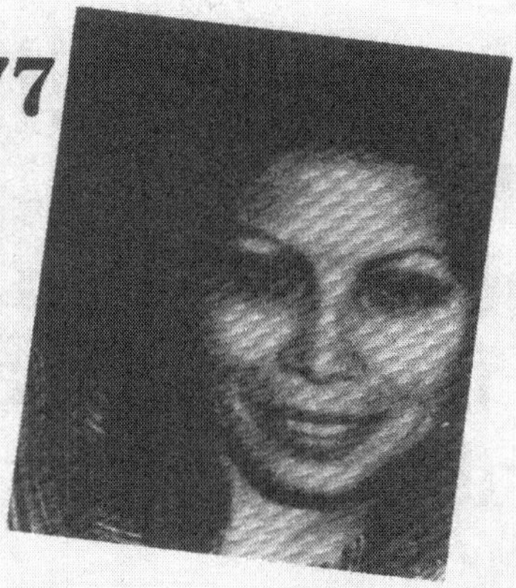

Rosie era una madre de 27 anos que vivia sola con su hija. Rosie tenia la esperanza de que sus estudios universitarios podian ayudarle a ella y a su hija a superar los problemas de la pobreza y del subempleo. Pero ella necesitaba un aborto. Su beca de $700 estaba asignada para sus estudios y nada mas, y la Enmienda Hyde (Hyde Amendment) habia eliminado el uso de fondos del Medicaid para los abortos. Ella logro ir a un abortador ilegal. Por el use de instrumentos no esterilizados le dio una infeccion que exigio su hospitalizacion al dia siguiente. En una semana Rosie se murio.

Rosie fue sola la *primera de muchas* victimas de los cortes en fondos requerido por la Enmienda Hyde. Massachusetts es uno de los pocos estados en que todavia hay fondos para ayudar a las mujeres que no pueden pagar por sus abortos. Sin embargo, ahora hay unos cambios propuestos de la constitucion del estado que constituyen una amenaza a estes fondos. La mayoria del cuerpo legislativo es contra el derecho de escoger: lo que paso a Rosie Jimenez puede pasar aqui. Tenemos que trabajar para mantener el aborto como un derecho para todas, no un privilegio para algunas.

¡ES URGENTE QUE ACTUEMOS AHORA!

VIGILIA

el lunes, 4 de octubre
4-6 p.m.
escaleras del State House

The Coalition for Reproductive Freedom
P.O. Box 686 Jamaica Plain, MA 02130

Para mas informacion: 524-2542.

Member

La **Cadena National de Derechos Reproductivos** es una organización de grupos locales de todas partes del país, cometidos a la libertad reproductiva para todos. Esto incluye acceso a abortos seguros y legales, proteción contra los abusos de esterilización, el fin a las políticas de control de la población, control de natalidad digno de seguridad, un fin al racismo y a la opresión contra el lesbianismo, mantenimiento del cuidado de niños, trabajos seguros, ingresos suficientes para mantener a la familia y educación sexual exacta.

Spanish-speaking audiences demonstrated the intended addressivity of back-alley appeals and the exclusionary rhetorical effects of this visceral public memory document. These two fliers demonstrated how "back-alley abortion" appealed almost exclusively to "white, monolingual"[109] English-speaking audiences and thus leveraged different memory demands upon that audience's relationship to the provider ethos and clinical space. Indeed, it was not a coincidence that "pro-choice" appeared only on the English version and not the Spanish. The English version referenced the event as a "pro-choice vigil," whereas the Spanish version read "vigilia." The absence of "choice" in the Spanish version was significant, for neither pro-"choice" nor "back-alley abortion" could produce a suitable translation. Instead, in de Onís's words, both "back-alley abortion" and "pro-choice" were each "transcreations" that were "forced, invented phrases . . . [whose] incompatibility exemplifies bordering in that it includes/excludes along particular lines."[110] Indeed, with no direct translation, English-language back-alley abortion and pro-choice appeals that elevated Rosie as an exemplar still spoke squarely to the position of English-speaking womanhood. Put simply, back-alley rhetoric simply could not fully address and include those who also shared Rosie Jiménez's positionality.[111]

Whereas Rosie Jiménez's visceral public memory of back-alley abortion attended most specifically to remembering the harm done to her viscera through spatialized sensory and border(ing) rhetorics, midwife denigration, and criminalized raids, the visceral public memory of Becky Bell's back-alley abortion implicated separate cultural dynamics. A different exigency (teenage pregnancy and parental notification requirements for abortion) with a different victim (a white youth), produced different back-alley contours. Becky's parents were the ultimate drivers of circulating her memory, illustrating how a white cis heterosexual nuclear family crisis was mediated through back-alley abortion rhetoric.

Teen Pregnancy, Parental Notification, and Becky Bell's Back-Alley Abortion

When Becky Bell, a white seventeen-year-old, discovered she was pregnant, she knew that she was not ready to parent. Although abortion was legal in her home state, Indiana's parental notification requirement demanded that she either alert her parents, Karen and Bill Bell, or seek a judicial bypass. Brian S. Amsden has argued people seeking judicial bypasses must often devalue their embodied knowledge, perform "age-appropriate emotions," and align themselves with a "devotion to patriarchy."[112] With circulating rumors that the judges she would encounter rarely granted bypass relief, Becky had the option of crossing state borders to Kentucky where such laws did not exist or of seeking an abortion with an unlicensed provider in her hometown. After realizing that she could not feasibly cross the state line, procure an abortion, and return without her family knowing, she opted for the second choice—something local. Becky's local abortion resulted in a septic infection, high fever, and pneumonia. Becky ultimately passed away from her injuries on September 16, 1988. Her autopsy report, which would later become a rhetorical site of contestation by anti-abortion activists, affirmed that an abortion indeed precipitated her death. Several documentaries and dramatized representations of her deadly abortion emerged. Becky's parents mobilized to remove parental notification requirements to honor her memory. Similar to what we saw with Jiménez, vivid sensorial descriptions of Bell's body were leveraged as explicit back-alley abortion appeals. What was different from Rosie's story was how Becky's deceased body became the rhetorical site of negotiation over the back-alley's impact on the dynamics of teenage pregnancy on white, cisgender, heterosexual nuclear family values, ultimately serving as a referendum on the (im)possibility of parental surveillance of children.

Becky Bell's untimely death occurred within larger contextual dynamics concerning national efforts to regulate teenage pregnancy. The rhetorical framing of teenage pregnancy as a national danger emerged in the second half of the twentieth century. While the *single* mother was long stigmatized as a " 'ruined' and 'fallen woman' "[113] who transmitted moral turpitude to her children, the age of this persona was unspecific. The so-called epidemic of *teenage* motherhood was a later twentieth century rhetorical creation that "rewrote concerns related to race and class through the prism of age."[114] In the context of the overwhelming unavailability of legal abortions mid-century, a too-common experience with white women's unwed pregnancy was banishment to religiously affiliated maternity homes to relinquish children after birth. This practice circulated shame, stigma, and long-term psychological damage.[115] Beginning in the 1970s, a wave of legislative achievements and Supreme Court decisions expanded reproductive-related rights for adolescent girls, preventing discrimination at school (Title IX), granting access to contraceptives (*Eisenstadt v. Baird*), and ensuring the protected right to abortion (*Roe v. Wade*).[116] Despite these victories, national narratives specifically articulated the threat of *teen* pregnancy as a national pathology.[117] Deliberations surrounding the 1975 National School-Age Mother and Child Health Act, for instance, circulated dominant narratives of teenage female bodies as "simultaneously in danger (of becoming pregnant) and dangerous (as potentially producing children who would damage the economy and lives)."[118] This reciprocal sense of risk—that the embodied threat of teenage pregnancy would also threaten the larger body politic—braided with long-standing racial discourses of abortion as a sign of social decay. These dual rhetorics of danger ultimately warranted parental control over teenagers' reproductive capacity, naturalizing a hierarchy of age and authority that "bears striking resemblance to social hierarchies in U.S. society overall."[119] In other words, parental control of their teens' abortion access was a key site of regulating not only teen pregnancy but the larger connection between familial and national health.

Although iterations of parental notification and consent requirements were written into many states' abortion laws even prior to the *Roe v. Wade* decision, the 1980s saw the enforcement of these laws flourish under the heading of "traditional family values."[120] When Becky Bell died at the end of the decade, the United States was just emerging from the Reagan administration. The Christian right's well-organized defense of "traditional" (white heteronuclear) families through the 1980s included sustained attacks on abortion access and welfare distribution for low-income families, as "Black mothers and teen mothers became the face of America's teen pregnancy crisis."[121] The Evangelical Christian Right's rhetorical resources gained purchase in the movement's framing of anti-abortion politics less as an attack on personal rights and more as "defense of the family."[122] For example, two years before Becky Bell died, the anti-LGBT anti-abortion fundamentalist evangelical organization Focus on the Family funded more than 1,500 crisis pregnancy centers.[123] It is no accident to see these attempts to regulate teenage pregnancy emerge in tandem with support of crisis pregnancy centers, as both leverage the presumed immaturity of youth to impede reproductive choices. Natalie Fixmer-Oraiz echoes a common infantilizing refrain CPC volunteers use: "protecting women from abortion as 'an adult tells a child not to touch a hot stove.'"[124] Becky Bell's parents authorized several visceral public memory rhetorics to resist infantilizing anti-abortion discourses.

The Visceral Public Memory of Becky Bell's Back-Alley Abortion

After Becky died, her parents participated in a 1990 documentary entitled *Abortion Denied: Shattering Young Women's Lives*. Eleanor Smeal and Toni Carabillo produced the documentary, which circulated vivid descriptions of Becky's viscera to accomplish two goals: to remember the era when abortion was a crime and describe the "back-alley" endpoints associated with then-contemporary access restrictions like parental notification and consent requirements. Narrator Christina Pickles introduces Becky's case, explaining that in states requiring parental notification, minors must either tell their guardians, travel to a non-restrictive state, or seek a judicial bypass. Pickles laments that fear paves the path to danger: "Many girls unable to do any of these freeze and drift further into pregnancy until it's too late or, like Becky, turn to the back-alleys."[125]

Juxtaposing the visceral memories of both the Bell family and Dr. Kenneth Edelin, the documentary situated the relationship between past abortion criminality and present threats to access by focusing upon the similar ways bodies were harmed by back-alley abortions across time and space. Dr. Edelin, a physician convicted of administering an abortion after *Roe v. Wade*, speaks from his position as the chair of the Planned Parenthood Federation of America from 1989 to 1992. He recalls a personally transformative moment from the mid-1960s when he treated a woman whose illegal abortion left her with deadly sepsis.[126] *Abortion Denied* toggles between testimonies of Edelin and the Bells, as they closely attend to the interiority of the bodies they are remembering:

Kenneth C. Edelin: I remember very vividly when I was a third-year medical student down in Nashville, Tennessee. It was 1965 or 1966, a young seventeen-year-old woman came into the emergency room of Hubbard Hospital.

Bill Bell: At 4:00 in the afternoon, we took her to this doctor. They x-rayed her, and her left lung was full of pneumonia.

Dr. Edelin: . . . her face was distorted and swollen.

Karen Bell: . . . and they said get her to the hospital *now*. She's bad.

Dr. Edelin: . . . her temperature was 105. She was in shock. She was clearly very, very sick.

Bill Bell: . . . the pneumonia and the infection in Becky . . . was running so rampant throughout her body, it virtually destroyed her lungs.

Dr. Edelin: . . . when he opened up her abdomen, it was full of the most awful-looking yellowish-green pus I had ever seen.

Karen Bell: She laid, and she died. I held her hand. I kept saying, Becky, what's wrong? Tell mommy. . . . She just wouldn't say anything.

Dr. Edelin: The catheter had gone through the backside of her uterus and carried all the bacteria and toxins. Not only into her uterus but into the rest of her body.

Bill Bell: The cause of death was listed as a septic abortion with pneumonia as a contributing factor.

Dr. Edelin: It was very sad. It was very moving. And probably the signal event in my professional career that made me understand that such a loss of life is so useless. That women sometimes during their lives will be so desperate when they find themselves pregnant and do not want to be pregnant will put their lives and health on the line to terminate that pregnancy.

Karen Bell: I just want people to remember Becky. What happened to us.

Abortion Denied stages this juxtaposition as an explicit act of remembrance, referring to a past almost twenty-five years earlier with Edelin's self-described "vivid" memory. Shifting to the Bells provided viewers with a visual, olfactory, and tactile exposure of Becky's internal organs as her parents describe her left lung full of pneumonia. Both patients' conditions were dire enough to render their emergencies almost interchangeable, collapsing the distance between past and present. Dr. Edelin recalls his patient's face as "distorted and swollen," while Becky's condition is more simply described as "bad." The film cuts from Becky's pneumonia traveling throughout her body and destroyed her lungs to Edelin performing surgery on his patient's fluid-infected abdomen. From narrating Becky's death, the camera returns to Edelin describing the catheter that had punctured his patient's uterus. The "bacteria and toxins" could not be contained to the uterus, invading the internal organs of her body. For Edelin, this was an indelible memory that inspired his career trajectory. As these recollections collapsed the distance between past and present abortion restrictions, the vivid descriptions that externalized each patient's viscera made the effects of a criminalized abortion transcendent. In this moment, it did not matter whether encounters with the back-alley were occurring in the 1960s or 1980s; the resulting harms brought on by abortion restrictions would inevitably harm reproductive viscera in similar ways.

In addition to this documentary, Becky's viscera were externalized for public remembrance and political contestation through the circulation of the coroner's report of her autopsy. Coincidentally, although Becky passed away on September 16, and the autopsy was completed the next day, the coroner report of the autopsy was completed on October 3, 1988—the anniversary of Rosie Jiménez's death and the perennial day of her remembrance. In the report, Dr. Dennis J. Nicholas confirmed her cause of death was "SEPTIC ABORTION with PNEUMONIA."[127] As is typical of any coroner's report, it painstakingly described the state of Becky's uterus. Although the report indicated that her uterus had not been punctured with a tool and that cervical dilation was even, the autopsy insisted that there was "evidence of recent pregnancy with recent partial abortion . . . the amniotic membrane has been ruptured."[128] As Toni Carabillo completed her documentary research, she acquired Becky Bell's coroner's report to accurately contextualize the harm of her unsafe abortion. The thick description common to the genre of the coroner's report served as crucial evidence for the documentary's back-alley rhetoric.

Anti-abortion activists seized on the coroner's report and drew upon a medicalized definition of miscarriage as "spontaneous abortion" to delegitimize Karen and Bill Bell's fight against parental notification laws. Abortion and miscarriage have been etymologically linked since the 1500s and have long been equated in medical contexts.[129] The president of the National Right to Life News, Dr. John C. Willke, leveraged his medical credentials to interpret the vocabulary in the coroner's report. He made extensive viscerally grounded arguments of alleged incongruence between the report and the public discourse being deployed about it. Translating the report to a nonmedical audience, Willke argued that deadly infections could occur only if there were a uterine puncture by some improperly deployed tool. Citing Dr. Bernard Nathanson, a physician who worked with NARAL until he embraced anti-abortion politics, Willke used Nathanson's experience to say that Becky's vagina and uterus would necessarily be "shaggy and discolored." In contrast, he insisted that the report indicated "no areas of perforation and pus."[130] By externalizing Becky's viscera and bodily fluids for critical assessment and contestation by "outside expert testimony" and public deliberation, the National Right to Life News invited audiences to reject a back-alley abortion narrative as her cause of death by leaning on technical, medicalized definitions of abortion as "induced" versus "spontaneous." Willke's line of reasoning was not only echoed throughout the National Right to Life News; contestation over the coroner's report—and, therefore, whether Becky died of an abortion gone wrong—made its way through legal deliberations such as opinion editorials in more mainstream media.[131] As mediated through her autopsy, Becky's viscera became public terrain, circulating in politically motivated ways that enabled her body to testify against a policy that would have prevented her death.

Dynamics of back-alley abortion's threat to normative nuclear families were perhaps most acute in a 1992 televised dramatization entitled *Families in Crisis: Public Law 106; The Becky Bell Story*.[132] The program inverted the script surrounding the law's intent: although parental notification was designed to foster communication between parents and their children, it actually tore families apart. *Public Law 106* opens at the height of Becky Bell's medical emergency: a family station wagon speeds down the main street of a small town. A young white girl asks to put her head on her mother's lap. As they arrived at the emergency room, her father heroically carries his daughter inside. With her case triaged as an immediate danger, doctors rush Becky back into surgery, as the camera angles upward from her vantage point to display several medical professionals looking over her with worry. As Becky's parents peer helplessly through a glass window, she fades in and out of consciousness. A doctor approaches Becky's parents and describes her internal organs: "Your daughter has a massive infection. It's everywhere. . . . It could be a kidney infection that spread to the blood. It could be any number of things. She's stabilized but not out of the woods yet." Without confirming to viewers whether Becky would pull through the ordeal, the scene cuts to the past so viewers might better understand the fearful present. Viewers return to a mundane moment weeks prior: a middle-class white family sits around their kitchen table. Demonstrating an intact and happy family, viewers hear Bill Bell on the phone with his father, securing last-minute plans for the family vacation to Florida as Becky, her brother, and her mother finish their meal at the family dinner table.

Before confirming her pregnancy, the show constitutes Becky's morality as she attempts to maintain her family's reputation in her small Indiana town. Becky goes to the local pharmacy to purchase a pregnancy test, and the pharmacist makes small talk by asking about her family, intimating a close community connection. Not wanting small-town gossip to circulate back to her parents, Becky steals a pregnancy test but leaves a twenty-dollar bill hidden near the cash register. This pharmacy exchange lends Becky an upstanding moral stature. Despite hiding her purchase of a pregnancy test, she is shown refusing to engage in criminal behavior. Becky's fear of exposure and disappointing her parents permeates the entire episode, especially as she struggles to figure out how she would travel to the Kentucky state line to have her abortion and get home without anyone knowing. Out of options, Becky and her friend take a late-night detour to the entrance of a dimly lit apartment building. The fearful and consigned looks that Becky and her friend give one another reflect a journey through the small town's *bas-fonds*—along with it was an acceptance of whatever care would come next—so long as her parents do not find out.

Like so many iterations of back-alley rhetoric, the program negotiated gendered and racialized morality in its framing of the public lessons related to Becky's death. Ending with Becky's death, the screen momentarily goes black, and the real Bill and Karen Bell appear and address two audiences: youths seeking abortion and their parents. The Bells contextualize that the previous story was about how the law put their daughter in danger. As they describe, *Roe v. Wade*'s guarantee of legal abortion presented Becky with just two legal options: tell her parents or a judge. By lamenting that "Becky could not bring herself to do either," the Bells forewarn others: "Know your options so you don't find yourself in a back-alley where an illegal abortion can take your life as swiftly as it took our Becky's." With their daughter functionally unable to exercise a full range of choices, they position back-alley abortion as the only choice available under current legal strictures. Reflecting on their daughter's tragedy as a parenting lesson for others, they appeal to their memories by encouraging other parents to rethink support for notification and consent laws. With twin appeals to the recollection and protection of youth, Karen asks viewers, " How do you protect a daughter as loving, as wonderful, as good as Becky?" Karen urges parents to "try to remember what it was like when you were young. When you couldn't talk to your parents about certain things. Make sure your daughter knows that if she can't talk to you, she should find someone else to help guide her. . . . All you want for your child is for her to come home safely. Our daughter didn't: she loved us as much as we loved her. She wanted to protect us." Inverting the protective scripts implied by the law—that parental notification/consent would somehow enable caregivers to protect their children—the Bells make an a fortiori argument to demonstrate how if the law did not protect even the "strongest" families like theirs, other "weaker" families would certainly experience harrowing outcomes. However, this possibility of inverting the law's protective scripts was only fully intelligible in the context of white heteronormative family structures. The discourse surrounding teen motherhood is racially framed, with white youth are more likely to be framed as "good girls who make a mistake,"[133] while Black pregnant youth are hypersexualized and framed as "a drain on the system."[134] Unlike cases of child abuse that impacted someone's ability and willingness to confer with parents, the Bells' appeal was grounded in an otherwise robust and intact family that would be torn asunder by the shame of not living up to a shared ideal.[135] In conjunction with legal strictures, the shame of family disappointment was the primary appeal Bill and Karen used when memorializing their daughter's motivation for seeking a back-alley abortion.

The sticky durability of Becky Bell's visceral memory of back-alley abortion over the next decade testified to its rhetorical power to mediate threats to a nuclear family by the crossing of state lines within a hermetically sealed US national imaginary. This is perhaps best seen in the 1997 Child Custody Protection Act, passed almost ten years after Becky died.[136] References to Becky Bell *and* back-alley abortion appeals were pervasive throughout this bill, specifically from Representatives Nita Sue Lowey, Diana DeGette, James Maloney, and Michael Pappas. As Lowey described, "Parental consent laws did not force Becky to involve her parents in her hour of need. Just the opposite. At her most desperate hour,

Indiana's parental consent law drove Becky away from the arms of her parents and straight into the back alley."[137] Further, Representative DeGette declared her "strong opposition to the deceptively titled Child Custody Protection Act. I am a mother, too. I have two young daughters. And I would hope and pray that my two young daughters would come to me if they got into the tragic situation of an inadvertent pregnancy. But if they could not come to me, I certainly do not want them in a back alley having an unsafe abortion."[138] Representative Maloney appealed similarly: "It will succeed only in making it more difficult for young women to gain safe, legal abortions. If she refuses to involve her family and the law prohibits her from looking to another responsible adult for help, she may be forced to travel alone to a clinic, adding delays which increase the risk to her health, or worse, resort to 'back alley' or even self-induced abortion."[139] Finally, Representative Pappas proclaimed, "Supporters of this bill claim that this legislation will strengthen the lines of communication between young women and their parents when actually the opposite will result. Fearful of putting a trusted family member at risk, who knows what a young, frightened teenager might do? Forced to make a decision on her own, she may make the journey across State lines by herself, traveling by bus or, even worse, hitchhiking. She may turn to an illegal back alley abortion where she puts her young life in unnecessary danger."[140] Drawing on Becky Bell almost ten years after her death, the visceral memory of her back-alley abortion was a continual means of generating affective detachment from restrictive parental notification requirements. As a barometer for the health of the white nuclear family, visceral back-alley appeals surrounding Becky Bell were a durable commemorative resource for generating an enduring sense of crisis.

Conclusion

Post-*Roe* back-alley abortion appeals to "never go back" to when abortion was a crime belied the extent to which laws, funding restrictions, and practices of medical dehumanization persisted and sutured normative white cisgender family production while excluding non-English-speaking activists. Rosie Jiménez's and Becky Bell's visceral public memories were exemplary. They both represented a larger trend and stood alone as figures for invocation, serving as enduring sites of rhetorical invention. Back-alley appeals to their bodies shaped public discourse in differential modes. While Jiménez's body invited regressive national border rhetorics that misremembered the complex pre-*Roe* era, Bell's body negotiated white cisgender nuclear family dynamics and mobility across state lines. While Bell's body was exposed for debate and public deployment in national abortion politics, Jiménez's body was acted upon as the "first" of many harmed bodies to come and absorbed racist projections of Mexican-origin women.

This chapter would be incomplete without reflecting on how Rosie Jiménez and Becky Bell's back-alley visceral memories circulated *together* for reproductive advocacy. For instance, the 1995 event Rock for Choice resulted in a compilation album, *Spirit of '73*, produced by 550 Music Epic Records to benefit the Feminist Majority's Becky Bell / Rosie Jiménez fund. Articulating together the exigencies of federal funding and parental consent, this album included twenty-four songs and skits, with the inner sleeve reading, "Rock for Choice dollars support the Feminist Majority's **Becky Bell / Rosie Jiménez Campaign** to lift lethal parental consent laws and federal funding restrictions that are forcing young women and poor women to turn to back-alley abortions."[141] In line with the foundation's work, proceeds also funded the "National Clinic Defense Project and Emergency Clinic Survival Fund," which provided legal assistance, security, and surveillance cameras in the wake of increased clinic violence by groups like Operation Rescue. The National Organization for Women produced paraphernalia for the Rock for Choice concert to remember Jiménez and Bell. As I completed this book's archival work, I found dog tags etched with their names displayed together at the Schlesinger Library in Cambridge. When not on public display, their archival box includes just four items: a doll with light skin, red hair, and blue eyes, a gold bracelet inscribed with "Becky Bell" and "Indiana PL-106," as well as two Rock for Choice dog tags that list both names and "Repeal the Hyde Amendment / Repeal Indiana PL-106."

Jiménez and Bell were also commemorated together during speeches at the 2004 March for Women's Lives, with both deaths marked by explicit back-alley appeals. Originally named "March for Freedom of Choice," this event was significant for several reasons. For one, Planned Parenthood, the National Organization for Women, the Feminist Majority Foundation, and NARAL Pro-Choice America initially planned the event "without any significant input" from "grassroots constituencies."[142] However SisterSong, the Black Women's Health Imperative, and the National Latina Institute for Reproductive Health pushed back, joined the planning team, broadened the scope of the march, and shifted the framing far "beyond choice."[143] The result was a turnout of over a million people on the National Mall. During the march, actor Tyne Daly first introduced Bill Bell with a moralizing appeal: "[Becky] was not a bad girl who never talked with her parents. She was so close to her parents she would have done anything not to disappoint them. . . . She died after that back-alley abortion. Her doctors said her lungs had literally come apart from infection."[144] In these brief sentences, viewers witness the persisting articulation of Becky's back-alley abortion to her harmed viscera and the morality of white family values. Immediately after Bill Bell's short speech, Charlene Ortíz of the Colorado Organization for Latina Opportunity and Reproductive Rights rose on behalf of Rosie Jiménez, opening that she died "of an illegal abortion, *a back-alley abortion*."[145] Ortíz, however, continued to discuss the specific issues Latina women experienced obtaining reproductive care. Despite more than a decade between their deaths, Becky and Rosie's persistent commemoration together invites critical attention to how their respective viscera are differentially—yet continually—rearticulated to meet evolving exigencies with back-alley abortion rhetoric.

Thus far, back-alley abortion appeals have primarily been in the hands of abortion rights and access advocates who have sought to render visible the harms of criminalized abortion. There were notable exceptions, including Mediclinic's ambulatory surgical lobbying efforts discussed in chapter 2 and the anti-abortion contestation over Becky Bell's autopsy in this chapter. On balance, back-alley abortion has served interests related to abortion access and legality even as it has often done so through regressive discursive logics and accompanying public feelings. However, the affective residue of the back-alley planted seeds for regressive rhetorical uptake. In the next chapter, I demonstrate precisely how anti-abortion activists thoroughly weaponized the back-alley. By introducing the case of Kermit Gosnell, I illustrate how, between 2010 and 2023, anti-abortion advocates took up back-alley appeals in the service of clinic and provider restriction.

CHAPTER FOUR

Kermit Gosnell and the Anti-abortion Uptake of Back-Alley Abortion

On June 27, 2016, the US Supreme Court issued a landmark decision on abortion access in the case of *Whole Woman's Health v. Hellerstedt.* In a 5–3 decision, the court deemed Texas House Bill 2 (HB2), which would require the state's abortion clinics to function as ambulatory surgical centers, unconstitutional. Under the guise of protecting people seeking abortions from unsanitary clinical conditions, HB2 required clinics to undertake expensive and medically unnecessary renovations while expecting providers to hold hospital admitting privileges. With the Hyde Amendment's perennial reauthorization, federal money could not fund the $2 million cost per clinic to undertake those renovations. Before the court's ruling, HB2 attracted significant nationwide attention when Senator Wendy Davis filibustered the bill for more than eleven hours in the summer of 2013. The court majority opinion ultimately agreed in 2016 that HB2 would shutter more than half of Texas's clinics, placing a then-unconstitutional "undue burden" on those seeking to terminate their pregnancies. According to the Center for Reproductive Rights, the organization that helped to shepherd the constitutional challenge, "This decisive rejection of clinic shutdown laws marks the most significant abortion-related ruling from the Court in more than two decades, and will have national impact in states where similar laws threaten to shutter abortion clinics with medically unnecessary red tape."[1] Despite the favorable ruling for abortion rights, HB2 illuminated the rhetorical power that public discussions of sanitary clinical space could hold in the anti-abortion lobby's relentless effort to eliminate access.

Embedded within HB2's legal justification was the case of former Pennsylvania physician Kermit Gosnell, whose clinical space and medical practices were framed by mainstream press as a contemporary "back-alley."[2] In 2010, a multiagency law enforcement team raided Gosnell's Philadelphia clinic, the Women's Medical Society, for reasons seemingly unrelated to abortion. Police suspected that his clinic was a "pill mill" circulating a massive quantity of opiates into West Philadelphia. According to the grand jury report:

> When the [search] team members entered the clinic, they were *appalled*, describing it to the Grand Jury as "filthy," "deplorable," "very unsanitary, very outdated, horrendous," and "by far the worst" that these experienced investigators had ever encountered. There was blood on the floor. A stench of urine filled the air. A flea-infested cat was wandering through the facility, and there were cat feces on the stairs. Semi-conscious women scheduled for abortions were moaning in the waiting room or the recovery room, where they sat on dirty recliners with blood-stained blankets.[3]

Demonstrating the residual stickiness of the back-alley's affects discussed in chapter 1, the grand jury report painstakingly described how the unsanitary clinical space assaulted the senses and detailed what it saw as Gosnell's moral failings and criminal activity. The report alleged that Gosnell used inexpensive, unpredictable sedatives like Demerol and employed unlicensed teenagers as nursing staff. In addition to several instances of patient morbidity, Gosnell's practices were found responsible for the deaths of twenty-two-year-old Philadelphia resident Semika Shaw and forty-one-year-old Nepali refugee Karnamaya Mongar. Without interrogating the medical racism and histories of segregated care that rooted the issues manifest in Gosnell's clinic, the report excoriated the Pennsylvania Department of State and Department of Health for failing, respectively, to oversee abortion clinics and investigate historical complaints. In addition to recommending indictments for Gosnell, his wife, and several staff members, the grand jury report proffered regulatory solutions that encouraged all of Pennsylvania's abortion clinics to function as ambulatory surgical centers and all abortion providers to be board-certified OB-GYNs with hospital admitting privileges.

While chapters 2 and 3 argued that back-alley abortion rhetoric appealed to expand abortion access, this chapter holds that the Gosnell case marked a contemporary inflection point when anti-abortion activists systematically hijacked appeals to back-alley abortion by circulating the grand jury report with the aim to regulate clinics out of existence.[4] As Linda Greenhouse and Reva B. Siegel argue, "Regulations that close clinics in the name of women's health, but without health-related justification, do not persuade: they prevent."[5] Investigating this relationship between persuasion and prevention, I take the grand jury report of

Kermit Gosnell as my focal object of analysis because of how widely it circulated through multiple sites of public discourse. I argue that the report's content and its overwhelming anti-abortion uptake drew on the Gosnell case *as* a back-alley "health-related justification" to warrant both clinic closures and provider censure, even though the phrase never appeared in the report. As is already evident from the previously quoted excerpt, the grand jury report's visceral sensory appeals to vision, olfaction, and tactility circulated feelings of horror, disgust, and outrage that adhered to Gosnell, his clinical space, and the governing apparatuses regulating abortion oversight in Pennsylvania. Ultimately, while back-alley abortion was attached to Gosnell in subsequent media coverage, the back-alley's affective residue was durable enough to not even need explicit reference to the phrase in the report to do its rhetorical work.

The grand jury report's subsequent anti-abortion uptake occurred through activist deliberations surrounding the case. Because the report framed the Gosnell case as a rare point of convergence between traditionally understood pro-life and pro-choice positions, it was taken up as ideologically "neutral" evidence for two films: *Gosnell: America's Biggest Serial Killer*, a dramatization of the case, and *3801 Lancaster: An American Tragedy*, an award-winning documentary. By framing the report as transcendent across political affiliations, these filmic treatments ultimately nourished abortion stigma while tacitly approving clinic overregulation and ceding ground to anti-abortion activists. Considering that the Gosnell case provided both legal and rhetorical precedent for the Texas legislation that led to the *Whole Woman's Health v. Hellerstedt* decision, an in-depth analysis of the Gosnell case illuminates the ever-evolving relationship between rhetorics of clinical space, monstrous provider *kakoethos*, and the saturation of sensorially resonant public feelings that grounded arguments to criminalize abortion clinics.

This chapter begins by narrating policy context relevant to understanding the Gosnell case. This context includes efforts by abortion access advocates to create clinic standards, laws that targeted restrictions on abortion providers, and Pennsylvania's Abortion Control Act of 1982, which had already rendered the state one of the most regulated in the nation. Next, I historicize the racially segregated medical care system in West Philadelphia, where Gosnell practiced. Then, I perform a close textual reading of the grand jury report that constituted the clinic as a "back-alley" operation and attend to how anti-abortion activists invoked the report and hijacked back-alley rhetoric to regulate clinics out of existence. I conclude by examining how a crisis pregnancy center became the "solution" to remember the visceral harms done to pregnant people in Gosnell's clinic.

Post-*Roe* Clinic Standards and Targeted Restrictions of Abortion Providers

Beginning in the early 1970s, debates surrounding whether abortions should occur in hospitals, freestanding clinics, or doctors' offices emerged as an important site of contestation for US medical professionals and feminist health advocates.[6] As abortion liberalization movements gained traction and *Roe v. Wade* was decided, outpatient surgeries, in general, became significantly more common. This was a double-edged sword: Improved technological advancements in general surgery, abortion techniques, and anesthetics led to fewer side effects and increased patient satisfaction. However, as chapter 2 identified, companies like Mediclinic, who stood to profit from manufacturing prefabricated "Surgiclinics," tried to influence the law by circulating back-alley fear appeals alongside pro forma restrictive policies.

Following *Roe v. Wade*, the task of regulating abortion clinic standards was front and center as the newly legal procedure invited questions about the propriety of clinical space and the organizational structure of clinics themselves. The impulse to standardize care expectations was partly due to the memories that physicians and patients had about the landscape of illegal abortion. To be sure, establishing a new system for abortion provision after *Roe* was fraught, reflecting splintering ideological contestation around medical expertise and authority. As historian Johanna Schoen found, "Male physicians found young women challenging and demanding while young women found male physicians patronizing and dismissive of their concerns."[7] Gathering at a 1975 national symposium, providers and advocates discussed various issues related to abortion techniques, counseling, birth control, and clinic management. A group of symposium attendees created the National Association of Abortion Facilities (NAAF) to exchange information, create standards for operating clinics, and engage in political lobbying. When NAAF members met two months later to craft their professional organization, disagreements emerged between nonprofit and for-profit interests. The splinter between these two groups led to the formation of the National Abortion Council (NAC). After months of negotiations between NAC and NAAF, the National Abortion Federation (NAF) was formed under the leadership of Francis Kissling, the activist who had written the afterword of *Rosie: An Investigation of a Wrongful Death*. In 1978, NAAF published *Standards for Quality Abortion Care*, which set new national standards for providers.[8]

The development of these standards was partially responsive to the public exposure of some low-quality clinics. The same year, the *Chicago Sun-Times* published a series of exposés about services in the city that, in Schoen's words, "was reminiscent of journalistic coverage before *Roe*."[9] This series of articles detailed the poor quality of care that pregnant people were experiencing in a handful of Chicago clinics. Harking back to characterizations of abortion mills, providers were described as paid per procedure, resulting in a greedy willingness to perform abortions rapidly and sometimes haphazardly. These articles detailed clinics neglecting sanitary procedures between clients, who were given insufficient time to recover, and poorly trained staff meeting them with callous attitudes. Not unlike what would come to occur in the Gosnell case, anti-abortion activists seized on the story to paint *all* abortion providers with the same brush. Concerned that the *Sun-Times* exposé would come to stand in for abortion provision in toto, the NAF created patient education brochures as outreach and deliberated upon clinical standards internally. Ultimately, abortion access advocates had a fine line to walk: "Caught between the twin evils of overregulation, on the one hand, and regulatory neglect, on the other, abortion providers hoped that standards would serve not only as guidelines to abortion clinics around the country but also as a model for politicians and public officials."[10]

Indeed, overregulation followed, as abortion providers became sustained targets for new legal restrictions. Just as outpatient clinics performed more abortions, mundane spatial restrictions became a covert way for local municipalities to circumvent *Roe*. Targeted restrictions on abortion providers (TRAP laws) constitute one of the more sustained limitations on abortion access, regulating both providers and clinical spaces. Significantly surpassing the sanitary and oversight requirements necessary to perform safe abortions, TRAP laws "impose physical plant and personnel regulations and requirements on abortion providers that exceed those imposed on comparable health care providers or outpatient medical facilities."[11] A decade before the *Dobbs* decision, economist Marshall H. Medoff declared in no uncertain terms that "the enactment of TRAP laws, under the guise of protecting women's health, represents a stealth strategy by anti-abortion activists to create an environment where the constitutional right . . . to have an abortion is moot because there are too few abortion providers offering services"[12] The technicalities of TRAP laws did not make for a consumable spectacle and therefore easily escaped media coverage and public condemnation. Importantly, TRAP laws did not seek to persuade pregnant people—they worked at the level of state and local ordinances to ultimately bypass any meaningful possibility of choice in the first place.[13]

While countless procedures ranging from colonoscopies to oral surgeries are performed outside the hospital setting, TRAP laws gained their name for stigmatizing and unduly *targeting* abortion. In a cross-sectional legal assessment of state facility laws for abortion providers and office-based surgeries (OBSs), a 2018 study in the *American Journal of Public Health* found that the number of laws targeting abortion providers was double that of other OBSs.[14] Abortion clinics and providers were targeted for restriction at a volume unlike those providing any other type of treatment. TRAP laws often specify surveillance of sedation unapplicable to other risk-comparable OBSs. They also produce more stringent restrictions than required for other OBSs, thus exceeding "necessary and accepted standards of practice and fail[ing] to provide countervailing benefits."[15] In outpatient procedures unrelated to abortion (such as endoscopy and oral and plastic surgery), regulatory processes generally have fallen to clinician-lead committees affiliated with professional associations and accreditation organizations to avoid putting an "unnecessary burden on clinicians in practice."[16] TRAP laws burden providers by amplifying their invisible labor, often requiring them to do more with fewer resources.[17]

In addition to TRAP laws, severe access restrictions and reporting requirements were imposed. The Abortion Control Act of 1982 was an essential structural feature of the Pennsylvania reproductive landscape that instantiated several omnibus bills and comprehensive restrictions that resulted in constitutional challenges, including *Thornburgh v. American College of Obstetricians and Gynecologists* and *Planned Parenthood of Southeastern Pennsylvania v. Casey*. The Pennsylvania Abortion Control Act (PACA) regulated issues related to informed consent, parental notification, clinical facilities, gestational limits, a requirement to "determine gestational age," prohibitions against infanticide, public abortion funding, and fetal experimentation. It promised both civil and criminal penalties. PACA retained the power to make rules "with respect to facilities in which abortions are performed, so as to protect the health and safety of women having abortions and of premature infants aborted alive. These rules and regulations shall include, but not be limited to, procedures, staff, equipment, and laboratory testing requirements for all facilities offering abortion services."[18] The act defined a medical facility broadly as "any public or private hospital, clinic, center, medical school, medical training institution, healthcare facility, physician's office, infirmary, dispensary, ambulatory surgical treatment center or other institution or location wherein medical care is provided to any person."[19] Pennsylvania underwent several iterations of the Abortion Control Act. However, the court found several of its provisions unconstitutional in *Thornburgh v. American College of Obstetricians and Gynecologists*.

A subsequent challenge to the Pennsylvania Abortion Control Act—*Planned*

Parenthood v. Casey—fundamentally transformed abortion jurisprudence in the United States. By 1989, three new justices had been seated, and Pennsylvania lawmakers strategically amended PACA to trigger a legal challenge before the Supreme Court. Sue Frietsche of the Women's Law Project makes this connection explicit: "The 1988–1989 Abortion Control Acts were a set of regulations that were designed specifically to get to the Supreme Court so that Pennsylvania would be the state that resulted in the overruling of *Roe*."[20] Planned Parenthood challenged several of the PACA assumptions mentioned previously. While *Roe*'s trimester system was marked by the "strict scrutiny" test that afforded the most substantial levels of constitutional protection when restricting abortion, *Casey* introduced the "undue burden" standard.[21] In this massive upheaval, *Casey* declared that even before fetal viability, states could institute laws and statutes to discourage abortion and promote full-term childbirth so long as regulations did not present an overwhelming "undue burden" for pregnant people in either intention or effect. Although *Planned Parenthood v. Casey* did not overturn *Roe*, it validated virtually every aspect of the PACA, except for the spousal notification law, on the grounds of domestic violence. However, none of the other restrictive statutes rose to the level of an undue burden in the majority opinion.

In addition to the loosened protections that resulted from the displacement of the "strict scrutiny" standard, the "undue burden standard" was a profound reproductive justice problem because it imagined the burden on a prototypically white, middle-class woman "by contemplating a mythical woman with unlimited human and economic resources, with no disabilities, no connections to anyone, and no responsibilities."[22] Reproductive activism that presented a homogenized view of women's subjectivity in *Casey* limited the possibilities for a broader coalition on behalf of reproductive justice by alienating women of color. Here, I offer just one example. Akiba Solomon, a journalist from West Philadelphia, was engaged in teen sexual education activism. When asked to publicly advocate against *Planned Parenthood v. Casey*, she declined. As Solomon later explained, she elected not to be more publicly vocal in this case because activism was privileging white-centric rhetoric and movement leaders at the expense of her community:

> I was not press-shy. I had already co-written a *Philadelphia Daily News* op-ed about the failure of sexuality education in city public schools, been quoted in the *Philadelphia Inquirer* about school violence and the devaluation of black life, and provoked television news coverage thanks to an anti-racism speakout my friends and I orchestrated at our school. But I drew the line at publicly aligning myself with

> "the abortion issue," *Roe v. Wade*, and the institutional white feminists popularly associated with the ruling.[23]

Solomon's words demonstrate just some of the residual reticence Black advocates have had with publicly associating with abortion advocacy. As a resident of West Philadelphia, Solomon's refusal to publicly advocate against *Planned Parenthood v. Casey* exemplified the fraught relationship between the disproportionately visible white activists of the post-*Roe* landscape and the long, historical disillusionment of the Black Philadelphia communities where the Women's Medical Society emerged and Gosnell operated his clinic.

From Black Bottom to University City: Histories of Health Care Segregation in West Philadelphia

The Women's Medical Society's location in West Philadelphia significantly conditioned its susceptibility to be defined by back-alley rhetoric. West Philadelphia refers broadly to land west of the Schuylkill River ending west of Cobbs Creek and south of Overbrook Park and Wynnefield Heights. It contains the area formerly known as Black Bottom, a predominantly African American neighborhood that is now known as University City, home to the University of Pennsylvania and its students, faculty, and staff. Within these soft boundaries, some museums occupy the former 1876 World's Fair grounds just slightly north of the Philadelphia Zoo. Although West Philadelphia is home to some of the world's preeminent research hospitals, it is also the historical and contemporary home to racially segregated medical care. The West Philadelphia area has a history of medical racism that demands contextualization to better understand the dynamics that not only contributed to the low quality of care that many experienced in Gosnell's clinic but also to its being one the few available options to access full-spectrum reproductive medicine. Most popular treatments of the Gosnell case omit the history of migration, deindustrialization, and gentrification projects that would illuminate dynamics of systemic and structural racism in the area where he practiced. The exposition of these dynamics in Philadelphia I offer here is abbreviated, but it draws attention to the health, well-being, and justified distrust Black West Philadelphia residents have about medicine in the city. In accounting for the Women's Medical Society's existence within this larger anti-Black dehumanizing ecology, I wish to hold the complexity of deploring Gosnell's unacceptable treatment of the pregnant people who visited his clinic while also considering his case as symptomatic of a larger matrix of medical racism.[24]

Writing almost a decade before Charles and Eugenia Weller surveyed Washington, DC, alley housing, W. E. B. Du Bois presciently anticipated slum clearance efforts in *The Philadelphia Negro: A Social Study*. After he traveled across Philadelphia and spoke with residents, DuBois wrote, "A slum is not a simple fact, it is a symptom, and to know the removable causes . . . requires a study that takes one far beyond the slum districts. For few Philadelphians realize how the Negro population has grown and spread."[25] A "natural gateway between the North and the South," Philadelphia was a region that received formerly enslaved people and freed Black families.[26] However, between 1833 and 1842, white residents violently demolished a Black church and twenty homes.[27] Du Bois also tethered racial disparities in Philadelphia health and death rates to the housing conditions that Black families endured, including unsanitary dwellings. As Marcus Anthony Hunter aptly summarizes, "Urban Black Americans, however, were not simply victims of the vast changes impacting American cities throughout the twentieth century—urban renewal, deindustrialization, and the New Deal, the War on Poverty, and general urban divestment. Nor were they passive bystanders who watched the city change from the windows of their row homes. Black Philadelphians were and are agents of urban change—citymakers."[28]

Much like other cities that received the influx of Black Americans after the Great Migration, Black Philadelphians held a notable distrust of white physicians, who had a reputation for medical racism. This distrust was by no means a problem confined to the Philadelphia area. Before the Civil War, Southern medical schools frequently looked to plantations for "clinical material" and publicized their need for "servants laboring under Surgical diseases."[29] While the Southern economy for the stolen remains of Black people supplied medical schools, this was not a problem confined to Southern states. For more than ten years, students and staff at Philadelphia's Thomas Jefferson Medical School procured cadavers by stealing human remains from Lebanon Cemetery, a historically Black burial site in Philadelphia, until the *Philadelphia Press* exposed the practice in 1882.[30] David C. Humphrey notes a pronounced collective outrage that ensued: "Philadelphia's black community responded so angrily that city medical leaders and Pennsylvania politicians agreed on a second anatomy law, requiring public officials throughout the state to turn over all unclaimed bodies to a state anatomy board."[31] These historical events, among countless others, have contributed to an understandable distrust of white-led medical care. This distrust circulated through oral folklore, which spread through the community during the Great Migration and beyond.[32]

Racial segregation in medical societies and hospitals was permitted nationwide, and Black physicians were excluded from membership in the American Medical Association. In Philadelphia, this segregation was met with the development of a robust Black hospital movement.[33] In 1895, Dr. Nathan F. Mossell established the Frederick Douglass Memorial Hospital after he was denied admission to a medical residency program in Philadelphia and had to travel to England to complete his education. The hospital served the African American population of Philadelphia and provided an educational space where Black doctors and nurses could train. It experienced underfunding and frequently relied on community help to procure clean linens and food. After younger doctors grew frustrated at the administration's unwillingness to allow interns hands-on experience, several left the institution and created Mercy Hospital in 1907, just a few blocks away.

Although Mercy Hospital flourished for several years, both hospitals experienced significant financial struggles during World War II because of the few patients privately paying for care and a dearth of governmental support. Underfunding often forced an impossible choice between paying the mortgage or purchasing enough sanitary supplies. By 1947, a joint committee representing both hospitals and the Philadelphia Community Chest recommended a merger. However, there was a poison pill: Section F of the merger agreement required Mercy and Douglass hospitals to relinquish control of administration, staff, and technical training to the University of Pennsylvania, Temple University, and Jefferson Medical College. Directors of Mercy and Douglas recoiled at the prospect of white institutions holding such power over the hospital, fearing it would lead the institution to become a space of medical experimentation. Of course, these concerns were hardly unfounded; not only was there the visceral memory of Lebanon Cemetery's desecration, but Black physicians "regardless of their credentials, found it difficult to obtain hospital admitting privileges."[34] Ultimately, staff members sought self-determination and "said that they didn't want to be dictated to by people who did not recognize racial equality."[35]

Mercy and Douglass ultimately merged in 1948 to become Mercy-Douglass Hospital and became a mainstay fixture for Black Philadelphia residents during Jim Crow's hospital segregation. As medical historian Vanessa Northington Gamble explains at the beginning of her monograph on the Black hospital movement: "As a child growing up in the late 1950s and early 1960s in predominantly Black West Philadelphia, Mercy-Douglass Hospital . . . was very much a part of my life."[36] Not only did members of the Philadelphia Black community entrust Mercy-Douglass with their care; it was considered a significant community cultural center for healing amid the larger context of Jim Crow. Segregated hospital care was permitted until the 1963 Fourth Circuit Court decision *Simkins v. Moses H. Cone Memorial Hospital* applied the holdings of *Brown v. Board of Education* to the inherent injustice and inequality of separated hospital spaces. However, owing to protracted financial issues, Mercy-Douglass was forced to close in 1973, just months after *Roe* was decided.

The University of Pennsylvania (known regionally as "Penn") transformed the social and economic dynamics of West Philadelphia, generating discord between students and the surrounding community while disrupting established members of the Black community. Benjamin Franklin chartered the university in 1749 to prepare white men for public service and commerce.[37] Penn moved the location of its school three times, twice within the center city, and ultimately landed in its current West Philadelphia location in 1870, moves often motivated by the perceived "creep" of the city into the university bubble. Harley Etienne explains how "a growing population of African Americans from the American South found their way into West Philadelphia. The deindustrialization that followed World War II set the city on a path toward population loss and urban poverty for the next sixty years."[38]

With deindustrialization siphoning economic opportunities from West Philadelphia after World War II, the area universities transformed Black Bottom. With the postwar GI Bill funding college tuition for white veterans, the University of Pennsylvania teamed up with the Drexel Institute of Technology, the University of the Sciences in Philadelphia, and the Presbyterian Hospital in 1959 to form the West Philadelphia Corporation. This corporation sought to redevelop the area into University City, acquiring properties by eminent domain, demolishing homes, and displacing hundreds of residents. As Etienne observes, "Largely, Penn succeeded in leveraging its medical school and strengths in information technology and life sciences to spawn the University City Science Center and what has become the hospital of the University of Pennsylvania complex—consistently one of the nation's leading recipients of funding from the National Institutes of Health." Penn's self-interest was often made clear by the racist ways it socialized students and engaged in economic revitalization practices, dubbed "Penntrification." For many years, Penn would hand out city maps to students as part of orientation that placed a thick black boundary line to demarcate Fortieth Street—a place where students should ostensibly not travel and which was predominantly populated by Black residents.[39]

Although the neighborhoods and the larger Philadelphia community are home to some of the preeminent medical care facilities in the world, significant racial health disparities remain today. Although the passage of Medicaid expansion as part of the Affordable Care Act brought 90 percent of Black Philadelphians and 96 percent of children insurance, they were not able to use that insurance at Philadelphia's many medical complexes.[40] Despite the abundance of health and medical resources, the West Philadelphia neighborhoods, composed of high percentages of African Americans, lack access to obstetrical and primary care.[41] Given the lack of available care—especially for minoritized pregnant people—it should not come as a surprise that clinics like Gosnell's were able to flourish. Chillingly, at 3801 Lancaster Avenue, Kermit Gosnell's clinic, the Women's Medical Society, sat just two blocks from Penn Presbyterian Medical Center, an affiliate of the Penn Hospital system, just north of the upper boundary of what was formerly known as Black Bottom.

Crafting Back-Alley Abortion in West Philadelphia

The grand jury report of the Kermit Gosnell case bore the name of R. Seth Williams, Philadelphia's first Black district attorney. More than 260 pages long, with four appendixes, it was filed on January 14, 2011, and divided into eight sections: (1) "Overview," (2) "The Raid," (3) "Gosnell's Illegal Practice," (4) "The Intentional Killing of Viable Babies," (5) "The Death of Karnamaya Mongar," (6) "How Did This Go On So Long?" (7) "The Criminal Charges," and (8) "Recommendations of the Grand Jury." Whereas the legal function of the grand jury report was to recommend indictments against Gosnell and several employees at the Women's Medical Society, I argue that one of the document's *rhetorical* functions was to depoliticize back-alley abortion in ways that enabled its uptake by anti-abortion advocates. It was important that the grand jury explicitly situated itself outside the scope of abortion politics. However, the pretense of political neutrality laid the groundwork for back-alley abortion rhetoric and the report's policy recommendations to later be uncritically deployed as apolitical, uncontroversial conclusions. Early on, the report acknowledged the sensitivities involved in presiding over a case about abortion but framed Gosnell's clinic as an elusive point of ideological convergence between pro-choice and anti-abortion interests. Grand jurors described the case as having transcended the political polarities of abortion in the United States: "We realize this case will be used by those on both sides of the abortion debate. We ourselves cover a spectrum of personal beliefs about the morality of abortion. For us as a criminal grand jury, however, this case is not about that controversy; it is about disregard of the law and disdain for the lives and health of mothers and infants. *We find common ground in exposing what happened here,* and in recommending measures to prevent anything like this from happening again."[42] This "common ground" was located in a shared moral revulsion that repudiated Gosnell's medical techniques, unsanitary clinic, and uncaring orientation to patients. At first glance, back-alley dynamics—routed through values of legal objectivity—seemed to have dislodge an immovable US controversy.

Much like the other back-alley rhetorics this book has examined, the case's copious descriptions brought the unsanitary conditions before the readers' senses and evoked horror grounded in a situated engagement with the clinical space. The vividness was related to not simply the shared assessment of disgusting clinical conditions but also the more considerable negotiation of proper surgical procedure, technique, protocol, and oversight. As Julia Kristeva argues, "It is not lack of cleanliness or health that causes abjection but what disturbs identity, system, order. What does not respect borders, positions, rules."[43] In this case, health, cleanliness, and the disturbance of boundaries intertwined: multisensory appeals to disgust not only cast this individual practice as outside of the boundaries of legitimate medicine but also leveraged attributions of disorder within institutions of the state, threatening its legitimacy. Indeed, Pennsylvania had to reckon with its own surveillance failures given the already restrictive features of the Abortion Control Act. Ultimately, the grand jury report's back-alley abortion rhetoric marked the *kakoethos* of Gosnell's monstrosity, the clinic's abject space, and a more extensive structural disorder of failed surveillance that enabled the back-alley to exist as a space of absent oversight within the state itself.

Kermit Gosnell, Abortion Monster

The grand jury report crafted Kermit Gosnell as an abortion monster: the malicious, careless, greedy, and callous antagonist of a back-alley horror story marked by provider *kakoethos* and saturated with visceral repugnance. Following Cassidy D. Ellis, it is crucial to pinpoint the "material quotidian effects/affects of this monsterization" to determine what made its framing so amenable to anti-abortion uptake.[44] Rhetorician Kendall Phillips writes that the monster's existence "violates natural categories such as living and dead [and] . . . must be treated as threatening and frightening."[45] As an abortion provider, Gosnell was already rhetorically imbued with the agency to traverse the contingent boundaries of life: its before, beginning, and end. Marina Levina and Diem-My T. Bui note that "what is at stake in the representational analysis of monster images is the definition of humanness, or, rather, a discursive production of subjectivity." In Gosnell's case, the "monster" conformed to a familiar typology of doctors whose natural operating space was saturated with unsanitary ambiance.[46] Yet

Gosnell's clinical subjectivity was also and already rhetorically shaped by the material influences of racism, classism, and patriarchal state formations: "The monster dwells at the gates of difference [which comes to] represent race, nationality, class, gender, ability, and sexuality."[47] By circulating the aversive affective residue of the back-alley—specifically disgust related to Gosnell's morality and criminality as a physician—the grand jury report generated the intentionally bad character of a rogue practitioner operating outside of the boundaries of legitimate medicine.

Gosnell's monstrous *kakoethos* also resulted from his dual status as a hypocritical "community servant" with a callous and greedy disposition toward patients and as a reckless medical practitioner who regularly used atypical and experimental surgical instruments. William Ian Miller states hypocritical behavior is acutely related to disgust elicitation, as hypocrites are "parasites on the moral order."[48] Whereas Dr. Edgar Keemer dissociated himself from the back-alley through his community engagement, refusal to explicitly profit from abortion provision, and systematic research, descriptions of Gosnell painted the opposite picture, depicting his willingness to operate in a self-serving manner for personal profit.[49] Specifically, the grand jury report claimed Gosnell to be a once esteemed member of the local community whose practice ultimately proved to be a sham. For years, Gosnell had been celebrated for his service to the community, maintaining a respected public persona.[50] According to the report, his monstrous character emerged from this contradiction, describing the newly discovered lacuna that had separated his public face from his actual practice: "The image of himself that Gosnell promoted had no truth to it. In newspaper and television interviews, he portrayed himself as a hard-working, conscientious doctor doing the best he could for his community. . . . Any contributions he may have made to the community are undermined by the substandard treatment that he passed off as medical care for the indigent."[51] Gosnell's duplicitous and prevaricating persona pervaded descriptions of his conduct. As further elaborated by the report, Gosnell had defrauded insurance companies and abortion funds, casting both his character and the professional space in which he operated as immoral.

Throughout several sections of the report, grand jurors argued that Gosnell's greed impacted the quality of care he provided: the money he allegedly skimmed should have been used to hire appropriately licensed staff. The grand jury report argued that such transgressions were both willful and intentional. For instance, Gosnell would take in approximately $10,000 to $15,000 per night, totaling $1.8

million per year, although he was rarely present for procedures in the clinic.[52] Instead, he allowed untrained staff to mix and administer intravenous sedatives: "The pain, suffering, and death that he and his employees perpetrated were not the result of accidentally botched procedures. It was Gosnell's standard business practice."[53] Purposefully doling out pain and suffering, the doctor was alleged to be a calculative actor whose typical medical practices and treatment of his staff demonstrated his greed. Gosnell "deliberately" hired unlicensed, unqualified staff to perform the procedures, including a fifteen-year-old student, because, as the grand jury editorialized, "he could pay them low wages often in cash."[54] The report indicated that Gosnell went through several registered nurses and cleaning orderlies because he did not pay them on time. Yet the police raid of Gosnell's home and clinic uncovered $250,000 in cash.[55] The report's strategic juxtaposition of stockpiled money with his refusal to pay employees foregrounded the blameworthy traits of a "back-alley butcher."

The report accused Gosnell of participating in racially discriminatory practices and specifically lacking concern for the low-income women of color who came to his clinic. He allegedly refused to supervise the administration of anesthesia "unless the patient was white."[56] Tina Baldwin, one of Gosnell's employees, testified to the grand jury that Gosnell explicitly gave substandard care to women of color: "So he didn't mind you medicating your African American girls, your Indian girl, but if you had a white girl from the suburbs, oh, you better not medicate her. You better wait until he go in and talk to her first. And one day I said something to him and he was like, that's the way of the world.[57] The report characterized Gosnell's invocation of this "way of the world" not as a reflection of Philadelphia's racially stratified health care systems or historical legacy of medical segregation but rather as an affirmation of Gosnell's own racial bias and individual moral failings. As the report put it, "Every aspect of that practice reflected an utter disregard for the health and safety of his patients, a cruel lack of respect for their dignity, and an arrogant belief that he could forever get away with the slovenly and careless treatment of the women who came to his clinic."[58]

The report also constructed Gosnell's monstrosity through his callous bedside manner and lack of empathy. He was characterized as having displayed cruelty toward patients' health outcomes by ignoring their wishes and minimizing their pain. The grand jury reported that one woman changed her mind after Gosnell had inserted a laminaria to dilate her cervix and promote contractions. When she asked him to stop the procedure, Gosnell allegedly refused to remove the laminaria. After the woman left Gosnell's clinic, she went to the hospital where she gave birth to a premature child who was "now a healthy kindergartener."[59] The report described another similar case and alleged that Gosnell ignored the woman's wishes not because it was too late to stop the procedure, but because he did not want to refund her payment. Moreover, the report described how Gosnell would over-sedate patients so that he did not have to hear them in pain during recovery. Even Gosnell's employees were unwilling to seek the doctor's assistance when they needed similar services: "When two of Gosnell's staff members sought abortions, they knew better than to go to him."[60]

Last, the report constituted Gosnell's monstrosity as a *butcher,* detailing how he mutilated patient and fetal flesh using improper, nonmedical tools. As Niall Scott has argued, "Like a Midas effect, all that the monster touches, wields, and or generates becomes monstrous."[61] Some of the more visceral back-alley narratives recounted across this book have referred to the use of household items in self-induced abortions, such as coat hangers and knitting needles. In the case of this grand jury report, Gosnell's monstrosity emerged through what it described as his "bizarre" use of scissors.[62] The report's fourth section, "The Intentional Killing of Viable Babies," described Gosnell's practice of using scissors to sever the spinal cords of fetuses once they were expelled from patient uteruses. The vivid descriptions of the practice were bookended by a graphic image of the back neck of a fetus.[63] The report denounced the use of scissors, distinguishing it from best practices in abortion care. Quoting a "medical expert with 43 years of experience in performing abortions" as being "appalled," while Gosnell told his staff that "this barbaric conduct was standard medical practice," the report asserted that the expert quickly assessed that "it was not. It was criminal behavior."[64]

The report also described how Gosnell's tools harmed vulnerable pregnant women. A representative hallmark in the report was the grand jury's association of Gosnell with what it called the "Mother's Day Massacre" and use of Harvey Karman's supercoil. In 1972, a year before the *Roe* decision, Gosnell was working with Harvey Karman, who had run an illegal practice in California since the 1950s and had also worked with the Jane Collective in Chicago. The supercoil was a ball of sharp plastic coated in a temperature-activated gel that would expand and end a pregnancy when inserted into a uterus. The inventor of the Karman cannula, which had transformed the safety and efficacy of early abortions in pre-*Roe* abortion care—and a participant in the Society for Humane Abortion's Office Abortion symposium in 1970—Karman was trying to develop a similar advance for those whose pregnancies were further developed.[65] When fifteen patients, mostly Black women, seeking abortions were bussed from Chicago to Philadelphia after the Jane Collective was raided, Karman and Gosnell performed the supercoil procedure. Nine of the fifteen women suffered severe complications, with two requiring hysterectomies. The report's description of the supercoil was thoroughly monstrous: "What also fills the spectator and future patient with terror, however, is the interlocking of the devices used with the agency of the hands that wield these objects, often represented by the scalpel or syringe."[66] Through its framing of abortion procedures conducted using inappropriate methods, Gosnell's tools became a criminalized extension of his bad character. Cumulatively, the report generated appraisals of Gosnell's moral, sanitary, and criminal character by alluding to his hypocrisy, poor bedside manner, and racially biased care. These factors, decontextualized from Philadelphia's history of medical racism, deftly shaped Gosnell into an abortion monster, the *kakoethotic* back-alley butcher.

3801 Lancaster Avenue: Main Street's Back-Alley

The grand jury report's characterization of Gosnell's clinic as a "house of horrors" allowed this space to function as a particularly sticky site for back-alley rhetoric. Readers encountered the clinic's squalid qualities through the report's texturing of the space to bring the conditions before readers' senses. I begin this section by describing how sensory appeals constituted various elements of the clinic's texture before tracing how these textures were deployed as narratives describing patients' experiences in the clinic. I close it by explaining how the architectural layout of the clinic served as a way to blame Gosnell for the death of Karnamaya Mongar.

As the grand jury report opened its vivid tour of 3801 Lancaster Avenue, references to noxious olfaction intertwined with the off-putting sights, grimy surfaces, and the distasteful presence of animals at the facility. The report attributed bad smells to visible contaminants in the environment and indicated the sensory overload physically assaulted those conducting the raid: "[Investigators] described the odor that *struck* one immediately upon entering—a mix of smells emanating from the cloudy fish tank where turtles were fed crushed clams and baby formula."[67] While this sentence made it clear that discrete senses were registering the atmosphere (smell, sight, touch, and even the taste of reptile food), the vivid rhetorical force emerged from the space's entanglement of the entire sensorium.

The report not only testified to these senses functioning at once but also attributed the texture to a spatial boundary violation—the inappropriate presence of animals in a medical facility. By the second page of the report, readers quickly learned "the clinic reeked of animal urine, courtesy of the cats that were allowed to roam and defecate freely."[68] This visual and olfactory affective alignment led into an extensive description of the clinical raid in section 2. During this initial raid, a search team reported a "stench of urine filled the air . . . and there were cat feces on the stairs."[69] The report drew on a logic of miasmatic contamination as it repeatedly returned to the odor of the cats and the presence of their excrement.[70] As this book has repeatedly shown, before and after its association with abortion, cats have been a peculiar mainstay of back-alley rhetoric. By reintroducing cats and their waste into the description, the report claimed a violation of the boundary between the human and nonhuman, rendering judgment on Gosnell's violation of the sanitary boundaries between humans and animals in medical space.

The report's textured description of blood and other bodily fluids provided a vivid tableau that also integrated sight, touch, and smell, making it a haunting space to practice medicine. As Eve Sedgwick reminds us, when we speak of "texture," we recognize that which cannot be reduced to a single sensory engagement. Instead, texture operates as an articulation of multiple senses, narrating how an object (or objects) emerged. Blood is always-already marked by cultural and discursive impressions.[71] As such, it matters where and how blood appears in clinical descriptions. In Gosnell's clinic, blood appeared in multiple forms, signaling disarray and chaos. For instance, the report describes blood as "leaking," "caked," "dried," "splattered," "stained," and "everywhere."[72] Blood textured medical instruments that were reused on multiple patients because they were too large to soak in a container of sterilizing solution.[73] Blood was also stained on blankets, caked on stirrups, and dried on walls, sinks, and toilets. By attending to how fluids were textured in the grand jury report, we might better understand how Gosnell's monstrosity was reinforced by the disgusting space in which he operated.

These textural formations narrated a sense of embodied boundary contamination that went beyond a characterization of Gosnell's monstrosity by marking the women who underwent procedures in his clinic as worthy of pity because they were unaware of the dehumanizing medical encounter to which they were subjected. For instance, the same "flea-infested cats" that had defecated on the floor often came into proximity with unknowing patients by sleeping on the facility's beds when they were not in use—leaving a contaminating residue.[74] The medical equipment, described as "dust-covered" with "corroded tubing," was reused for multiple patients.[75] Former employee Kareema Cross testified that the unsterilized, reused instruments were likely the culprit for the number of complaints from women who contracted chlamydia and gonorrhea while at Gosnell's clinic.[76] However, unlike the immediate harm the women could gauge from Gosnell's callous bedside manner, the report made it seem like patients were not privy to the bigger picture of cross contamination. Much like alley clearance literature discussed in chapter 1, passages like these enabled readers to encounter the conditions from a removed bird's-eye view. By summarizing the clinical space as a breeding ground for disease, the report allowed readers to imagine the patients violated in these spaces as becoming unknowingly contaminated by their proximity to pathogens during their medical encounter. Given the economic, racialized context and ambient abortion stigma, such depictions generated a distanced affective attachment to the patients insofar as they enabled more privileged readers to feel bad *for* them—and not necessarily imagine themselves in a similar circumstance. By creating a hierarchical relationship of distanced pity based on physical proximity to inappropriate tools and medical practice, actionable redress of "protecting women's health" could emerge as a persuasive solution—even if it meant that a more dignified clinic offering abortions would not exist.

Just as nineteenth-century sanitation reformers were concerned with the design of hospitals and charged architects with moral violations, the grand jury made moral condemnations of the clinic's confusing layout, which was punctuated by descriptions of "cluttered hallways" and "padlocked emergency doors." The grand jury at least partially blamed the death of Karnamaya Mongar on these layout issues. "Another violation of Pennsylvania law . . . clinics must have doors, elevators, and other passages adequate to allow stretcher-borne patients to be carried to a street-level exit. Gosnell's clinic, with its narrow, twisted passageways, could not accommodate a stretcher at all. And his emergency street-level access was bolted with no accessible key. Any chance Mongar had of being revived was hampered by the time wasted looking for keys to the door."[77] On the next page, the report showed photographs of the barricaded emergency access with peculiar historical resonances. Recall how, in chapter 2, cartoon representations of back-alley abortion frequently alluded to the interior of clinics without showing them, instead featuring a foreboding perspective of their entryways from the outside street. With Gosnell's clinic, caged security bars on the door and neighboring windows reinforced the clinic's impermeable boundary, signifying that danger lay inside. When attempting to admit emergency personnel, one assistant testified, she tried more than thirty keys on six different padlocks. Between the building's sensorial texturing and confusing layout, the Women's Medical Society clinic was a particularly potent site for moral judgment about sanitary conditions to occur in the grand jury report.

"See No Evil": Pennsylvania's Jurisdictional Back-Alley

It is significant that the phrase "see no evil" appeared as a section heading in the grand jury report because, as argued in chapter 1, before its association with abortion, back-alley rhetorics often referred to city spaces that the state could not fully see, surveil, or manage. The grand jury was not content with merely identifying Gosnell's character flaws and medical incompetence. The report capped its back-alley narrative by blaming the State of Pennsylvania's abortion oversight apparatuses. Despite Pennsylvania having some of the country's more stringent abortion restrictions with the Abortion Control Act, the report made two allegations. First, the grand jury asserted that regulators ignored issues that emerged. Second—and important for how we understand how back-alley logics can morph—they suggested that split jurisdiction in oversight responsibilities was why Gosnell's practice operated for as long as it did. Zornitsa D. Keremidchieva argues that "jurisdiction matters because it entails questions of who gets to act and what rules apply."[78] Contestations over jurisdictional authority are crucial to the state management of health care providers, and Gosnell's legal case made apparent how neither state agency could "see" the totality of the situation to intervene. The grand jury report's back-alley rhetoric blamed the Department of Health (DOH) for not regulating Gosnell's clinical space and the Department of State (DOS) for continuing to license Gosnell despite copious complaints. It thus materialized what I term Pennsylvania's *institutional back-alley* as the effect of an impervious jurisdictional boundary between oversight bodies.

Although the DOH was responsible for regulating clinical spaces to ensure sanitary practices, the grand jury report asserted that it skirted its responsibilities by rendering abortion regulation invisible and allowing clinics to essentially oversee themselves. Capturing residual appeals of Progressive Era alley surveillance, the inability of the state to fully surveil Gosnell's clinic structured this back-alley appeal. First, the grand jury report indicated that the DOH employed a "bizarre" classification for abortion clinics: rather than defining them under the Division of Acute and Ambulatory Care, which was designated for outpatient surgery and anesthesia, it was nestled into the DOH's Division of Home Health. The report charged that this classification rendered abortion clinics invisible and made oversight "impossible":

> The [DOH] website published phone numbers to call for various types of complaints: the Division of Acute and Ambulatory Care for ambulatory surgical facilities, the Division of Home Health's "hotline" for home health agencies, hospices,

> and End State Renal Disease facilities. There is no mention, however, that DOH even oversees abortion facilities, or that it accepts complaints about them. In light of this, the policy that the DOH would inspect facilities only in response to complaints goes beyond bad management. It appears to reflect purposeful neglect.[79]

The report moralized this issue by taking this regulatory "blind spot" and casting the produced jurisdictional nonspace as intentional "by design." The report continued its indictment of the agency by questioning its character, claiming that members "abdicated" their responsibility: "Pennsylvania officials have created what amounts to an honor system, a system conspicuously lacking in regulatory oversight or enforcement."[80] Ultimately, the grand jury circulated moral judgment by rebuking the regulatory body for failing to see what should have been under its jurisdiction.

The grand jury also juxtaposed Gosnell's clinical conditions to what they perceived as particular DOH agents' intentional neglect. First, the report critiqued the DOH for not having recently inspected Gosnell's clinic. After providing an abbreviated chronology of the few times the DOH did inspect the clinic, the grand jury report rhetorically amplified Gosnell's misdeeds in the sixteen-year gap in the department's performance of its inspection duties:

> During the next *16 plus years*—as Gosnell collected fetuses' feet in jars in his office and allowed medical waste to pile up in the basement; as he replaced his few licensed medical assistants with untrained workers and a high school student; as his outdated equipment rusted and broke and he routinely reused instruments designed for single-use; as he allowed unqualified staff to administer anesthesia and to deal with babies born before he arrived at work for the day; and as he caused the deaths of two patients while continuing to perform illegal third-trimester abortions and kill babies outside their mothers' wombs—DOH never conducted another on-site inspection at the Lancaster Avenue facility.[81]

Bookending appeals that evoked disgust at Gosnell's medical practice with the DOH's culpability, the affective residue of the back-alley adhered not only to the figural butcher but also to the regulatory body that had ignored complaints by deferring to the DOS, "believ[ing] they didn't have the legal authority" to intervene.[82]

While the Department of Health was mandated to inspect clinical facilities, the Department of State was responsible for overseeing physician licensure. In other words, the DOS was accountable for overseeing Gosnell's own certifications and for the employees in his practice who would administer anesthesia.

After identifying individual DOS actors responsible for ignoring complaints about Gosnell, the grand jury asserted that the issue was a systemic failure: "The Grand Jury is convinced . . . that the problem does not lie with the individual attorneys. There are clearly problems with procedures, training, management, and motivation within the Department of State's Bureau of Professional and Occupational Affairs."[83] The report levied outrage at the DOS's unresponsiveness to complaints, transforming their inaction into a moral judgment: like Gosnell, members of the DOS were alleged to not *care* about abortion patients.

The report also blamed the Department of State's failure to censure Gosnell after the death of twenty-two-year-old Philadelphia resident Semika Shaw. After Shaw died from sepsis following a botched abortion, autopsy reports indicated that her uterus had been perforated. Although Shaw's family was awarded $400,000 from a liability insurance company in 2002, the DOS deemed that further investigation was not necessary. The grand jury report expressed disbelief at the department's justification, reprinting its internal summary to demonstrate that Shaw was being unfairly demonized for acquiring an abortion:

> Brief Factual Summary: The file was opened as a result of a Medical Malpractice Payment Report. The underlying malpractice case involved the death of a 22-year-old female following the termination of her 5th pregnancy. Following a seemingly routine procedure on 3/1/02, the patient was taken to the E.R. at the University of Pennsylvania with complaints of pain and heavy bleeding. The patient underwent surgery but the surgeon was unable to locate any perforation and the patient died from infection and sepsis. Although the incident is tragic, especially in light of the age of the patient, the risk was inherent with the procedure performed by the Respondent [Gosnell] and administrative action against respondent's license is not warranted.[84]

By claiming that the information about Shaw's fifth termination was "irrelevant, but pointed," the grand jury also noted that the DOS report ignored the autopsy results that *did* indicate perforation in Shaw's uterus. The grand jury reported at least one other woman's story and several other examples of the department's failure to investigate. The DOS did, however, get involved when Gosnell's victims fell within the affiliative boundaries of agency members: "It is curious, therefore, that the only complaint against Gosnell that did lead to any disciplinary action by the Board involved a non-certified physician's assistant who treated a child for pink eye in 1990. As it happens, the child's grandmother, the complainant, worked for the Bureau of Professional and Occupational Affairs."[85] By reporting this information, the grand jury levied accusations of hypocrisy and preferentialism at the Department of State. If a case of *pink eye* could rally department censure while death was considered an "inherent risk" of an abortion procedure, the DOS could be construed as speaking out both sides of its regulatory mouth by setting inconsistent oversight boundaries. By creating and maintaining a regulatory lapse that resulted in the state's formation of its very own back-alley, the report laid the groundwork for further regulation and surveillance—an argument that would be picked up in subsequent anti-abortion advocacy efforts

The Anti-abortion Uptake of Back-Alley Rhetoric in the Grand Jury Report

Although grand juries are shrouded in secrecy and granted the bounded task of considering evidence to recommend indictments, the grand jury report of the Women's Medical Society received remarkable public circulation. Escaping its legal confines, the report was taken up in popular journalism, with the case eventually being cited in the Supreme Court's decision in *Whole Woman's Health v. Hellerstedt*. Despite the grand jury's hope that the case could serve as an elusive point of agreement, the case was overwhelmingly channeled to remove abortion as a category of legitimate medical care by justifying clinic closures and provider restrictions. To track the grand jury report's rhetorical life as a back-alley rhetoric is to simultaneously recognize how fragments of the document participated in what Jenny Edbauer names "an ongoing circulation process" for competing and contradictory purposes over time, producing an "extended half-life in its range of circulation and visibility" while "chang[ing] the shape, force, and intensity" of the original rhetorical appeal.[86] Beyond the internal dynamics of the grand jury report, its popular uptake is rhetorically significant because it demonstrates how back-alley appeals—historically a rhetorical resource for abortion activists—held the capacity to be taken up for regressive anti-abortion advocacy. While chapter 1 argued that the rhetorical history of the back-alley before abortion capacitated that possibility from the start, the grand jury report of the Gosnell case represented a flashpoint, marking how the back-alley's potential for anti-abortion mobilization and uptake became kinetic.

The rhetorical concept of *uptake* has largely been used to gesture to the movement of texts across the boundaries of genres, shaping subjectivities in the process. Kimberly K. Emmons has helped to further clarify the embodied relationship of uptake between legal and medical genres, a connection that is crucial for thinking about how a legal document like the grand jury report shaped readerly subjectivities about reproductive medical care and spaces like abortion clinics.[87] Particularly, Emmons encourages us to "redefine uptake not as the relation between two (or more) genres, but as the *disposition* of subjects that results from that relation. Genres as social actions are powerful only when they direct or forestall human interaction."[88] If we consider what Emmons calls "disposition" as an affective quality or characteristic, we might also understand historically circulating genres like back-alley abortion rhetoric to be imbued with a regressive residue that had circulated for more than a century. Such affective residue, I wager, risks normalizing anti-abortion positions to which subjects might not otherwise assert.

To fully investigate how uptake can produce these transformative yet regressive adherences, I turn to the *Oxford English Dictionary*, which provides definitions of "uptake" that are useful for understanding how the report's back-alley rhetoric was captured by anti-abortion activists. "Uptake" refers to the process by which one takes possession of or occupies something else, alluding to the way that back-alley abortion can be dis- and repossessed by interested parties who occupy this rhetorical space. The architectural meaning of "uptake" becomes even more interesting to the historical context of sanitary reform movements and their reliance on miasmatic explanations of disease: "a ventilating shaft by which foul air ascends." Finally, "uptake" is defined as a biological process of "absorption or incorporation by a living system. Also *transferred*."[89] Understanding that any social movement is dynamic, we may understand back-alley abortion as the transfer of a rhetorical appeal from one advocacy domain to another.

Anti-abortion activists' possessive absorption (or uptake) of back-alley appeals can at least partially be understood by considering the grand jury report as a recurring legal genre that enabled situated social judgment when recommending indictment.[90] Within the forensic register that traditionally defines the scope of criminality, the report's function was to investigate the past, search for the "truth," and, as a written composition, generate jury agreement in its recommendations to the district attorney—even as diverging opinions existed as to the "moral propriety" of abortion. As rhetorical critics Amy D. Propen and Mary Lay Schuster have recognized, legal genres like victim impact statements can often become a "tool for advocacy" inside the courtroom.[91] Yet, with the more expanded circulation of the grand jury report beyond the courtroom, I am particularly taken with their claim that "genres might serve to reflect and sustain the ideologies of the contexts in which they exist while also allowing room for expansion and growth."[92] Not only did the report sustain the ideological legitimacy of a carceral, legal solution to a long history of racialized health care injustice in Philadelphia; once back-alley abortion was "occupied" by anti-abortion activists, it expanded and transformed into an affectively potent inventional resource that stigmatized abortion to warrant intensified clinic access restrictions.

Through its circulation, the sticky residue of back-alley rhetoric firmly adhered to Gosnell in the legal and cultural domains. The grand jury report inspired films, think pieces, and anti-abortion legislative action—many with the regressive aim to limit abortion access on a larger scale. Some abortion rights activists' posttrial rebukes of Kermit Gosnell tried to prevent regressive uptake by staging a discussion about how legal dynamics could force pregnant people into the back-alley. Several organizations for abortion rights have adopted a similar approach, at times to the dismay of activist-scholars informed by a reproductive justice framework. In a statement following his May 2013 conviction, Ilyse Hogue, then president of NARAL Pro-Choice America, declared, "Justice was served to Kermit Gosnell today and he will pay the price for the atrocities he committed. We hope that the lessons of the trial do not fade with the verdict. Anti-choice politicians, and their unrelenting efforts to deny women access to safe and legal abortion care, will only drive more women to back-alley butchers like Kermit Gosnell."[93] Hogue's explicit back-alley reference projected a future where criminalized abortion would return to the *bas-fonds*. Yet, as J. N. Salters reminded us, without proceeding through a reproductive justice framework, homogenizing *women* as a category risked erasing the structural realities and histories of racist and segregationist medical practices that allowed a clinic like Gosnell's to flourish in the first place. Indeed, Salters's observations about the Gosnell verdict affirmed that "more women" would only encounter back-alley butchers within a reproductive configuration where the humanity of Black, Brown, and Indigenous women living in poverty went unrecognized by doctors and lawmakers.[94] By placing the phrase "Back Alley" in the title in scare quotes, Salters rejected the mythic *bas-fonds* in favor of a grounded analysis of the unjust health care realities faced by women of color.

Although some invested in reproductive rights and justice discussed the case in the back-alley frame, anti-abortion activists incorporated the report as an affective resource to occupy and reframe back-alley abortion by condemning *all* abortion as being of the *back-alley* variety. As Leandra Hinojosa Hernández and Sarah De Los Santos Upton have argued, such invocations of Kermit Gosnell dissociated abortion from the boundaries of "legitimate" medicine, associating his practice as "representative of *all* health care organizations and clinics that provide abortion procedures."[95] Anti-abortion activist Charmaine Yoest made this damaging hasty generalization explicit: "Legal abortion is the back alley of

American medicine, with which fewer and fewer doctors are willing to be associated."[96] Proclaiming abortion as incompatible with "American medicine," Yoest encouraged a wholesale dissociation of abortion from medicine and set the stage for abortion providers to be further stigmatized and socially ostracized from the medical community. Marjorie Dannenfelser of the Susan B. Anthony List echoed Yoest by likening abortion providers to back-alley butchers: "[Gosnell] is not an outlier."[97] The Elliott Institute, a group that researches the so-called adverse effects of abortion, touted the aphorism "Legal abortions, back alley ethics," which depicted *all* abortions as being performed by immoral, unskilled providers in unsanitary environments. Ultimately, the Gosnell case has served as a synecdoche for abortion writ large. As the report continued to circulate, it did not simply remain in the legal domain or a limited sphere of opinion-editorials. Rather, it was taken up as a visceral interventional resource for two films, spurring fundraising efforts for *Gosnell: America's Biggest Serial Killer* and providing embedded "evidence" for *3801 Lancaster: An American Tragedy.*

Gosnell: America's Biggest Serial Killer

Hailing from the abortion-restrictive nations of Northern Ireland and Poland, *Gosnell: America's Biggest Serial Killer* producers were conservative documentarians Phelim McAleer, Ann McElhinney, and Magdalena Segieda. These filmmakers set out to combat what they described as a nonresponse from mainstream media outlets.[98] After initiating what they called a "historic" campaign on the crowdfunding website Indiegogo, the producers raised more than $2.2 million between March 28 and May 12, 2014, with twenty-six thousand contributors and "most of the money coming from the United States."[99] The producers' use of the grand jury report to raise money for the film demonstrated the uptake, possession, and continual rhetorical occupation of back-alley abortion rhetoric by citing some of the most visceral elements of the report itself.

To raise funds for *Gosnell: America's Biggest Serial Killer,* the producers created seven promotional vignettes of McElhinney performing some of the more visceral excerpts from the grand jury report, many of which are quoted elsewhere in this chapter. Each promotional video follows an identical form: McElhinney begins with a brief phrase or sentence from the report to pique the audience's attention. The screen then goes black and cuts to white-lettered text: "Extract from the Grand Jury Report on the crimes of Kermit Gosnell." After the text fades to black, McElhinney returns and dramatically reads portions of the report, replete with dramatic pauses and eye contact with the camera to connect with viewers. Once complete, viewers hear haunting piano music as the video fades to black with the words "Help us make this movie; Go to GosnellMovie.com." Viewers then hear a jarring sound reminiscent of a prison door closing, affectively conveying Gosnell's criminal conviction. The movie's poster appears with a faded image of Gosnell, and the camera pans down until one can see only from his cheekbones to shoulders. Over his mouth appears a bloody image akin to an infant-sized handprint with bloodstains splattered across the screen reminiscent of the descriptions of blood in the grand jury report. Unsettling music further amplifies feelings of dis-ease, modeling what the film's producers deemed an appropriate emotional reaction to the vivid and graphic material. They also explicitly invoke the jury's assessment of the Gosnell case as an opportunity for cross-ideological consensus, that his criminality was a point they could all agree upon. Drawing on the report as an impartial legal document, they proffer an argument about legal legitimacy by situating a shared repudiation of back-alley abortion as the elusive "common ground" between abortion's advocates and adversaries. While the final film itself did not draw on the grand jury report, it is significant that the fundraising efforts used the document to amplify back-alley affects and occupy back-alley abortion rhetoric to argue for the supposed evils of abortion in toto.

3801 Lancaster: An American Tragedy

The documentary *3801 Lancaster: An American Tragedy* similarly invoked the grand jury report. Critically acclaim as the recipient of the 2013 Best Short Film Documentary at the Justice Film Festival, the film referenced the exact address of the Women's Medical Society: 3801 Lancaster Avenue. By allowing the grand jury report to serve as the inspirational grounding document for the film, it engaged a journalistic, documentary style to generate agreement about the need for clean clinical space as a universally shared value without fully interrogating the racist and classist dynamics embedded within the Philadelphia health care context. Like *Gosnell: America's Biggest Serial Killer, 3801 Lancaster* enabled anti-abortion activists to stealthily gain possession of back-alley abortion topoi by centering patients' moral agony and elevating law enforcement opinion to the same level as scientific and medical expertise.

In promotional interviews for the film, the phrase "back-alley abortion" was depoliticized and abstracted by statements that Gosnell's clinic was on a main street and *not* physically located in an alley. Targeting anti-abortion internet communities when promoting the documentary, filmmaker David Altrogge positioned Gosnell's clinic as distinct from other instances of back-alley abortion because it was physically located at a highly trafficked intersection: "Gosnell didn't operate out of a back alley. His clinic was on a busy street in West Philadelphia, just a stone's throw away from Drexel University."[100] The appeal to the clinic's prominent placement on the street suggested that dehumanizing abortions were not a hidden practice but highly visible and out in the open. Additionally, describing the Women's Medical Society's geographic proximity to reputable medical institutions granted Altrogge ground to amplify the grand jury's arguments about the institutional "back-alley" of failed oversight while ignoring the history of segregated health care. Although he admitted that he did not believe that all clinics are as "filthy and unsanitary as Dr. Gosnell's," he repudiated the Supreme Court's striking down Texas's HB2 by dissociating abortion access from abortion safety: "This Supreme Court decision makes it clear our country hasn't learned what happens when we make women's access to abortion a higher priority than women's safety." Indeed, it was not only promotional interviews that appeared on anti-abortion websites; the content of the documentary itself offered several moments that undermined Altrogge's assertion that his film was not motivated by a desire to stigmatize abortion and limit access.

The film made copious use of the grand jury report, both in the structure of the documentary and by displaying the report's images and text across the screen, supplemented with voice-over interviews with journalists and jurors. For critics who have read the entirety of the report, the documentary was incredibly familiar, mostly repeating what could be found in the three-hundred-page document. More than simply structuring the film, however, visual text from the grand jury report appears onscreen throughout the film, emphasizing discussions of the "Mother's Day Massacre," the noncommunication between the Department of State and Department of Health, reports of ignored complaints about Gosnell's practice, and the deaths of Semika Shaw and Karnamaya Mongar. The film also amplified the report's unsanitary affects by displaying a pair of scissors that were surmised—but never proven—to be the instrument that Gosnell used in his termination practices. Many of the film's still images, which showed overflowing waste, broken and dusty medical equipment, fish tanks, and dirty surroundings, were taken directly from the report. Shaky camcorder footage amplified the horror aesthetics of the clinic, giving viewers the impression that they were active bystanders to the raid that led to Gosnell's arrest.

The 3801 Lancaster documentary was a unique articulation of back-alley rhetoric because it was one of the few times that Gosnell's former patients spoke for themselves, rather than being spoken for. The inclusion of patient voices departed from simply re-presenting the content of the grand jury report. However, these personal narratives fed moral arguments for restricting abortion rather than offering a case for abortion access in safer, more dignified conditions. To be sure, each testimony reflected dehumanizing experiences in the clinic ranging from being chastised to "stop being a big baby" on the examination table, to awakening from anesthesia alone in the middle of the night, to being discharged while still heavily bleeding. While interviewees understandably had difficult feelings about their medical encounter and struggled to share their medical trauma, the documentary prioritized moments when they described their moral feelings about having an abortion at *all*.

The patients featured in *3801 Lancaster* described their experiences through what Mari Boor Tonn would call a rhetoric of "moral agony" and anguish, which in the context of abortion rights, "casts women as morally diminished individuals who violate their own moral code."[101] One woman, Davida, softly discusses having become pregnant after she was sexually assaulted, while another woman, Marquieta, laments how, at seventeen years old, she could not bear to tell her mother that she was pregnant. She described how growing up active in a church made her abortion "a hard decision." She questions the status of her moral compass, lamenting that "I don't know if I'm going to hell having an abortion and killing my baby." The thread of moral agony and implied abortion regret continues to build as the scene immediately cuts to Desiree: "I kept asking myself is this the right thing to do? Should I be doing this? Should I hate myself for doing this?" Desiree's agony is compounded by her mother's reflections: "I think about it everyday because these are choices we all live with. . . . I do know that when I die I have to answer for that because I'm not the one who says—none of us are—to say who stays and who goes." Each of these narrations suggested that abortion seekers and their families experienced agony because *any* abortion would provoke complicated feelings, regardless of the quality of the clinical surroundings and the provider's bedside manner. To be clear, I am not trying to dictate the proper responses of people after having an abortion. It is *always* important to hold space for a person's abortion experiences, as complicated as their feelings might be. From a feminist rhetorical and health equity standpoint, however, it is also important to not lose sight of the larger political implications of coupling a contemporary back-alley narrative with accompanying feelings of abortion regret and moral anguish. As Tonn elaborates, "The tales of abortion decisions by women who share their emotional struggles also provide ammunition to abortion critics."[102] Following Tonn, I am wary of the rhetorical resources that these narratives provide to anti-abortion activists who wish to see the procedure legislated out of existence. Considering that TRAP laws claim their argumentative ground by virtue of "protecting" patients, these narratives of patient vulnerability craft their subjectivity as *morally* vulnerable and in need of protection. However, it is important to critically interrogate the root causes of vulnerability for these patients. For example, consider that Desiree Manning was referred to Kermit Gosnell by a clinic in Hagerstown, Maryland, because they would not perform an abortion at twenty-two weeks gestation. Manning was not vulnerable owing to some intrinsic moral deficiency but rather because of the structural conditions that made safer access to an abortion impossible. All told, I seek to carefully consider these narratives of guilt, shame, and anguish in the context that they reinforced anti-abortion goals of restriction rather than addressing the need for greater health equity and access.

Further distancing the documentary from values of health equity, the film elevated a form of carceral expertise over scientific and medical expertise, constructing a version of fetal viability inconsistent with agreed-upon understandings of viability among scientific and medical communities. As just one example, at the end of *3801 Lancaster,* we meet not a physician or other medical expert but rather a police officer who synthesized the film's lessons by reframing the temporality of pregnancy: "At twelve weeks they look like babies. At sixteen weeks, they look *more* like babies. At nineteen weeks, they *are* babies." This makeshift construction of fetal personhood failed to align with even the highly restrictive Pennsylvania abortion statutes operative at the time. Ultimately, by allowing the grand jury report to serve as affective inspiration and evidentiary grounding, both films channeled the avowed ideological neutrality of the report by claiming universal agreement on the need for clean clinical space—even if it meant regulating abortion clinics out of existence. Indeed, that was precisely a question the Supreme Court would take up in *Whole Woman's Health v. Hellerstedt.*

Kermit Gosnell and *Whole Woman's Health*

While these two films dramatized fragments of the grand jury report to create a sense of depoliticized shared moral judgment about "back-alley practitioners," the report was traversing judicial discourse and influencing anti-abortion legislation across the United States.[103] Although several states drew upon Gosnell to restrict clinical space or provider credentials, I focus on Texas because it was the site of HB2, whose legal challenge led to *Whole Woman's Health v. Hellerstedt.* Texas already had laws in place that anticipated many of the characteristic restrictions of HB2. Back in 2004, the Woman's Right to Know (WRTK) Act had an "immediate and dramatic" impact.[104] Offering a precedent for the spatial restrictions enshrined by the 2013 HB2, the WRTK required abortions after sixteen weeks gestation to be performed in an ambulatory surgical center. When WRTK went into effect, none of the nonhospital providers in Texas met the ambulatory surgical center requirements. The number of abortions after sixteen weeks in Texas dropped by 69 percent, as residents left the state to pursue care.

As HB2 encountered legal challenges through the district and appeals courts, it finally reached the Supreme Court, where the grand jury report of Kermit Gosnell appeared again in defense of the law. In an amicus brief on behalf of the defendant(s), the governors of Texas, Alabama, Arkansas, Iowa, Kentucky, Louisiana, Maine, Mississippi, Nebraska, and South Dakota asserted that Gosnell's clinic (as represented in the grand jury report) was a central justification for the legislation. Indeed, the second sentence in the "Summary of the Argument" read, "HB2 was enacted in response to recommendations from the grand jury that indicted Kermit Gosnell."[105] Their solutions parroted the grand jury report's own recommendations: "By ensuring that doctors are affiliated with local hospitals and by improving safety standards at clinics, HB2 aligns abortion clinics more closely with mainstream medical practice."[106] Of course, this statement does not reflect the history of conservative activists and politicians systematically dissociating abortion from "legitimate" medical practice. As Gamble reminds us, provider admitting privileges have historically been a fraught negotiation that has systematically excluded Black doctors. Another amicus brief from Senators Ted Cruz (R-TX) and John Cornyn (R-TX) and Representatives Vicky Hartzler (R-MO), Pete Olson (R-TX), and Lamar Smith (R-TX) leveraged appeals to "women's health" and denigrated abortion rights advocates for not supporting HB2 in light of the Gosnell grand jury report. As Cruz summarized the brief: "[Gosnell] subjected the women in his care to unsanitary, degrading, and inhumane treatment, undermining their dignity and health, and even taking one of their lives."[107] As a unified category, *women* who encountered his clinic were mobilized as being "under threat" and in need of legal protection. A press release from the Texas Attorney General's Office echoed the centrality of the grand jury's report in its justification for seeking to restrict abortion to ambulatory spaces: "The grand jury that indicted Gosnell called on state legislatures to find the fortitude to pass regulations to ensure such a thing doesn't happen again, including ensuring clinics meet minimum standards of ambulatory surgical centers."[108]

Despite a favorable ruling for abortion accessibility in *Whole Woman's Health v. Hellerstedt*, the use of Kermit Gosnell and his grand jury report as a justification for abortion clinics closures remains enshrined in Supreme Court legal discourses—both in plurality and dissent. Justice Samuel Alito's dissent "did not dispute that H.B. 2 caused the closure of some clinics" and argued that a beneficial purpose of the law was to specifically shut down unsafe clinics—which did not constitute an undue burden. Invoking the grand jury's recommendation that all abortion clinics comply with ambulatory surgical protocols, Alito wrote, "The law was one of many enacted by the States in the wake of the Kermit Gosnell scandal." Alito and the other dissenters were unpersuaded by the plurality's argument that "the record contains nothing to suggest that H.B. 2 would be more effective than pre-existing Texas law at deterring wrongdoers like Gosnell from criminal behavior."[109] Indeed, Pennsylvania already had the highly restrictive Abortion Control Act on its books. However, it is notable that the plurality framed Kermit Gosnell as "deplorable" and "terribly wrong" while citing the grand jury report directly to argue "there is no reason to believe that an extra layer of regulation would have affected that behavior." While that particular case was not successfully mobilized to restrict abortion spaces and providers, the condemnation of Gosnell remains historically and synchronically uncontextualized, allowing back-alley residue to live on in reproductive jurisprudence.

Conclusion: From "Back-Alley" Clinic to Crisis Pregnancy Center

After Kermit Gosnell and several others employed at the clinic were sentenced, 3801 Lancaster Avenue became the target of a new deliberation—over the case's memory. An article declared, "And six years after Gosnell's conviction, a thorny question remains: how to memorialize the victims of his crimes . . . at his now-abandoned clinic at 38th Street and Lancaster Avenue?" With more than $56,000 in back taxes having accrued on the property since Gosnell's arrest, the building was listed for sheriff's sale four times, but no sale was ever completed because of perpetual legal issues. As Mantua Civic Association president De'Wayne Drummond acknowledged, "It's been a lot of trauma that took place in that building, and I think it's time for this area to go through some kind of healing and some kind of positive change."[110] These nuanced and localized discussions among community members reflected divergences about the now-abandoned clinical space. While some neighboring business owners, such as consignment shop owner Phyllis Carter, wished for the new use to be utterly unrelated to reproductive health to "draw people from other neighborhoods," resident Gail Floyd—a supporter of abortion rights who saw her friends experience lingering health problems after visiting Gosnell's clinic—struggled to think of the best use for the space but instead sought wider recognition of how pregnant patients had been treated there.[111]

Anti-abortion activists had their own plan for a "new chapter"—opening a crisis pregnancy center in the space Gosnell had once operated. Crisis pregnancy centers (CPCs) are most often religiously affiliated spaces that seek to dissuade pregnant people from seeking abortion. "Legal, but unethical," as the American Medical Association describes them, CPCs use deceptive practices and lack patient-centered care.[112] Nonetheless, Karen Hess and Kim Bennett opened AlphaCare, a CPC, just two doors from the former clinic at 3807 Lancaster Avenue. Not content to merely share a wall with the former Women's Medical Society, these "clinic" operators[113] "won't consider their vision to have come full circle until Alpha expands to 3801–05 Lancaster Avenue, the multi-unit office formerly occupied by Kermit Gosnell and his staff. At Heartbeat International's Annual Conference in 2011, Hess, Bennett, and a handful of their key staff and board members watched '3801 Lancaster' for the first time. Immediately, Bennett . . . envisioned a goal the organization has chased ever since."[114] Inspired by the rhetorical uptake of the grand jury report as presented in *3801 Lancaster*, Hess and Bennett declared, "The redemption has begun." AlphaCare advertised its prime location as "close to Drexel and UPenn's campus in University City and the Mantua and Powelton Village neighborhoods." Clicking on a thumbnail image below the description will direct one to images of a freshly painted waiting area, a clinical space with new exam tables, a state-of-the-art ultrasound machine, and an exterior image of the clinic with vibrant window box plants and a contemporary-looking logo. A far cry from the images that the grand jury report circulated with dead plants and corroded medical equipment, AlphaCare appeared clean, modern, and inviting. AlphaCare sanitized the presence of past reproductive injustice and decoupled full-spectrum reproductive care from the image of a clean clinic with caring staff.

As this chapter has argued, one cannot understand the rhetorical reach and significance of Kermit Gosnell being constructed as a "back-alley" butcher without attending both to the histories of medical racism and distrust among Black Philadelphians alongside the rhetorical circulation and uptake of the grand jury report. With a community still experiencing the injustices of segregation and dehumanization characteristic of so much institutionalized medical care, it is telling that community members recalled knowing friends who sought out Gosnell because they did not have other options. In channeling the discursive and affective residues of the back-alley before abortion, the grand jury report intermingled visceral sensory rhetorics that brought the conditions at 3801 Lancaster Avenue before the eyes, hands, and noses of readers. The visceral sensory resources allowed the report to constitute back-alley abortion without ever using the phrase, marked by the monstrosity of Gosnell's clinical *kakoethos*, the corporeal threats of an unsanitary and dangerous space, and the anxieties surrounding the legitimation crises of a state oversight system. Back-alley abortion rhetoric circulated in the Gosnell case was taken up in several different modes and domains.[115] Filmic treatments of the case, replete with plentiful appeals to the grand jury report either for fundraising or as part of the script, amplified the visceral dimensions of an already visceral case, inspiring anti-abortion activists to rally in the service of "clean clinical space," something that the report surmised that everyone could agree upon. As AlphaCare transformed the ruins of Gosnell's practice with fresh paint and new equipment—but no access to abortion—reproductive justice advocates now face a devastating new structural hurdle: the fall of *Roe v. Wade*.

(Never) Going Back

The Back-Alley When Abortion *Is* a Crime

As abortion legalization progressed throughout the 1960s and culminated in the 1973 *Roe v. Wade* decision, "back-alley abortion" has circulated during moments of reproductive precarity. The phrase has dictated the clinical and personnel boundaries of legitimate care provision, constituted public memory about a past to which we should never return, and nurtured anti-abortion clinical restrictions. Although I began this book years before *Dobbs v. Jackson Women's Health* went before the courts, concluding it in the wake of this Supreme Court decision has forced me to consider how the phrase has mutated according to new contextual demands. The June 2022 repeal of *Roe v. Wade* has ushered in a stark reality, literally returning us to a jurisprudential past and shifting the rhetorical work of "back-alley abortion" from a past threat to an imminent present and future. For instance, a 2022 review of HBO Max's *The Janes* declared that the documentary was "a crystal ball, a time machine, and a warning."[1] Noting how it "opened with a harrowing account of a back-alley abortion," the documentary series was described as having issued a demand for "audiences to recall a time before *Roe v. Wade* while grounding us firmly in the terrifying present." Implied by post-*Dobbs* back-alley appeals is that the threat of *Roe*'s overturning is gone, the past is present, and the future promises forced reproduction, without immediate—and urgent—action. Although feminist legal scholars and reproductive justice advocates have long critiqued *Roe* for tethering abortion rights to a narrow doctrine of individual privacy, the massive upheaval in abortion jurisprudence has sent veritable shockwaves through public culture.[2] The terrain of abortion shifts almost daily in a post-*Dobbs* world—and increasingly toward the ends of reproductive injustice. While reproductive justice advocates had long anticipated this moment based on the prevailing political winds, many others have struggled to

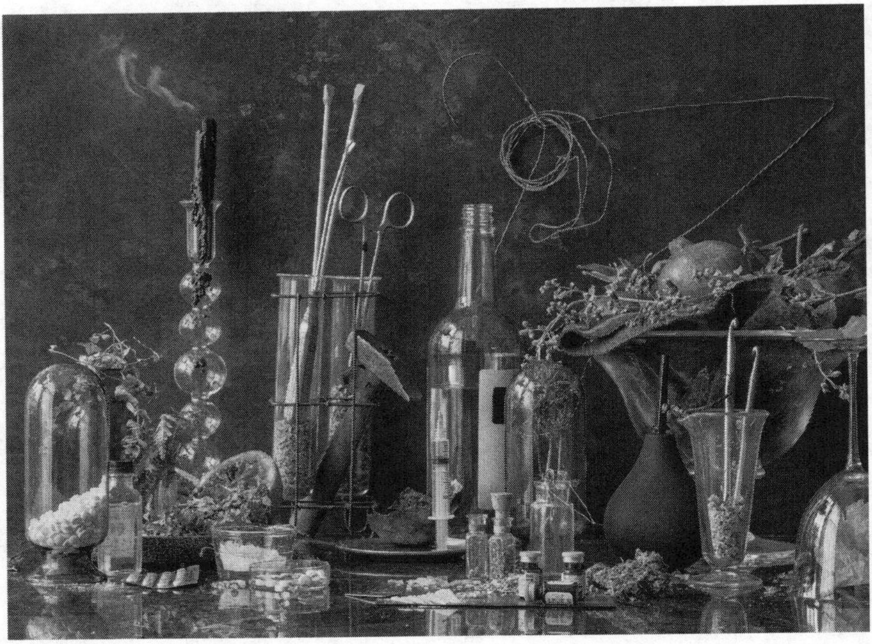

Figure C.1. Objects Used to Abort. Photograph by Beth Galton

make sense of how a newly removed constitutional right to privacy impacts pregnant people moving forward.

Capturing this sense of public disorientation and panic after *Dobbs*, photographer Beth Galton released a photography series titled Aftermath, which invited contemporary audiences to grapple with the future without safe, legal access to abortion.[3] Ironically, she imagined the future using an aesthetic borrowed from the past: the still life. Seventeenth-century Dutch still-life paintings frequently featured tablescapes of half-eaten foods that implored viewers to imagine the actions, behaviors, and lives lived to result in the haphazard configuration of objects. Many famously made use of the memento mori, a reminder of death, by more and less subtly including insects, skulls, and other symbols of physical decay. Invoking this style, Galton photographed a colorful array of tools and abortifacients, arranging grapefruit, pomegranate, and dried herbs under glass alongside inorganic items such as scissors, knitting needles, and coat hangers. Galton's vivid yet disorienting tablescape is titled *Objects Used to Abort* (figure C.1). Described by Dana Goodyear as "macabre," these items are intended to "confront the viewer with the tools and tactics that the desperate used to end unwanted pregnancies before abortion was an enshrined right and are once again using in a post-*Roe* world." In a personal conversation, Galton shared the logic behind her photographic choices. She began Googling ways to terminate a pregnancy, reasoning that people seeking to terminate in our post-*Dobbs* world without access might proceed similarly.

As a synecdoche for how the larger ecology of criminalized abortion is imagined, *Objects Used to Abort* presents an array of options to end a pregnancy, gesturing to a multitude of potential experiences. However, much in the vein of the still life genre, there are no people pictured and no stories being told. These images instead work through the capacity of phantasia, which allows the viewer to envision the potential for embodied harm in the mind's eye. With the sharp and rusted textures of a coat hanger juxtaposed to fragrant herbs, an extinguished candle, and delectable fruits, these carefully placed objects arouse the senses and instill profound dread. Without bodies present to tell their story, viewers must work at the level of the visceral imagination, with some of these tools piercing flesh while others are ingested to induce contractions. As Ryan Mitchell argues, appealing to this capacity to imagine the visceral—be it harmed flesh or the embodied panic of needing to end a pregnancy—"supports speculative, non-technical arguments about health and medicine."[4] In other words, while these may all be objects people have used to terminate a pregnancy, the safety and efficacy of the techniques are not given and viewers are invited to fill in the missing context, perhaps without knowing which will be fatal and which will not. This tablescape invites viewers to coalesce in outrage against the *Dobbs* decision by imagining how each of these objects will potentially be incorporated into women's fearful bodies experiencing an unwanted pregnancy when they are resolved to terminate it.

Among her series of other tablescapes—*Drugs, Herbs*, and *Bodily Harm*, one image stands apart. Galton's photograph *Back-Alley Abortion* arranges medical instruments, including a curette, an empty syringe, surgical scissors, forceps, plastic tubing, bloody gauze, and bagged white pills that she received from her own OB-GYN (figure C.2).

The caption perhaps offers a clue as to how back-alley abortion molds the memory of earlier eras of criminalized abortion for contemporary US audiences: "These objects traditionally used by medical professionals are also used illegally to perform abortions." The grammatical structure of Galton's caption is instructive for pondering how back-alley abortion rhetoric is newly and differentially animated in the post-*Dobbs* world today. Her use of the passive voice ("are also used illegally") invites us to ask, Who are the people using these medical instru-

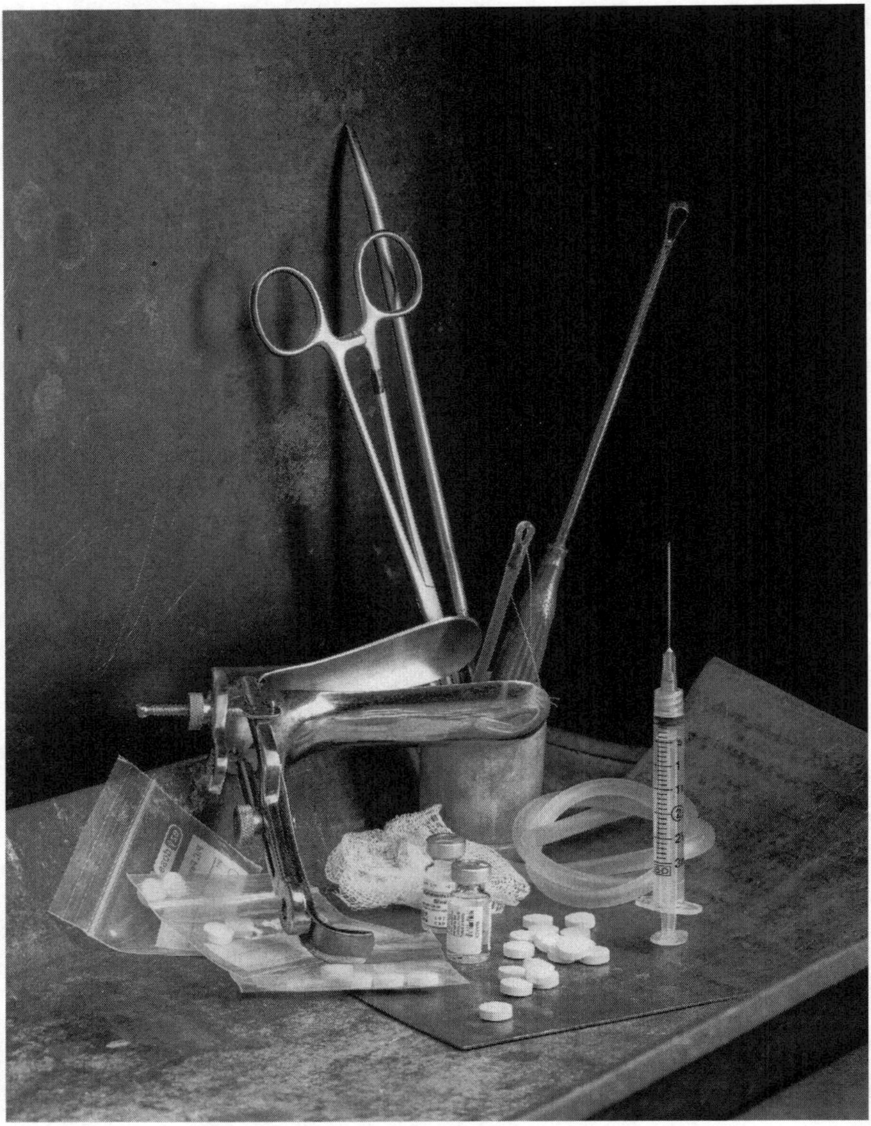

Figure C.2. Back-Alley Abortion. Photograph by Beth Galton

ments to perform "back-alley abortions"? Are they the "doctors of conscience" who have "traditionally used" them?[5] Are they medical "irregulars" or the so-called quacks who elicited the ire of the American Medical Association in the nineteenth century?[6] Are they part of a for-profit criminal syndicate looking to cash in on pregnant people's desperation?[7] Or could they be the pregnant people themselves, self-managing their abortions? The phrasing offers little clarity on the agent using these tools; it is only certain that they were used for a back-alley abortion. The caption thus offers an open-ended detour to viewers, relying on their *phantasia* to bring the available rhetorical pathways and affective residue of the back-alley *bas-fonds* before their mind's eye.[8] Peppered between these medical instruments used when abortion *was* a crime is an aperture into how advocates and commentators anticipate pregnant people will circumvent draconian laws moving forward in jurisdictions where abortion now *is* a crime—a pharmaceutically induced abortion. The caption of Galton's *Back-Alley Abortion* tableau reads, "Also represented is the abortion pill, shipped to states where abortion is now illegal." When considered alongside the tablescape's title, *Back-Alley Abortion*, this part of the caption draws our attention to how many state laws conflate pharmaceuticals that can safely end a pregnancy with the tools of an unsafe abortion.

It is crucial to reject the rhetorical association of pharmaceutically induced pregnancy termination with back-alley abortion, especially considering how back-alley abortion appeals have recently fueled anti-abortion activists' rhetorical repertoire. While mifepristone and misoprostol are two drugs taken in tandem to halt the circulation of progesterone and empty the contents of the uterus, respectively, each also has additional medical purposes. Misoprostol induces labor and halts postpartum hemorrhage and, beyond the labor and delivery context, manages stomach ulcers. Mifepristone treats high blood sugar in Cushing syndrome when patients have type 2 diabetes and are not ideal candidates for surgery.[9] To be clear, I specify these alternative uses not to further stigmatize abortion or these medications but to gesture to the wider ripple effects any potential bans would set in motion. Such bans would be akin to a population-level autoimmunity in which the US social body attacks itself, further depriving its people of crucial health care resources. Put another way, the rhetorical association of these medications to "back-alley abortion"—even in contexts where they might be procured extralegally—situates them as separate from "legitimate" medical care.

Some abortion activists resist this rhetorical collapse. Amelia Bonow, one of the #ShoutYourAbortion campaign founders, renders pharmaceutically induced pregnancy termination as a future distinct from "back-alley" techniques in her comments on Michele Pred's fifty-foot snow drawing of mifepristone and misoprostol at the Sundance Film Festival: "If the coat hanger symbolizes the devastation of pre-*Roe* back-alley abortion, abortion pills have come to represent the fact that safe, early abortion care is in the hands of the people and always will be, regardless of what any Court decides."[10] Bonow is correct: these drugs are safer than Viagra and Tylenol.[11] Relatedly, following the *Dobbs* decision, Planned Parenthood actively discouraged people from engaging coat hanger iconography, citing *Mel Magazine*'s article "Can We Stop with the Coathanger Imagery?"[12] Magdalene Taylor reasons that most abortions are completed with medication, making the coat hanger inaccurate: "And if abortion does become fully illegal for some, these pills should continue to be their first choice for abortion care—not this image of a back-alley abortion conducted with a wire coat hanger, as the current narrative suggests."[13] However, Bonow's assertion that these medications would allow abortion care to remain in the hands of the people and Taylor's assertion that the medications are very separate from back-alley abortion have recently come into crisis.

Similar to anti-abortion activists latching onto back-alley abortion rhetoric to shutter clinics in the Kermit Gosnell case and Mediclinic attempting to advance overwrought clinical standards, anti-abortion activists have also begun using back-alley abortion appeals to generate undue fear about pharmaceutically induced terminations since *Dobbs*. For example, the Stanton Public Policy Center responded to a January Food and Drug Administration decision to approve pharmaceutical retail sales of mifepristone and misoprostol with a national campaign called #BanChemicalAbortions. CEO and founder Brandi Swindell circulated disinformation about the medications: "Chemical abortions now account for more than half of all abortions in the U.S. and have significantly higher complication rates than that of surgical abortions. *What the FDA and the abortion lobby are now promoting is a new type of 'back-alley abortion' with no medical oversight and care.* We will not be silent when it comes to standing for the safety of women's health and wellness."[14] Naming the transit of these medications a "back-alley" allows anti-abortion activists to weaponize a sense of care to place that health and wellness further out of the grasp of people seeking to terminate their pregnancies. The association of these medications with "chemicals" *and* "back-alley abortion" further hardens the long-standing rhetorical connection between chemicals, pollution, and the morality of sexual (im)purity.[15] Much like how the Gosnell grand jury report constituted a back-alley in the jurisdictional space between the Department of State and the Department of Health in Pennsylvania, Swindell here constitutes the back-alley as a function of inadequate state oversight of abortion medication.

These efforts are inching ever closer to fruition. In March 2023, a conservative legal advocacy group, the Alliance for Hippocratic Medicine, led by the Alliance Defending Freedom, filed an injunction in the US district court in Amarillo, Texas, to demand the Food and Drug Administration repeal its authorization of mifepristone. Although the drug was approved in 2000, Trump-appointed federal judge Matthew Kacsmaryk entertained arguments that the approval process was hasty—that the FDA did not engage in proper due diligence and oversight in its approval process. Furthermore, under the pressure of twenty-one state attorneys general, Walgreens pharmacy declared in March 2023 that it would not dispense mifepristone. Following immense public blowback and plummeting stock prices, the corporation partially walked back its decision and ultimately restricted mifepristone distribution only in those jurisdictions that had already declared the drug to be illegal.[16] The Texas case *Alliance for Hippocratic Medicine v. FDA* made it to the Supreme Court but, on June 13, 2024, a unanimous decision held that the providers who brought the lawsuit did not have the standing to bring their claim forward. As Jess Braverman, legal director at Minnesota's Gender Justice, warned, "Unfortunately, in the process of resolving this case, the Court used overly broad language that threatens access to medical care for all patients throughout the country, suggesting that doctors with religious objections to any care may allow any patient to die rather than provide them with treatment."[17] Indeed, it remains to be seen how the court will rule should future plaintiffs be found to have standing.

Galton's artwork representing back-alley abortion and the term's newfound negotiation regarding misoprostol and mifepristone take me back to the questions I posed at the beginning of this book. If back-alley abortion does not reflect the relational nuances in the pre-*Roe* period when abortion was a crime, what exactly *is* back-alley abortion? How has its deployment in public culture navigated reproductive exigencies? How does it function today in a rapidly changing landscape of reproductive injustice? In the remainder of this conclusion, I weave together insights from the analyses in the previous chapters while also looking toward its implications for a post-*Dobbs* world.

First, back-alley abortion triangulates space, provider, and technique to shape the historical progression of criminalized abortion and reproductive injustice, organizing publics that grapple with our present reproductive exigencies. Rather than stop at the observation that back-alley abortion is misaligned with the history of pre-*Roe* criminalized abortion, this book has demonstrated analytic and cultural value in disarticulating this history from its rhetoric. Tracing back-alley abortion through the lens of rhetorical history has enabled us to understand precisely how the intersections of back-alley abortion as a cultural artifact shaped dominant understandings of the imagined racialized and classed relationships among medicine, law, gender, and national identity that have long undergirded abortion politics.

This association began even before back-alleys had any significant association with abortion. As the poem that opens chapter 1 demonstrates, back-alley abortion carries the residue of how city planners, medical professionals, and eugenic discourses pejoratively discussed alleys' sanitary, moral, and criminal features even before pregnancy termination entered the linguistic picture. Throughout the cartoons and thick descriptions that were focal artifacts of analysis in the remaining chapters, we glimpse the return of rats and cats—dwelling where they should not: too close to the imagined spaces of abortion care. Chapter 1 identified how alley discourses imbued discussions of criminalized abortion with the inherited affective residue of fear, disgust, and pity. Based on the notion that alleys were always-already unsanitary—and thus disgusting—spaces that were ostensibly right to feared by middle- and upper-class white city dwellers, alleys (and the people living therein) were represented as the breeding ground for the destruction of the morality of white womanhood. Those who had no choice but to live in alley spaces were pitied, feared, or denigrated, producing a racist and paternalistic distance between the observer and the observed. Because alleys evaded state surveillance, the publics who had no relational ties to these spaces could only experience them through voyeuristic muckraking journalism that relied on vivid rhetorical appeals to phantasia to keep relational distance from people who consumed the exposés of those living in alley homes.

Because back-alley discourse had a long history before it ever intersected with abortion, alleys became ripe metaphoric vehicles to grapple with spaces where pregnancy termination occurred. As this book and other scholars have shown, they were not the only spatial metaphors that addressed the unseen elements of criminalized abortion. Metaphors of mills, rackets, and rings enabled publics to imagine the moral scourge of pregnancy termination from within relational frames that made sense to their everyday living—such as the abortion mills in the "mill city" of Minneapolis, Minnesota. Stigmatizing abortion spaces notably imbued the providers with varying levels of bad character, forcing resignations in some cases and criminal convictions in others. While Charles H. Hunter, a white medical school professor, never served prison time for his role in the Minneapolis "abortion mill," Edgar Keemer, a second-generation African American physician with an impeccable office practice, certainly did, demonstrating a racialized stratification in who was held responsible under these laws.

As the human fallout of criminalized abortion became more visible, journalistic exposés incorporated alley aesthetics to sensitize prime-time television audiences to public conversations that predominantly male physicians had in the late 1950s to mid-1960s. Back-alley abortion appeals mediated the relationship between clinical space, the law, and advocacy for compassionate care provision. Such appeals enabled some "doctors of conscience" like Kenneth Edelin, Edgar Keemer, and T. R. M. Howard to claim a moral high ground for abortion providers by specifically dissociating themselves (and their immaculately clean offices) from unskilled and greedy "back-alley men." However, in the same state of Michigan, back-alley appeals were used in the courts in the case of Robert Stanley Nixon to draw the boundaries around careful and sanitary medical practice. Once abortion laws were narrowly reformed, alley appeals lamented the inevitable outcomes of failing to institute more radical repeals.

As abortion began to enjoy piecemeal decriminalization across the United States, back-alley abortion morphed, taking on a unique temporality to negotiate our relationship with the past. Appeals to "never forget" and "never go back" amplified significantly after the 1973 *Roe v. Wade* decision. Through graphic photographs and vivid descriptions, the visceral public memory of back-alley abortion aligned the traversal of racialized reproductive bodies with national and state borders when federal abortion funding and parental notification requirements became roadblocks to abortion access. Post-*Roe* back-alley abortion appeals misremembered how hundreds of pregnant people safely traversed the Mexico-US border for care. Remembering Rosie Jiménez, Becky Bell, and Geri Santoro served unique functions for advocacy in their respective contextual moments, even as they were remembered together as time progressed.

The rhetorical temporality implied in "We'll never go back" situates us within the legal frame of reproductive *rights* because *Roe v. Wade* orients it. While legal protections for abortion are essential when we consider *how bad* it is without those protections in place, the phrase has been defined by privacy doctrines and individual choice making. Because the exhortation that "We'll *never go back*" (as Senator Elizabeth Warren frequently declares in stump speeches and articles) implies *Roe* as the temporal threshold—and codifying *Roe* serves as a Democratic political platform—the decision becomes the rhetorical pivot by which we define progression and regression. Never going back implies that *Roe* resolved the exigency of the legal protection of abortion and that it was sufficient to guarantee the procedure could be accessible, safe, dignified, and free of coercion. However, privacy was always far from perfect. Traveling alongside a newly won legal right to privacy was the still intact North Carolina Eugenics Board that authorized forcible sterilizations on more than seven thousand Black women.

Involuntary sterilization laws remained on the books in North Carolina until 2013.[18] And as the story of Rosie Jiménez reminds us, the Hyde Amendment guaranteed that rights were never enough to ensure safe abortion care.

As we increasingly wade into post-*Dobbs* waters, Natalie Fixmer-Oraiz has urgently warned that "there is no going back," because post–September 11 homeland security culture amplified surveillance technologies in ways wholly unimaginable in the years before *Roe*.[19] Fixmer-Oraiz's observation is a particularly notable antithesis to back-alley rhetoric, considering that back-alleys (and back-alley abortions) have long been marked by an *inability* to surveil them. As the alley clearance efforts detailed in chapter 1, alleys were dangerous *because* of the unseen. We are in a remarkable moment where almost everything can be surveilled. Pregnancy tests can be tracked by the simple use of a Walgreens reward card, menstrual apps create a likely story of pregnancy, and smartphones trace movement across state lines (which was not relevant in Becky Bell's case, for instance).[20] As such, we must be further wary of post-*Dobbs* back-alley appeals. Appeals to the unseen warrant and invite surveillance, which has been normalized by homeland security culture.

As a necessary corrective to the temporal hegemony that the phrase "We'll never go back" institutes, theoretical insights from Black feminist rhetorical theory enable reproductive justice advocacy to look forward even as it takes a thorough accounting of past and present reproductive injustices. Loretta Ross confirms, "Reproductive justice provokes and interrupts the *status quo* and imagines better futures through radical forms of resistance and critique."[21] Indeed, walking toward this forward-looking horizon requires present-oriented strategies of resistance and care that remain cognizant of a long history of reproductive injustice. As I have echoed Fixmer-Oraiz elsewhere: "The fearful and paralyzing adage of 'never going back' to the era of back-alley abortions cannot comport with the long-urgent and unmet demands of reproductive injustice's racial and economic distribution of precarity."[22] In other words, "back-alley abortion" carries a history of racial injustice with it. As Logan Rae Gomez has persuasively argued, it is far more crucial and difficult to orient ourselves to how seemingly discrete moments of reproductive injustice "reoccur, accumulate, and overlap."[23]

Because Black feminist theories undergird the reproductive justice framework, Tamika L. Carey's *rhetorical impatience* offers a temporal orientation attuned to the cyclical and repeated nature of reproductive injustice that can help to enact reproductive justice in real time. According to Carey, "Rhetorics of impatience are performances of frustration or dismissal and time-based arguments that reflect or pursue haste for the purpose of discipline."[24] As "the disciplining arm of a Black woman's self-care project" necessary for survival, rhetorical impatience counters the pre-*Dobbs* white mythos of hermetically sealed, but threatened, abortion rights with the assumption that "equity and justice are late."[25] Reproductive justice is late because the histories of enslavement, eugenics boards, and long-acting reversible contraception abuse compound with ongoing practices of obstetric violence and rising Black maternal mortality rates.[26] With deft and flexible tactics for managing the "temporal hegemony"—the feigned linearity of reproductive progress—rhetorical impatience accounts for the need to dismiss irritants, enact "indignant agency," and engage in actionable redress depending on how the situational nuances threaten the well-being of Black women, specifically.[27] Rhetorical impatience challenges temporal hegemony by locating situated apertures for agency amid concretized reproductive regimes.

Rhetorical impatience has notably contributed to the historical battle for abortion rights. For instance, in an alternative timeline, we might not be marking the death of *Roe v. Wade* but rather *Abramowicz v. Lefkowitz*. This 1969 class-action lawsuit argued in the Southern District of New York made constitutionally grounded arguments and brought people who had pre-*Roe* unwanted pregnancies to testify. In the face of a disrespectful dismissal by the state's attorneys, Florynce Kennedy engaged in each of the temporal tactics of rhetorical impatience that Carey theorizes to counter the delegitimizing interruptions of her witnesses' narratives.[28] Doing so ensured the court record included their voices, even though New York's narrow repeal of abortion laws rendered the case moot. Kennedy frequently engaged in such spectacles to enact impatience, enabling her to "not rely completely on the courts."[29] It is striking to reflect on the absence of the phrase "back-alley abortion" in the courtroom tactics Kennedy used. Rather than invoke a disembodied speculative victim, she made space for a group of women who experienced the fallout of unwanted pregnancies in the 1960s.

Those navigating a post-*Dobbs* future need reproductive impatience in the ways that Carey theorizes. For instance, clinic defense workers who escort patients in the face of anti-abortion protestors may feel tempted to respond to dehumanizing epithets. However, because defense workers are there to support patients' emotional and physical needs rather than debate, engagement with anti-abortion "sidewalk counselors" would decenter the individuals most requiring community care and put them at risk for potential violence.[30] In this case, impatient dismissal to keep patients moving will most likely produce an outcome aligned with reproductive justice's sensibilities. Other cases can benefit from different impatient tactics. Because crisis pregnancy centers are subject to few, if any, national regulations, activists enact indignant agency and help people seeking abortions repossess valuable time in early pregnancy by providing Yelp and Google reviews to warn people about deceptively named clinics that do not provide abortions.[31] Rhetorical impatience recognizes the endurance necessary to fight for reproductive justice and encourages a forward horizon while recognizing that the past practices of reproductive injustice continue to have a residual influence. Appeals to "never go back" to back-alley abortions, although evocative of harrowing and unsanitary circumstances, maintain regressive temporal orientations to a past that continues to unfold.

Second, back-alley abortion is a politically fungible rhetorical appeal—easily weaponized for anti-abortion goals while evading more significant structural issues in medicine. Many people describe their experiences of pre-*Roe* criminalized abortions as back-alley procedures—this provided a sensemaking mechanism for some to grapple with their experiences of reproductive injustice. In part because of the affective residue of back alleys *before* abortion and partly because the history of back-alley appeals centers on the vulnerability of white womanhood, we should not be surprised to see back-alley appeals weaponized to limit abortion access and shutter clinics. Chapter 4—the case of Kermit Gosnell—exemplifies this phenomenon. By positioning Gosnell as a rare point of agreement between abortion advocates and adversaries, clinical restrictions like ambulatory surgical centers and provider licensure requirements become seemingly apolitical, even "reasonable responses" to some. However, rather than ensuring the safety of pregnant people and opening new clinics that provide a full spectrum of reproductive care at 3801 Lancaster Avenue, a crisis pregnancy center becomes the "sanitary" and "moral" answer to the reproductive injustices caused by the former occupant.

To be clear, no one should ever experience medical care in an unsanitary clinical space from a provider who is not present for procedures, is overly financially motivated, and does not exhibit compassion for patients. However, before characterizing this type of care provision as typical of *abortions* (as the back-alley framing can encourage), it is worth considering how some of these same dynamics are present in all health care contexts and disproportionately harm people of color. While it may be tempting to deplore the grimy, disgusting "back-alley" clinic, we must first consider inadequate infection control in "legitimate" health care facilities. Nosocomial infections (or health care–associated and originary infections) are not present when a patient presents themselves for treatment but instead are acquired when receiving care at a hospital or ambulatory surgical clinic. Affecting *at least* 3.2 percent of hospitalized patients in the United States, viral, bacterial, and fungal nosocomial infections are "the most common adverse event in health care that affects patient safety. They contribute to significant morbidity, mortality, and financial burden on patients, families, and healthcare systems."[32] COVID-19 precautions such as mandated masking have been sunset in many hospitals, allowing an aerosolized, disabling virus to spread unhindered in such settings as well. As legislators concern themselves with the surveillance of abortion spaces, perhaps a consistent mechanism to track hospital-acquired infections would be a better place to start.

Rather than consider monstrous health care providers as a feature of "back-alley" abortion, we must also home in on the structural dynamics and inequities that feed into the production of uncaring or cruel providers. The monstrous framing of abortion providers—greedy and indifferent to the well-being of patients—is structurally encouraged in a for-profit health care system where there is a shortage of providers and where profit (not healing) mandates standardized well visits be limited to approximately fifteen or twenty minutes. Greed, a quality of *kakoethos* imputed to providers like Kermit Gosnell, is baked into the systemic expectations of even the best-intentioned provider.

Along with profit motives that incentivize brief encounters, we must also imagine how medical racism produces what we might define as "back-alley" experiences of cruel providers for Black, Brown, and Indigenous people, as well as other people of color. Consider, for instance, persistent and unrelenting racial bias in pain assessment.[33] As Oluwafunmilayo Akinlade wrote in the *New England Journal of Medicine*, "myths, disparities, and pervasive systemic inequities in health care have fostered bias and distorted perceptions of Black people's pain, leading to catastrophic outcomes."[34] The charge that sickle cell disease patients are "frequent fliers" when seeking pain medication from emergency rooms often results in a dehumanizing callousness from providers.[35] The features of the back-alley butcher—as callous and cruel—are a structural feature of racialized disparities of medicine in the United States when pain is not heard.[36] In the Gosnell case, the back-alley framing diverted attention from histories of economic deprivation and medical segregation in West Philadelphia in favor of a "rogue" doctor who was out to enrich himself.

In the post-*Dobbs* context, cruel, surveillant hospital providers were thrown into sharp relief with the dehumanizing experience that Brittany Watts had while managing a miscarriage in Warren, Ohio, where abortions are banned after twenty-two weeks. Watts was twenty-one weeks pregnant when her water broke and her pregnancy was deemed nonviable. She waited for hours in the hospital for doctors to end her pregnancy but left that evening. She returned the next day and continued waiting to be seen by a doctor. Unbeknownst to her, because Watts had used the language "abortion," which is synonymous with miscarriage,[37] a provider referred her case to the hospital ethics committee. She left again and miscarried at home two days later. When she returned to the hospital and updated her case to her attending nurse, the nurse called the police to report that there were fetal remains at Watts's home. As Watts recalled in a CBS interview with Gayle King, "Little did I know that the nurse who was comforting me . . . was the one who called the police." In 911 footage that CBS procured, the nurse equated a nonviable fetus with a baby: "I had a mother who, um, had a delivery at home and came in without the baby and I need to have someone go find this baby or direct me on what I need to do." When the 911 dispatcher asked whether there was any sign of life, the nurse responded: "She said she didn't want to look. She didn't want the baby, and she didn't look." Watts recoiled at the suggestion she would say that she did not want her baby: "I would have never said something like that. It just makes me angry that someone would put those types of words in my mouth to make me seem so callous and so hateful." Of course, such an assumption is grounded in the legacy of enslavement, as Harper reminds us: "Black mothers were not considered women; therefore, it was thought they were unable to demonstrate the same virtues of nurture and emotional care that White women extended to their families."[38] Not unlike the 1970 case of Carmen Rodríguez elevated by the Young Lords Party discussed in chapter 2, Watts's nurse did not even bother to check her medical chart and rhetorically equated her miscarriage with infanticide. Police raided Watts's house and arrested her under charges of abusing a corpse. Although the grand jury eventually declined to indict, Watts in no uncertain terms attributes the cause of this issue to medical racism: it was, she said, "because of my skin color."[39] While the exact phrase "back-alley abortion" has not been used in media coverage surrounding her case, it should give us pause that this dehumanizing event occurred in a hospital, a setting that was long differentiated from back-alleys in advocacy by clean clinical space and capable providers. Watts's experience also echoes the inept and cruel care that Edgar Keemer recalled Mrs. X experiencing in a Detroit hospital.

Third, back-alley abortion rhetoric has historically erased the voices of those who have succumbed to unsafe abortions, either by ignoring them as stakeholders or by speaking for them. Notably missing from this book is a full narration of individuals' stories of criminalized abortion—a feature that repeatedly gave me pause as I wrote it. After poring over countless archival boxes of NARAL, NOW, the Society for Humane Abortion, Florynce Kennedy, Bill Baird, and Planned Parenthood Federation of America, scanning for the three words—one phrase—that define the contours of this study, it became more apparent that with the few exceptions noted throughout, back-alley abortion rhetoric was so *rarely* spoken from the first-person experiential perspective. Rickie Solinger made this observation decades ago, but it bears repeating.[40] First-person accounts of people seeking abortions rarely deployed back-alley appeals when they, for instance, wrote Robert Spencer from Ashland, Pennsylvania—one of the doctors of conscience Joffe profiles—begging for an abortion. Nor did I encounter the phrase from any of the patients Patricia Maginnis and Rowena Gurner referred to when combing through hundreds of reviews of clinics in Mexico.

In a sense, public rhetoric cannot help but mediate the experiential. Consider so many of the exemplars in chapter 2—*CBS Reports*' "Abortion and the Law" spent the balance of its time interviewing physicians, clergy, and legal experts—all people removed from the embodied pregnancy experience. Although a few pregnant people and their partners were part of the program, their experiences were narrated *for* them. This framing contributes to Katie L. Gibson's critique that *Roe v. Wade* was grounded in the expertise and best judgment of physicians—not pregnant people.[41] Although its creator recognized his problematic distance from the true stories of people experiencing unwanted pregnancies, California's "Abortion and the Law" used seemingly catch-all imagined subject positions to break down classed experiences. The stories of Rosie Jiménez, Becky Bell, and Gerri Santoro were similar in that their experiences were narrated *for* them—sometimes by friends, other times by family. The grand jury report of Kermit Gosnell rendered each patient's story a case exhibit that ultimately resulted in a crisis pregnancy center setting up shop at 3801 Lancaster Avenue. Something similar happened when tertiary news sources and subsequent documentaries elevated perspectives of the family and friends of Karnamaya Mongar and Semika Shaw. Stories of dehumanizing abortions certainly appear in published anthologies such as *The Worst of Times*, which is peppered throughout this book's epigraphs. These gripping compendiums of interviews—sometimes gut-wrenching stories but other times empowering recollections of receiving dignified care—are worthy of reading, analyzing, and amplifying in future studies.

Although storytelling is crucial to the reproductive justice movement and RJ theory, I am conscious of Ross's reflection that the RJ movement could not be built "only based on stories of individual women's experiences."[42] Instead, she argues that an "intersectional episteme" is necessary to examine how some would define their "back-alley abortions" as existing at multiple axes of legal and social oppression. I take Ross's assertion to also establish that uncritical and extractive storytelling cannot be a foundation for reproductive justice. Quite the opposite; a consistent practice to establish trust helps to ensure that stories reflecting the needs of those who exist at the margins are told to help guide activism and policy; this is a crucial undertaking. Building meaningful relationships to hear community needs is an exercise in what Rachel Bloom-Pojar and Maria Barker call creating confianza, a practice that is "much more dynamic than simply talking about whether someone trusts another person or not. It is not something that can be accomplished in one interaction, nor is it something that the promotores simply have with others because of how they look or talk. It is something that the promotores have developed an expertise with as they continuously work to build relationships and genuine connections with their communities. Confianza comes with great responsibility and, at times, additional pressure to help people."[43]

Intersectional analysis explains why a consistent process of creating confianza is necessary to building post-*Dobbs* capacities for storytelling. As Bloom-Pojar and Barker contextualize, US Latinx communities face profound reproductive injustices related to immigration status. An understandable reticence to seek hospital care for fear of surveillance and deportation, low-quality care leading to miscarriages in detention centers, and amplified stress related to ICE raids all require a consistent community-oriented approach to trust building to hear the stories that can help inform reproductive justice efforts. As chapter 3 indicated, because it is monolingual, back-alley abortion rhetoric is not as likely to cast a wide net for coalition as other strategies, as it focuses on the story itself rather than the process it takes to allow narratives to safely emerge on their own terms. As post-*Dobbs* reproductive injustices inevitably occur in the context of abortions, whether they reflect pregnant people traveling out of criminalized states or experiencing callous miscarriage care in hospitals, it is crucial to be attuned to dynamics of confianza to prevent back-alley framing with its historical and rhetorical baggage.

Returning to the collection of vignettes that opens this book, that of congressional representative Barbara Lee, a Black woman, it is difficult not to be moved by her experience, even as she defined it within the back-alley frame. Her appeal to phantasia—"I know what that back alley looked like . . . I see it right now"—reflects a strong sense of knowing based upon her visceral memories, deeply embodied experiences that remain impossible to forget. Unlike Elizabeth Warren's repeated statement, "We've all heard the stories," Representative Lee took her audience with her as she described knowing "what that dark light looked like."[44] At the same time, I would like to hope that I and readers of this book would be as moved by her story even if it did not use the phrase "back-alley abortion." The important feature of her narrative is that Lee shared her story in several instances to reflect several political initiatives, such as attempts with Cori Bush and Alexandria Ocasio-Cortez to repeal the Hyde Amendment, which disproportionately harms women of color on Medicaid. The role of storytelling is not distinct from rendering structural change; in fact, it undergirds the reproductive justice movement as such. Back-alley abortion stories are, as this book has demonstrated, *fraught*. We must imagine new containers for these awful, and deeply personal, experiences of terminating an unwanted pregnancy in the criminal context. As we move forward after *Dobbs*, we should be reminded of the power of rhetorical histories to shape spaces that remind us of our past while gesturing toward futures that can be better—if we are *impatient enough* to resolve the underlying structural dimensions of reproductive injustice.

NOTES

Introduction

1. Phyllis, Virtual Volunteer Storyteller, "I Had an Illegal Abortion before *Roe v. Wade,*" Planned Parenthood, March 15, 2022, //www.plannedparenthood.org/blog/i-had-an-illegal-abortion-before-roe-v-wade.

2. Patricia G. Miller, *The Worst of Times: Illegal Abortion—Survivors, Practitioners, Coroners, Cops, and the Children of Women Who Died Talk about Its Horrors* (New York: Harper Collins, 1994), 15.

3. Elizabeth Warren, "America Can Never Go Back to the Era of Back-Alley Abortions," *Time,* January 21, 2018, https://www.warren.senate.gov/newsroom/op-eds/2018/01/21/time-op-ed-america-can-never-go-back-to-the-era-of-back-alley-abortions-1.

4. *Root* (@TheRoot), "These U.S. Reps Want to End the Hyde Amendment Now," Twitter, September 30, 2019, https://twitter.com/theroot/status/1178730705322418176.

5. April Ryan, "Black Women Leaders 'Mad as Hell' after Supreme Court Overturns Abortion Rights, Vow to 'Fight,'" *Grio,* June 24, 2022, https://thegrio.com/2022/06/24/black-women-supreme-court-overturn-abortion/.

6. Carole E. Joffe, *Doctors of Conscience: The Struggle to Provide Abortion before and after "Roe v. Wade"* (New York: Beacon Press, 1995), vii.

7. Leslie J. Reagan, *When Abortion Was a Crime: Women, Medicine, and the Law in the United States, 1867–1973* (Los Angeles: University of California Press, 1997).

8. Rickie Solinger, *Beggars and Choosers: How the Politics of Choice Shapes Adoption, Abortion, and Welfare in the United States* (New York: Hill and Wang, 2001), 55.

9. Lina-Maria Murillo, "*Espanta Cigüeñas*: Race and Abortion in the US-Mexico Borderlands," *Signs: Journal of Women in Culture and Society* 48, no. 4 (2023): 798.

10. Sara Ahmed, *Living a Feminist Life* (Durham, NC: Duke University Press, 2017).

11. Solinger, *Beggars and Choosers,* 37.

12. Solinger, *Beggars and Choosers,* 60.

13. Celeste Michelle Condit, *Decoding Abortion Rhetoric: Communicating Social Change* (Champaign: University of Illinois Press, 1990), 28.

14. Jenell Johnson, *American Lobotomy: A Rhetorical History* (Ann Arbor: University of Michigan Press, 2014), 7.

15. Within rhetorical studies, there have been several notable and lasting contributions to thinking about rhetoric as constitutive of national subjectivities in constituting

"a people." See Maurice Charland, "Constitutive Rhetoric: The Case of the *Peuple Québécois*," *Quarterly Journal of Speech* 73, no. 2 (1987): 133–150. In terms of rhetorical history, I am also drawing upon James Jasinski, "A Constitutive Framework for Rhetorical Historiography: Toward an Understanding of the Discursive (Re)constitution of the 'Constitution' in the *Federalist Papers*," in *Doing Rhetorical History: Concepts and Cases*, ed. Kathleen J. Turner (Tuscaloosa: University of Alabama Press, 1998), 72–92.

16. I recognize that the position I bring to this book and its accompanying critical examination of the circulation of "back-alley abortion" could easily be weaponized by anti-abortion activists to argue that advocates of abortion and reproductive justice more broadly are generating false histories to dupe people into supporting abortion rights and reproductive justice more broadly. I explicitly foreground this statement because one of this book's findings is that anti-abortion activists and lawmakers *have* deployed back-alley abortion rhetoric to amplify targeted restrictions on providers and clinics.

17. Although I do name these periods throughout this section, it can be helpful to see coordinates of the larger epoch in advance. Reagan begins the epoch of illegal abortion in 1880, once rolling statewide statutes resulted in nationwide prohibition. The first fifty-year period (1880–1930) reflects "continuity." Abortions were accepted, performed in homes and physician and midwife offices. Within this period, a more sustained "crackdown" occurred between 1890 and the 1920s when medical professionals began to assist with criminal law enforcement. The second period (1930s) aligned with the Great Depression and reflected a "structural transformation" when abortions moved into hospitals and were more visible for regulation. The third (postwar) period (1940–1973) reflected amplified medical strictures, law enforcement raids, and racialized and classed stratified care. The fourth period (mid-1950s–1973) reflected a period of movement toward decriminalization, initially begun by physicians but conjoined by a nascent feminist movement. For more detail, see Reagan, *When Abortion Was a Crime*, 15.

18. Reagan, *When Abortion Was a Crime*, 10.

19. Janet Farrell Brodie, *Contraception and Abortion in Nineteenth-Century America* (Ithaca, NY: Cornell University Press, 1994), 43.

20. Linda Kerber, "The Republican Mother: Women and the Enlightenment—an American Perspective," *American Quarterly* 28, no. 2 (1976): 187–205. For an example of how republican motherhood ideologies exert a more contemporary influence, see Natalie Fixmer-Oraiz, *Homeland Maternity: US Security Culture and the New Reproductive Regime* (Champaign: University of Illinois Press, 2019).

21. Kerber, "The Republican Mother," 202.

22. Dorothy Roberts, *Killing the Black Body: Race, Reproduction, and the Meaning of Liberty* (New York: Vantage Books, 1997); Michele Goodwin, *Policing the Womb: Invisible Women and the Criminalization of Motherhood* (Cambridge: Cambridge University Press, 2020), 52.

23. Rickie Solinger, *Pregnancy and Power: A Short History of Reproductive Politics in America* (New York: New York University Press, 2005), 29.

24. Loretta J. Ross, "African American Women and Abortion: A Neglected History," *Journal of Health Care for the Poor and Underserved* 3, no. 2 (1992): 274–284. In addition to preventing birth as a form a resistance, Kimberly C. Harper importantly writes that enslaved Black women also resisted reproductive injustice by engaging in emotional

expressions of care, as moral motherhood attributions were often denied to them. Mourning, as Harper explains, "was a way of reclaiming a sense of power and control over the lives of their children," amid profoundly dehumanizing regimes of power. See Kimberly C. Harper, *The Ethos of Black Motherhood in America: Only White Women Get Pregnant* (Lanham, MD: Lexington Books, 2020), 5–6.

25. James C. Mohr, *Abortion in America: The Origins and Evolution of National Policy* (Oxford: Oxford University Press, 1979), ebook loc. 3/332. This is a parliamentary law titled England's Ellenborough Act of 1803.

26. Kristin Luker, *Abortion and the Politics of Motherhood* (Berkeley: University of California Press, 1984), 20.

27. Brodie, *Contraception and Abortion in Nineteenth-Century America*, 44.

28. Mohr, *Abortion in America*, loc. 21/332.

29. Carroll Smith-Rosenberg, *Disorderly Conduct: Visions of Gender in Victorian America* (Oxford: Oxford University Press, 1986), 225.

30. Marvin Olasky, "Advertising Abortion during the 1830s and 1840s: Madame Restell Builds a Business," *Journalism History* 13, no. 2 (1986): 50.

31. Olasky, "Advertising Abortion," 53.

32. Tanfer Emin Tunç, "Unlocking the Mysterious Trunk: Nineteenth-Century American Criminal Abortion Narratives," in *Transcending Borders: Abortion in the Past and Present*, ed. Shannon Stettner, Katrina Ackerman, Kristin Burnett, and Travis Hay (London: Palgrave Macmillan, 2017): 35–52.

33. Tunç, "Unlocking the Mysterious Trunk," 39.

34. Tunç "Unlocking the Mysterious Trunk," 39.

35. Tunç, "Unlocking the Mysterious Trunk," 40.

36. Tunç, "Unlocking the Mysterious Trunk," 41.

37. Tunç, "Unlocking the Mysterious Trunk," 42

38. Amy Gilman Srebnick, *The Mysterious Death of Mary Rogers: Sex and Culture in Nineteenth-Century New York* (New York: Oxford University Press, 1995), 10.

39. Daniel Stashower, *The Beautiful Cigar Girl: Mary Rogers, Edgar Allan Poe, and the Invention of Murder* (London: Penguin Press, 2007), 5.

40. Mohr, *Abortion in America*, loc. 98–99/332.

41. Srebnick, *The Mysterious Death*, 11.

42. Tunç, "Unlocking the Mysterious Trunk," 43.

43. Mohr, *Abortion in America*, loc. 47/332.

44. Guy Reel, *"National Police Gazette" and the Making of the Modern American Man, 1879–1906* (New York: Palgrave, 2006).

45. John Hoberman, *Black and Blue: The Origins and Consequences of Medical Racism* (Berkeley: University of California Press, 2012).

46. For a helpful history of medical professionalization, especially as it related to its gendered dimensions, see Regina Markell Morantz, "Introduction: From Art to Science; Women Physicians in American Medicine, 1600–1980," in *In Her Own Words: Oral Histories of Women Physicians*, ed. Regina Markell Morantz, Cynthia Stodola Pomerleau, and Carol Hansen Fenichel (Westport, CT: Greenwood Press, 1982), 3–44.

47. Goodwin, *Policing the Womb*, 54.

48. Goodwin, *Policing the Womb*, 52.

49. Keisha Goode and Barbara Katz Rothman, "African American Midwifery, a History and a Lament," *American Journal of Economics and Sociology* 76, no. 1 (2017): 65–94; Harper, *The Ethos of Black Motherhood*, 86–88.

50. Ross, "African American Women and Abortion," 276.

51. Smith-Rosenberg, *Disorderly Conduct*, 229.

52. Mohr, *Abortion in America*, loc. 37/332.

53. Nathan Stormer, *Articulating Life's Memory: U.S. Medical Rhetoric About Abortion in the Nineteenth Century* (Lanham, MD: Lexington Books, 2002), xiii.

54. Alicia Gutierrez-Romine, *From Back-Alley to the Border: Criminal Abortion in California: 1920–1969* (Lincoln: University of Nebraska Press, 2020), 26.

55. Stormer, *Articulating Life's Memory*, 31.

56. Nicola Beisel and Tamara Kay, "Abortion, Race, and Gender in Nineteenth-Century America," *American Sociological Review* 69 (2004): 498–518, 502.

57. Stormer, *Articulating Life's Memory*, 75.

58. Mohr, *Abortion in America*, loc.179/332.

59. Tunç, "Unlocking the Mysterious Trunk," 35.

60. Mohr, *Abortion in America*, loc. 176–332.

61. Mohr, *Abortion in America*, loc. 177–178/332.

62. Karen Weingarten, *Abortion in the American Imagination: Before Life and Choice, 1880–1940* (New Brunswick, NJ: Rutgers University Press, 2015), 24–25.

63. Reagan, *When Abortion Was a Crime*. Reagan reminds us that physicians and midwives did not practice in two separate worlds—any strict bifurcation must be reconsidered, as they operated in the same ecology.

64. Reagan, *When Abortion Was a Crime*, 47; see also Gutierrez-Romine, *From Back-Alley to the Border*, 23.

65. Reagan, *When Abortion Was a Crime*, 52.

66. Reagan, *When Abortion Was a Crime*, 54–57.

67. Reagan, *When Abortion Was a Crime*, 57.

68. Reagan, *When Abortion Was a Crime*, 60.

69. Reagan, *When Abortion Was a Crime*, 51.

70. Gutierrez-Romine, *From Back-Alley to the Border*, 21.

71. Reagan, *When Abortion Was a Crime*, 43.

72. Luker, *Abortion and the Politics of Motherhood*, 38.

73. Luker, *Abortion and the Politics of Motherhood*, 35.

74. Rickie Solinger, "'A Complete Disaster': Abortion and the Politics of Hospital Abortion Committees, 1950–1970," *Feminist Studies* 19, no. 2 (1993): 241–268; Reagan, *When Abortion Was a Crime*; Stormer, *Articulating Life's Memory*.

75. Reagan, *When Abortion Was a Crime*, 81.

76. Reagan, *When Abortion Was a Crime*, 89.

77. Reagan, *When Abortion Was a Crime*, 121.

78. Reagan, *When Abortion Was a Crime*, 131.

79. Reagan, *When Abortion Was a Crime*, 15.

80. Reagan, *When Abortion Was a Crime*, 138.

81. Johanna Schoen, *Choice and Coercion: Birth Control, Sterilization, and Abortion in Public Health and Welfare* (Chapel Hill: University of North Carolina Press, 2005), 145.

82. Miller, *Worst of Times*, 71.
83. Schoen, *Choice and Coercion*, 153.
84. Reagan, *When Abortion Was a Crime*, 160–162.
85. Reagan, *When Abortion Was a Crime*, 165.
86. Reagan, *When Abortion Was a Crime*, 167.
87. Maggie Jones Patterson and Megan Williams Hall, "Abortion, Moral Maturity and Civic Journalism," *Critical Studies in Mass Communication* 15, no. 2 (1998): 91–115, 94.
88. Reagan, *When Abortion Was a Crime*, 163.
89. Reagan, *When Abortion Was a Crime*, 197–199.
90. Solinger, "A Complete Disaster."
91. Solinger, "A Complete Disaster," 246.
92. Solinger, "A Complete Disaster," 242.
93. Reagan, *When Abortion Was a Crime*, 205.
94. Reagan, *When Abortion Was a Crime*, 207.
95. Reagan, *When Abortion Was a Crime*, 211.
96. Amy Helen Bell, "Abortion Crime Scene Photography in London, 1950–1968," *Social History of Medicine* 30, no. 3 (2017): 661.
97. Nathan Stormer, "A Likely Past: Abortion, Social Data, and a Collective Memory of Secrets in 1950s America," *Communication and Critical/Cultural Studies* 7, no. 4 (2010): 337–359.
98. Stormer, "A Likely Past," 349.
99. An EBSCOhost search through *Jet* magazine's digitized archives reveals 192 entries for Black providers (both medical and nonmedical) who were raided, prosecuted, or convicted between the magazine's inception and *Roe v. Wade* (1951–1973). To be sure, some of them are updates surrounding the same cases, but they offer a rich repository for future studies.
100. Leslie J. Reagan, *Dangerous Pregnancies: Mothers, Disabilities, and Abortion in Modern America* (Los Angeles: University of California Press, 2012).
101. Madison A. Krall, "Regulatory Rhetoric and Mediated Health Narratives: Justifying Oversight in the Sherri Chessen Finkbine Thalidomide Story," *Rhetoric of Health & Medicine* 6, no. 3 (2023): 304–334.
102. Leslie J. Reagan, "Crossing the Border for Abortions: California Activists, Mexican Clinics, and the Creation of a Feminist Health Agency in the 1960s," *Feminist Studies* 26, no. 2 (2000): 324.
103. Lina-Maria Murillo, "*Espanta Cigüeñas*," 804–805.
104. Laura Kaplan, *The Story of Jane: The Legendary Underground Feminist Abortion Service* (Chicago: University of Chicago Press, 1995).
105. Darrel Wanzer-Serrano, *The New York Young Lords and the Struggle for Liberation* (Philadelphia: Temple University Press, 2015), 97.
106. Jennifer A. Nelson "'Abortions under Community Control': Feminism, Nationalism, and the Politics of Reproduction among New York City's Young Lords," *Journal of Women's History* 13, no. 1 (2001): 174.
107. Howard Moody, "Abortion: Woman's Right and Legal Problem," *Theology Today* 28, no. 3 (1971): 337–346; Howard Moody, "Abortion: A Woman's Right and Legal Problem," *Christianity and Crisis* (1971), 340–341.
108. Gillian Frank, "The Miseries and Heartbreak of Backstreet Abortions: Before

and after *Roe,*" *NursingClio,* March 28, 2017, https://nursingclio.org/2017/03/28/the-miseries-and-heartbreak-of-backstreet-abortions-before-and-after-roe/.

109. Moody, "Abortion: Woman's Right."

110. Moody, "Abortion: Woman's Right," 344.

111. David Zarefsky, "The Four Senses of Rhetorical History," in *Doing Rhetorical History: Concepts and Cases,* ed. Kathleen J. Turner (Tuscaloosa: University of Alabama Press, 1998), 29, emphasis added.

112. Robin E. Jensen, *Infertility: Tracing the History of a Transformative Term* (University Park: Pennsylvania State University Press, 2016), 11–13.

113. Jenny Edbauer, "Unframing Models of Public Distribution: From Rhetorical Situation to Rhetorical Ecologies," *Rhetoric Society Quarterly* 35, no. 4 (2005): 20. For an understanding of constitutive rhetoric as subject making, see Charland, "Constitutive Rhetoric."

114. Michael Calvin McGee, "Text, Context, and the Fragmentation of Contemporary Culture," *Western Journal of Speech Communication* 54 (1990): 274–289.

115. Atilla Hallsby, "Recanonizing Rhetoric: The Secret *in* and *of* Discourse," *Journal for the History of Rhetoric* 25, no. 3 (2022): 346–370.

116. I thank Kimberly Singletary for making this keen observation.

117. Jael Silliman, Marlene Gerber Fried, Loretta Ross, and Elena R. Gutiérrez, *Undivided Rights: Women of Color Organize for Reproductive Justice* (Chicago: Haymarket, 2016), xvii. Loretta Ross explicitly names herself along with Toni M. Bond, Reverend Alma Crawford, Evelyn S. Field, Terri James, Bisola Maringay, Cassandra McConnell, Cynthia Newbille, Elizabeth Terry, "Able" Mabel Thomas, Winnette P. Willis, and Kim Youngblood as the "founding mothers of the concept of reproductive justice." Loretta Ross, "Reproductive Justice as Intersectional Feminist Activism," *Souls: A Critical Journal of Black Politics, Culture, and Society* 19, no. 3 (2017): 286–314.

118. Silliman et al., *Undivided Rights,* xvii; Ross, "Reproductive Justice."

119. Zakiya Luna, *Reproductive Rights as Human Rights: Women of Color and the Fight for Reproductive Justice* (New York: New York University Press, 2020), 5.

120. Shui-yin Sharon Yam, "Visualizing Birth Stories from the Margin: Toward a Reproductive Justice Model of Rhetorical Analysis," *Rhetoric Society Quarterly* 50, no. 1 (2020): 19–34; Savannah Greer Downing, "Toward Reproductive Justice Rhetorics of Care: State Senator Jen Jordan's Dissent of Georgia's Heartbeat Bill," *Quarterly Journal of Speech* 109, no. 4 (2023): 376–399.

121. Combahee River Collective, "The Combahee River Collective Statement," in *Home Girls: A Black Feminist Anthology,* ed. Barbara Smith (New Brunswick, NJ: Rutgers University Press, 1983), 264.

122. Jennifer Nelson, *Women of Color and the Reproductive Rights Movement* (New York: New York University Press, 2003).

123. Sherie M. Randolph, *Florynce "Flo" Kennedy: The Life of a Black Feminist Radical* (Chapel Hill: University of North Carolina Press, 2015).

124. Kimala Price, "What Is Reproductive Justice? How Women of Color Activists Are Redefining the Pro-choice Paradigm," *Meridians* 19 (2020): 340–362.

125. Angela Davis, "Racism, Birth Control and Reproductive Rights," in *Women, Race and Class* (London: Women's Press; New York: Random House, 1982), 354–355.

126. These issues are both historical and remain ongoing. For the issue of steriliza-

tion abuse, see Laura Briggs, *Reproducing Empire: Race, Sex, Science, and U.S. Imperialism in Puerto Rico* (Berkeley: University of California Press, 2002); Roberts, *Killing the Black Body*; Nelson, *Women of Color and the Reproductive Rights Movement*. For the relationship between environmental justice and reproductive justice, see Catalina M. de Onís, "Reproductive Justice as Environmental Justice: Contexts, Coalitions, and Cautions," in *The Routledge Companion to Motherhood* (New York: Routledge, 2019), 496–509. For the relationship between police contact and reproductive justice, see Rachel R. Hardeman, Tongtan Chantarat, Morrison Luke Smith, David C. Van Riper, and Dara D. Mendez, "Association of Residence in High–Police Contact Neighborhoods with Preterm Birth among Black and White Individuals in Minneapolis," *JAMA Network Open* 4, no. 12 (2021): e2130290–e2130290. For the relationship between childcare and reproductive justice, see Thia Cooper, "Achieving Reproductive Justice," in *Taking It to the Streets: Public Theologies of Activism and Resistance*, ed. Jennifer Baldwin (Lanham, MD: Lexington Books, 2018): 129.

127. "Intersectionality" was originally coined by legal scholar Kimberlé Crenshaw in 1989 to help disrupt "single-axis" analyses of *either* race, gender, or class, arguing that such an analytic frame was incapable of fully illuminating Black women's subordination and intelligibility, as major power systems of domination intersect. Intersectionality grew far beyond the scope of legal studies and has experienced important uptake in fields like rhetorical studies. Importantly, intersectionality is an indispensable analytic and political priority in reproductive justice theory. Scholars who mobilize this framework inside and outside rhetorical studies are cited throughout this book. See Kimberlé Williams Crenshaw, "Demarginalizing the Intersection of Race and Sex: A Black Feminist Critique of Antidiscrimination Doctrine, Feminist Theory, and Antiracist Politics," *University of Chicago Legal Forum* (1989): 139–167. Brittney Cooper provides an excellent overview and genealogy of intersectionality that locates some of its grounding antecedents in the rhetorical practices of Black feminists like Anna Julia Cooper and Mary Church Terrell. See Brittney Cooper, "Intersectionality," in *The Oxford Handbook of Feminist Theory*, ed. Lisa Disch and Mary Hawkesworth (New York: Oxford University Press, 2016): 385–406.

128. Thomas K. Nakayama and Robert L. Krizek, "Whiteness: A Strategic Rhetoric," *Quarterly Journal of Speech* 81, no. 3 (1995): 291–309.

129. Shui-yin Sharon Yam and Natalie Fixmer-Oraiz, "Against Gender Essentialism: Reproductive Justice Doulas and Gender Inclusivity in Pregnancy and Birth Discourse," *Women's Studies in Communication* 46, no. 1 (2023): 1–22.

130. Condit, *Decoding Abortion Rhetoric*, 27–28, emphases added.

131. Leandra Hinojosa Hernández and Sarah De Los Santos Upton, "Reproductive Justice and the Post-*Roe* Landscape: Chicana Feminisms, Coraje, and Collective Solidarity," *Journal of Autoethnography* 4, no. 4 (2023): 577–585; Natalie Fixmer-Oraiz and Shui-yin Sharon Yam, "Queer(ing) Reproductive Justice," in *Oxford Encyclopedia of Queer Studies and Communication*, ed. Isaac West, Emerson Cram, Frederick Dhanens, Pamela Lannutti, and Gust A. Yep (New York: Oxford University Press, 2024), 713–731. I also want to recognize Laura Briggs's argument that, in the context of constitutional challenges, the distinction between "pregnant people" and "nonpregnant people" was used to evade accountability for workplace sex discrimination claims. Because this book does not attend to this context, I am not as concerned about inadvertently bolstering

those conservative claims with my naming. See Laura Briggs, *How All Politics Became Reproductive Politics: From Welfare Reform to Foreclosure to Trump* (Oakland: University of California Press, 2017), 4–5.

132. Danielle Endres and Samantha Senda-Cook, "Location Matters: The Rhetoric of Place in Protest," *Quarterly Journal of Speech* 97, no. 3 (2011): 259–260.

133. Raka Shome, "Space Matters: The Power and Practice of Space," *Communication Theory* 13, no. 1 (2003): 41.

134. Erving Goffman, *Stigma: Notes on the Management of a Spoiled Identity* (New York: Simon & Schuster, 1963), 3.

135. Anuradha Kumar, Leila Hessini, and Ellen M. H. Mitchell, "Conceptualising Abortion Stigma," *Culture, Health, and Society* 11, no. 6 (2009): 629.

136. Kumar, Hessini, and Mitchell, "Conceptualising Abortion Stigma."

137. Thomas F. Gieryn, "Boundary-Work and the Demarcation of Science from Non-science: Strains and Interests in Professional Ideologies of Scientists," *American Sociological Review* (1983): 781–795; Colleen Derkatch, "Method as Argument: Boundary Work in Evidence-Based Medicine," *Social Epistemology* 22, no. 4 (2008): 371–388.

138. Coretta Pittman, "Black Women Writers and the Trouble with Ethos: Harriet Jacobs, Billie Holiday, and Sister Souljah," *Rhetoric Society Quarterly* 37, no. 1 (2006): 43–70; Harper, *The Ethos of Black Motherhood.*

139. Jenell Johnson, "The Skeleton on the Couch: The Eagleton Affair, Rhetorical Disability, and the Stigma of Mental Illness," *Rhetoric Society Quarterly* 40, no. 5 (2010): 465.

140. Alison Norris, Danielle Bessett, Julia R. Steinberg, Megan L. Kavanaugh, Silvia De Zordo, and Davida Becker, "Abortion Stigma: A Reconceptualization of Constituents, Causes, and Consequences," *Women's Health Issues* 3 (2011): S49–S54.

141. Lori A. Brown, *Contested Spaces: Abortion Clinics, Women's Shelters, and Hospitals: Politicizing the Female Body* (New York: Routledge, 2016), 2.

142. Cara A. Finnegan, "Doing Rhetorical History of the Visual: The Photograph and the Archive," in *Defining Visual Rhetorics*, ed. Charles A. Hill and Marguerite Helmers (Mahwah, NJ: Lawrence Erlbaum Associates, 2004), 198.

143. Cassidy D. Ellis, "'Doctors Don't Kill Babies! Monsters Do!': Using Performance and Personal Narrative to Identify the U.S. Abortion Monster," *Text and Performance Quarterly* 42, no. 1 (2022): 67–82.

144. Jeffrey Jerome Cohen, introduction to *Monster Theory: Reading Culture*, ed. Jeffrey Jerome Cohen (Minneapolis: University of Minnesota Press, 1996), 6.

145. Bernadette Marie Calafell, *Monstrosity, Performance, and Race in Contemporary Culture* (New York: Peter Lang, 2015).

146. Mary Douglas, *Purity and Danger: An Analysis of Concept of Pollution and Taboo* (United Kingdom: Routledge, 1966), 2.

147. Douglas, *Purity and Danger*, 2.

148. Alexis Shotwell, *Against Purity: Living Ethically in Compromised Times* (Minneapolis: University of Minnesota Press, 2016), 16.

149. Casey Ryan Kelly and Kristen Hoerl, "Shaved or Saved? Disciplining Women's Bodies," *Women's Studies in Communication* 43, no. 1 (2020): 1–22.

150. Shotwell, *Against Purity*, 15.

151. Karma R. Chávez, *The Borders of AIDS: Race, Quarantine & Resistance* (Seattle: University of Washington Press, 2021), 19–40.

152. Rima L. Vesely-Flad, *Racial Purity and Dangerous Bodies: Moral Pollution, Black Lives, and the Struggle for Justice* (Minneapolis: Fortress Press, 2017), xxiii.

153. Jessica Valenti, *The Purity Myth: How America's Obsession with Virginity Is Hurting Young Women* (Berkeley, CA: Seal Press, 2010), 41.

154. Stephanie R. Larson, *What It Feels Like: Visceral Rhetoric and the Politics of Rape Culture* (University Park: Pennsylvania State University Press, 2021), 16.

155. Kathleen Stewart, "Afterword: Worlding Refrains," in *The Affect Theory Reader*, ed. Melissa Gregg and Gregory J. Seigworth (Durham, NC: Duke University Press, 2010), 340.

156. Debra Hawhee, "Rhetoric's Sensorium," *Quarterly Journal of Speech* 101, no. 1 (2014): 5.

Chapter 1 • Before Abortion

1. Charles A. Singler, "Alleys—Past and Present," *Cement Era: Devoted to Cement, Concrete and Related Machinery* 15, no. 3 (1917): 35.

2. The concept of the sensorium here refers to Debra Hawhee's explication: "Sensorium therefore names a locus of feeling, and yet that locus is not confined to presumed bodily boundaries, especially when technology is considered." Debra Hawhee, "Rhetoric's Sensorium," *Quarterly Journal of Speech* 101, no. 1 (2014): 2–17.

3. Dawn Day Biehler, *Pests in the City: Flies, Bedbugs, Cockroaches, and Rats* (Seattle: University of Washington Press, 2013), 39.

4. Kate Siegfried, "Making Settler Colonialism Concrete: Agentive Materialism and Habitational Violence in Palestine," *Communication and Critical/Cultural Studies* 17, no. 3 (2020): 269.

5. For more information on the environmental impacts of concrete production, see Ian A. Wright, Peter J. Davies, Sophia J. Findlay, and Olof J. Jonasson, "A New Type of Water Pollution: Concrete Drainage Infrastructure and Geochemical Contamination of Urban Waters," *Marine and Freshwater Research* 62, no. 12 (2011): 1355–1361.

6. I ground this claim in a Google Ngram search, which, although imperfect, surveyed a large corpus of literature, journalism, and technical documents. I found that while "back-alley abortion" enjoyed more profound circulation after the 1973 *Roe v. Wade* decision, "back-alley" as both a noun and adjective circulated at least a century prior. I thank my research assistant Brandon R. Rogers for his brilliant idea to use this tool.

7. *Oxford English Dictionary Online* (Oxford University Press, March 2020), s.v. "Back, adj."

8. Chávez, *The Borders of AIDS*, 23.

9. Larson, *What It Feels Like*, 14.

10. Jensen, *Infertility*.

11. Edbauer, "Unframing Models."

12. As Dominique Kalifa argues, social imaginaries "describe the way in which societies perceive their components—groups, classes, and categories—and hierarchize their divisions and elaborate their evolutions. Thus, they *produce and institute* the social

more than they reflect it." Dominique Kalifa, *Vice, Crime, and Poverty: How the Western Imagination Invented the Underworld* (New York: Columbia University Press, 2019), 7, emphasis in original.

13. Edbauer, "Unframing Models," 13.

14. Lisa M. Burns, "Ellen Axson Wilson: A Rhetorical Reassessment of a Forgotten First Lady," in *Inventing a Voice: The Rhetoric of American First Ladies of the Twentieth Century*, ed. Molly Meijer Wertheimer (Lanham, MD: Rowman & Littlefield, 2004): 79–102.

15. Robin E. Jensen, "An Ecological Turn in Rhetoric of Health Scholarship: Attending to the Historical Flow and Percolation of Ideas, Assumptions, and Arguments," *Communication Quarterly* 63, no. 5 (2015): 522–526.

16. Debra Hawhee and Christa J. Olson, "Pan-historiography: The Challenges of Writing History across Time and Space," in *Theorizing Histories of Rhetoric* (Carbondale: Southern Illinois University Press, 2013), 90–105.

17. Kalifa, *Vice, Crime, and Poverty*, 21.

18. Krishna Savani, Satishchandra Kumar, N. V. R. Naidu, and Carol S. Dweck, "Beliefs about Emotional Residue: The Idea That Emotions Leave a Trace in the Physical Environment," *Journal of Personality and Social Psychology* 101, no. 4 (2011): 684–701.

19. Teresa Brennan, *The Transmission of Affect* (Ithaca, NY: Cornell University Press, 2004).

20. Deborah B. Gould, *Moving Politics: Emotion and ACT UP's Fight against AIDS* (Chicago: University of Chicago Press, 2009).

21. Savani et al., "Emotional Residue," 684. Ideas of contagion become easily connected to early literature on crowd psychology, like Gustav LeBon and the transference of emotions among bodies. For representative literature from social psychology, see Paul Rozin, Maureen Markwith, and Carol Nemeroff, "Magical Contagion Beliefs and Fear of AIDS 1," *Journal of Applied Social Psychology* 22, no. 14 (1992): 1081–1092; Andrea C. Morales, Darren W. Dahl, and Jennifer J. Argo, "Amending the Law of Contagion: A General Theory of Property Transference," *Journal of the Association for Consumer Research* 3, no. 4 (2018): 555–565; Zahra Zanjani, Hamid Yaghubi, Ladan Fata, Mohammadreza Shaiiri, and Mohammad Gholami, "The Mediating Role of Fear of Contagion in Explaining the Relationship between Disgust Propensity and Fear of Contamination," *Iranian Journal of Psychiatry and Clinical Psychology* 23, no. 4 (2018): 454–465; Christal L. Badour and Thomas G. Adams, "Contaminated by Trauma: Understanding Links Between Self-Disgust, Mental Contamination, and Post-traumatic Stress Disorder," in *The Revolting Self* (New York: Routledge, 2018), 127–149. Critical theorists and rhetoricians who have explored the connection between contagion and emotion include Jeffrey A. Bennett, *Banning Queer Blood: Rhetorics of Citizenship, Contagion, and Resistance* (Tuscaloosa: University of Alabama Press, 2015); Peta Mitchell, "Contagion, Virology, Autoimmunity: Derrida's Rhetoric of Contamination," *Parallax* 23, no. 1 (2017): 77–93; Shawn D. Ramsey, "Gustave Le Bon, Rhetoric as Mass Contagion, and 19th Century Rhetoric," *Celt: A Journal of Culture, English Language Teaching & Literature* 17, no. 2 (2017): 230–249.

22. Raymond Williams, *Marxism and Literature* (Oxford: Oxford University Press, 1977), 122.

23. Stuart Hall, "Lecture 8: Culture, Resistance, and Struggle," in *Cultural Studies*

1983: A Theoretical History, ed. Jennifer Daryl Slack and Lawrence Grossberg (Durham, NC: Duke University Press, 2016), 190.

24. Emerson Cram, *Violent Inheritance: Sexuality, Land, and Energy in Making the North American West* (Berkeley: University of California Press, 2022), 23.

25. Yannis Hamilakis, *Archaeology and the Senses: Human Experience, Memory, and Affect* (New York: Cambridge University Press, 2014): 13.

26. Sara Ahmed, *Cultural Politics of Emotion* (Edinburgh: Edinburgh University Press, 2004), 90.

27. Ahmed, *Cultural Politics of Emotion*, 92.

28. Kalifa, *Vice, Crime, and Poverty*, 22.

29. Hawhee, "Rhetoric's Sensorium," 6.

30. Emerson Cram, "Archival Ambience and Sensory Memory: Generating Queer Intimacies in the Settler Colonial Archive," *Communication and Critical/Cultural Studies* 13, no. 2 (2016): 109–129.

31. Cram, "Archival Ambience," 115–116.

32. Hamilakis, *Archaeology and the Senses*, 3, 6.

33. Literature on phantasia is vast. For a brief tour, see Martha Craven Nussbaum, *Aristotle's "De Motu Animalium"* (Princeton, NJ: Princeton University Press, 1985); Ned O'Gorman, "Aristotle's *Phantasia* in the *Rhetoric*: *Lexis*, Appearance, and the Epideictic Function of Discourse," *Philosophy & Rhetoric* 38, no. 1 (2005): 16–40; Michele Kennerly, "Getting Carried Away: How Rhetorical Transport Gets Judgment Going," *Rhetoric Society Quarterly* 40, no. 3 (2010): 269–291; Debra Hawhee, *Rhetoric in Tooth and Claw: Animals, Language, Sensation* (Chicago: University of Chicago Press, 2017); Allison M. Prasch, "Obama in Selma: Deixis, Rhetorical Vision, and the 'True Meaning of America,'" *Quarterly Journal of Speech* 105, no. 1 (2019): 42–67.

34. O'Gorman, "Aristotle's *Phantasia*," 22.

35. Debra Hawhee, "Looking into Aristotle's Eyes: Toward a Theory of Rhetorical Vision," *Advances in the History of Rhetoric* 14, no. 2 (2011): 153.

36. O'Gorman, "Aristotle's *Phantasia*," 22.

37. Prasch, "Obama in Selma."

38. Hsuan L. Hsu, *The Smell of Risk: Environmental Disparities and Olfactory Aesthetics* (New York: New York University Press, 2020), 6.

39. Yi-Fu Tuan, *Space and Place: The Perspective of Experience* (Minneapolis: University of Minnesota Press, 1977), 11.

40. Hsu connects rhetorical power to physiological processes by declaring, "Because olfaction is physiologically connected to the limbic system (a key neurological site of emotion and memory), descriptions of unwelcome smells exert immense rhetorical force." Hsu, *The Smell of Risk*, 5.

41. Emily Winderman, Robert Mejia, and Brandon Rogers, "'All Smell Is Disease': Miasma Sensory Rhetoric, and the Sanitary-Bacteriologic of Visceral Public Health," *Rhetoric of Health & Medicine* 2, no. 2 (2019): 115–146; Alain Cobrin, *The Foul and the Fragrant: Odor and the French Social Imagination* (Cambridge, MA: Harvard University Press, 1988); Melanie Kiechle, *Smell Detectives: An Olfactory History of Nineteenth-Century Urban America* (Seattle: University of Washington Press, 2017); Joel Lee, "Odor and Order: How Caste Is Inscribed in Space and Sensoria," *Comparative Studies of South Asia, Africa, and the Middle East* 37, no. 3 (2017): 470–90.

42. Cram, *Violent Inheritance.*

43. Darrel Enck-Wanzer, "Trashing the System: Social Movement, Intersectional Rhetoric, and Collective Agency in the Young Lords Organization's Garbage Offensive," *Quarterly Journal of Speech* 92, no. 2 (2006): 183.

44. Enck-Wanzer, "Trashing the System," 184.

45. Rhetorical scholars generally take in situ to examine developing social practices and material places. See Michael Middleton, Aaron Hess, Danielle Endres, and Samantha Senda-Cook, *Participatory Critical Rhetoric: Theoretical and Methodological Foundations for Studying Rhetoric in Situ* (Lanham, MD: Lexington Books, 2015); Kathleen S. Lamp, "Rhetoric in Situ," *Advances in the History of Rhetoric* 20, no. 2 (2017): 118–120; Heather Ashley Hayes, "Doing Rhetorical Studies in Situ: The Nomad Citizen in Jordan," *Advances in the History of Rhetoric* 20, no. 2 (2017): 167; Jean Bessette, "Queer Rhetoric in Situ," *Rhetoric Review* 35, no. 2 (2016): 148–164.

46. Eve Kosofsky Sedgwick, *Touching Feeling: Affect, Pedagogy, Performativity* (Durham, NC: Duke University Press, 2003), 17.

47. Sedgwick, *Touching Feeling,* 16.

48. Stephen Feld, "Places Sensed, Senses Placed: Toward a Sensuous Epistemology of Environments," in *Empire of the Senses: The Sensual Culture Reader,* ed. David Howes (Oxford: Berg, 2005), 179.

49. Kalifa, *Vice, Crime, and Poverty,* 24.

50. Gloria Anzaldúa, *Borderlands: The New Mestiza—La Frontera,* vol. 3 (San Francisco: Aunt Lute Books, 1987), 3. While Anzaldúa is clearly talking about the unnaturalness of the US-Mexico border, her insights also illuminate back-alley rhetorical dynamics.

51. Jenell Johnson, "'A Man's Mouth Is His Castle': The Midcentury Fluoridation Controversy and the Visceral Public," *Quarterly Journal of Speech* 102, no. 1 (2016): 2.

52. Kalifa, *Vice, Crime, and Poverty,* 18.

53. J. Johnson, "Skeleton on the Couch," 465.

54. Robert Chambers, *The Book of Days: A Miscellany of Popular Antiquities in Connection with the Calendar, Including Anecdote, Biography, and History Curiosities of Literature and Oddities of Human Life and Character* (London: W&R Chambers, 1863), 307.

55. Interdisciplinary literature that has examined various historical dimensions of sanitary reform includes but is not limited to Gerry Kearns, "Private Property and Public Health Reform in England 1830–1870," *Social Science & Medicine* 26, no. 1 (1988): 187–199; Gerry Kearns, "Cholera, Nuisances and Environmental Management in Islington, 1830–55," *Medical History* 35, no. S11 (1991): 94–125; Mary Poovey, *Making a Social Body: British Cultural Formation, 1830–1864* (Chicago: University of Chicago Press, 1995); Louise Penner, *Victorian Medicine and Social Reform: Florence Nightingale among the Novelists* (New York: Springer, 2010); Geof Rayner, "Conventional and Ecological Public Health," *Public Health* 123, no. 9 (2009): 587–591; Sabine Schülting, *Dirt in Victorian Literature and Culture: Writing Materiality* (London: Routledge, 2016); Michelle Allen, "From Cesspool to Sewer: Sanitary Reform and the Rhetoric of Resistance, 1848–1880," *Victorian Literature and Culture* 30, no. 2 (2002): 383–402.

56. Robert H. Bremner, *From the Depths: The Discovery of Poverty in the United States* (New Brunswick, NJ: Transaction, 1956), 7.

57. Stephen Halliday, "Death and Miasma in Victorian London: An Obstinate Belief," *British Medical Journal* 323, no. 7327 (2001): 1469.

58. Winderman, Mejia, and Rogers, "'All Smell Is Disease.'"

59. Even after germ theory displaced miasmatism among technical public health experts and scientists, miasmatism held residual cultural currency in what David S. Barnes calls a "sanitary-bacteriological synthesis." See David S. Barnes, *The Great Stink of Paris and the Nineteenth-century Struggle against Filth and Germs* (Baltimore: John Hopkins University Press, 2006).

60. Hamilakis, *Archaeology and the Senses*, 18.

61. Cobrin, *The Foul and the Fragrant*, 143.

62. Sonia Fleury, "Brazil's Health-Care Reform: Social Movements and Civil Society," *Lancet* 377, no. 9779 (2011): 1724–1725.

63. "Sewer Connections to Private Houses," *Sanitary Engineer* 6 (1883): 531.

64. Biehler, *Pests in the City*.

65. Linda Lorraine Nash, *Inescapable Ecologies: A History of Environment, Disease, and Knowledge* (Berkeley: University of California Press, 2006), 56.

66. J. Foster Jenkins, *Relations of the War to Medical Science: The Annual Address Delivered Before the Westchester County (N.Y.) Medical Society, June 16, 1863* (New York: Baillière Brothers, 1863), 4, http://resource.nlm.nih.gov/62730350R.

67. Jenkins, *The Annual Address*, 4.

68. Jenkins, *The Annual Address*, 4.

69. Ellis P. Townsend, "Back Alley Obstetrics," *Medical Visitor* (1894): 206. This was also published in *The Medical Sentinel*, demonstrating the piece's influential circulation.

70. Sandra W. Moss, *The Country Practitioner: Ellis P. Townsend's Brave Little Medical Journal* (self-published, Xlibris, 2011), 55.

71. Townsend, "Back Alley Obstetrics," 207.

72. Townsend, "Back Alley Obstetrics," 207.

73. Biehler, *Pests in the City*, 5.

74. Miriam King and Steven Ruggles, "American Immigration, Fertility, and Race Suicide at the Turn of the Century," *Journal of Interdisciplinary History* 20, no. 3 (1990): 347–369.

75. Nash, *Inescapable Ecologies*, 13.

76. James Borchert, *Alley Life in Washington: Family, Community, Religion, and Folklife in the City, 1850–1970*, vol. 82 (Champaign: University of Illinois Press, 1982), 27.

77. Borchert, *Alley Life in Washington*, 27.

78. Borchert, *Alley Life in Washington*, 14.

79. Nash, *Inescapable Ecologies*, 14.

80. Borchert, *Alley Life in Washington*, 14. "Moreover, fragmentary and incomplete evidence does seem to indicate that a variety of groups, ranging from white property-owners and neighborhood associations to real estate agents and bankers, conspired to limit certain neighborhoods to white residents in the last twenty years of the nineteenth century" (7).

81. Ellen H. Richards, *Euthenics: The Science of Controllable Environment—a Plea for Better Living Conditions as a First Step toward Higher Human Efficiency* (Boston: Whitcomb & Barrows, 1910).

82. Richards, *Euthenics*, viii.

83. Richards, *Euthenics*, viii.

84. Richards, *Euthenics*, 150.

85. Bremner, *The Discovery of Poverty*. Beginning in 1895, George Kober, chair of the Committee on Housing the People, the Women's Anthropological Society, and the Associated Charities of Washington each took interest in intervening in the alley space by gathering data. Biehler, *Pests in the City*, 36.

86. Jacob Riis has enjoyed extensive rhetorical circulation and commemoration as representative of the muckraking tradition. For instance, the Library of Congress has a digital exhibition to Riis's "now enduringly famous" literature. See *Jacob Riis: Revealing "How the Other Half Lives,"* Library of Congress, accessed April 23, 2020, https://www.loc.gov/exhibits/jacob-riis/writer.html.

87. Jacob A. Riis, *How the Other Half Lives: Studies among the Tenements of New York* (Mansfield Centre, CT: Martino, 2015).

88. Riis, *How the Other Half Lives*, 23.

89. Riis, *How the Other Half Lives*, 28.

90. Bremner, *The Discovery of Poverty*, 69; Reginald Twigg, "The Performative Dimensions of Surveillance: Jacob Riis' *How the Other Half Lives*," *Text & Performance Quarterly* 12, no. 4 (1992): 305–328.

91. In 1904, Jacob Riis was brought into Washington, DC, to view the alley system and report findings to Congress. Convinced by Riis, Theodore Roosevelt delivered a 1904 address to Congress in which he declared, "Hidden residential alleys are breeding grounds of vice and disease and should be opened into minor streets." Borchert, *Alley Life in Washington*, 48; Theodore Roosevelt, *State Papers as Governor and President* (New York: Charles Scribner's Sons 1925), 229.

92. Charles Frederick Weller and Eugenia Winston Weller, *Neglected Neighbors: Stories of Life in the Alleys, Tenements, and Shanties of the National Capital* (Philadelphia: J. C. Winston, 1909), 1–2.

93. The Progressive Era was marked by an ideology of expertise that believed that Progressivism would be ushered in by scientific experts generating specialized knowledge that could efficiently intervene in social life. Thus, the appeal in Wellers' text to a lay audience was a notable divergence from some Progressive reform ideology that ignored their role in instigating social change. For more about rhetorics of the Progressive Era, see J. Michael Hogan, ed. *Rhetoric and Reform in the Progressive Era: A Rhetorical History of the United States* (East Lansing: Michigan State University Press, 2003); Belinda A. Stillion Southard, *Militant Citizenship: Rhetorical Strategies of the National Woman's Party, 1913–1920*, vol. 21 (College Station: Texas A&M University Press, 2011); Leslie A. Hahner, *To Become an American: Immigrants and Americanization Campaigns of the Early Twentieth Century* (East Lansing: Michigan State University Press, 2017). In matters of sex education, some reformers did engage technical and lay expertise in tandem to accomplish their rhetorical goals. Robin E. Jensen, "Using Science to Argue for Sexual Education in US Public Schools: Dr. Ella Flagg Young and the 1913 'Chicago Experiment,'" *Science Communication* 29, no. 2 (2007): 217–241.

94. Winderman, Mejia, and Rogers, "'All Smell Is Disease.'"

95. Weller and Weller, *Neglected Neighbors*, 17.

96. Weller and Weller, *Neglected Neighbors*, 10.

97. Weller and Weller, *Neglected Neighbors*, 22.

98. Weller and Weller, *Neglected Neighbors*, 64.

99. "Urges Clean Alleys. J. M. Waldron Says Conditions Should Be Improved: Cites Menace to Health," *Washington Post*, July 27, 1910, 3.

100. "Alley Improvement Association, Washington D.C.," in *Organizing Black America: An Encyclopedia of African American Associations*, ed. Nina Mjagkij (New York: Routledge, 2010), 25.

101. For scholars who have examined Ellen Wilson's rhetorical work, see Shawn J. Parry-Giles and Diane M. Blair, "The Rise of the Rhetorical First Lady: Politics, Gender Ideology, and Women's Voice, 1789–2002," *Rhetoric & Public Affairs* 5, no. 4 (2002): 565–600.

102. Constance McLaughlin Green, *The Secret City: A History of Race Relations in the Nation's Capital* (Princeton, NJ: Princeton University Press, 1967), 175.

103. "Urges Clean Alleys," 3.

104. "Schools for Alleys: Poor Children to be Taught during the Summer," *Washington Post*, June 30, 1913, 12.

105. Alison Bashford, *Purity and Pollution: Gender, Embodiment, and Victorian Medicine*, Studies in Gender History (London: Palgrave Macmillan, 1998), 1.

106. Weller and Weller, *Neglected Neighbors*, 65.

107. Biehler, *Pests in the City*.

108. Weller and Weller, *Neglected Neighbors*, 28.

109. Borchert, *Alley Life in Washington*, 46–47.

110. Weller and Weller, *Neglected Neighbors*, 27.

111. Murali Balaji, "Racializing Pity: The Haiti Earthquake and the Plight of 'Others,'" *Critical Studies in Media Communication* 28, no. 1 (2011): 50–67; Anne-Kathrin Weber, "The Pitfalls of 'Love and Kindness': On the Challenges to Compassion/Pity as a Political Emotion," *Politics and Governance* 6, no. 4 (2018): 53–61.

112. Weller and Weller, *Neglected Neighbors*, 56, emphasis added.

113. Weller and Weller, *Neglected Neighbors*, 20.

114. Weller and Weller, *Neglected Neighbors*, 20.

115. Borchert, *Alley Life in Washington*, 108.

116. Daniel Makagon, "Sloths in the Streets," in *The Urban Communication Reader*, ed. G. Burd, S. J. Drucker, and G. Gumpers (Cresskill, NJ: Hampton Press, 2007), 151.

117. Weller and Weller, *Neglected Neighbors*, 29.

118. Weller and Weller, *Neglected Neighbors*, 51.

119. Weller and Weller, *Neglected Neighbors*, 51.

120. Elizabeth Clark-Lewis, *Living In, Living Out: African American Domestics in Washington D.C., 1910–1940* (Washington, DC: Smithsonian Institution Press, 1994).

121. Clark-Lewis, *Living In, Living Out*, 52, 76–77.

122. Dwight Conquergood, "Life in Big Red: Struggles and Accommodations in a Chicago Polyethnic Tenement," *Structuring Diversity: Ethnographic Perspectives on the New Immigration* (1992): 95–144.

123. Weller and Weller, *Neglected Neighbors*, 51.

124. Borchert, *Alley Life in Washington*, 132.

125. Makagon, "Sloths in the Streets"; Conquergood, "Life in Big Red."

126. Kalifa, *Vice, Crime, and Poverty*, 3.

127. Ned Buntline was the pen name for Edward Zane Carroll Judson. Buntline's *Mysteries and Miseries* series deserves special attention among a larger sea of revelatory works on poverty in part because of its profound uptake in the nineteenth century. *Mysteries and Miseries of New York* was adapted for the stage soon after it was published. See Bremner, *The Discovery of Poverty*, 90. Other scholars who have critically examined Buntline's *Mysteries and Miseries* series include voyeuristic treatments of minstrel themes in the book, where Black women in nightclubs were "the objects of male desire precisely because they were considered 'inferior and exploitable.'" See William J. Mahar, *Behind the Burnt Cork Mask: Early Blackface Minstrelsy and Antebellum American Popular Culture* (Champaign: University of Illinois Press, 1999), 318–319.

128. Margaret Jay Jesse, *Female Physicians in American Literature: Abortion in 19th Century Literature* (London: Routledge, 2023), 34.

129. Ned Buntline, *Mysteries and Miseries of New York: A Story of Real Life* (New York: W. F. Burgess, 1849), 59.

130. Buntline, *Mysteries and Miseries*, 60.

131. Buntline, *Mysteries and Miseries*, 76.

132. Buntline, *Mysteries and Miseries*, 107.

133. George Sinclair, "Actress' Ready-Press-Agent," *Green Book Album* 6 (August 1911): 368–372.

134. Marlis Schweitzer, "Surviving the City: Press Agents, Publicity Stunts, and the Spectacle of the Urban Female Body," in *Performance and the City* (London: Palgrave Macmillan, 2009), 134. For a more extended historical treatment about the life and anxieties of young white women in nineteenth-century cities, see Christine Stansell, *City of Women: Sex and Class in New York, 1789–1860* (Urbana: University of Illinois Press, 1987).

135. Sinclair, "Ready-Press-Agent," 370

136. J. Johnson, "Skeleton on the Couch."

137. "Dry Chief Visits Bootlegging Fleet off Ambrose Light," *New York Times*, April 20, 1923, 1.

138. "The Playboy Panel: Religion and the New Morality," *Playboy*, June 1967, 152.

139. "The Playboy Panel," 152.

140. "Sale Stirs Ghost of John Wilkes Booth: Barn where Assassin Stabled His Horse on the Night of Lincoln's Murder Is Put Up for Public Auction," *New York Times*, November 28, 1926, 10.

141. Henry Tanner, "Both Sides Fight a 'Dirty War' in Algeria," *New York Times*, April 12, 1959, E6.

142. Heidi Heller, "Minneapolis 'Alleywalkers' and the Campaign to End Prostitution," Historyapolis Project, July 1, 2024, https://historyapolis.com/2014/07/01/minneapolis-alleywalkers-and-the-campaign-to-end-prostitution/index.html.

143. Freda L. Fair, "Surveilling Social Difference: Black Women's 'Alley Work' in Industrializing Minneapolis," *Surveillance & Society* 15, no. 5 (2017): 659. The Bertillon system of criminal identification was created by French criminologist Alphonse Bertillon in 1879. Integrating mugshots and embodied, measurable "criminal characteristics," the system sought to standardize categories of criminality, contributing to a more modern policing system. By the late nineteenth century, it had been taken up in several cities in the United States. For a treatment of the rhetorical dimensions of the Bertillon

system, its mutation into crime scene photography, and eventual overtaking by fingerprinting, see Lela Graybill, "The Forensic Eye and the Public Mind: The Bertillon System of Crime Scene Photography," *Cultural History* 8, no. 1 (2019): 94–119.

144. Fair, "Surveilling Social Difference," 655.

145. J. Johnson, "Skeleton on the Couch."

146. Mark Twain, *Pudd'nhead Wilson* (Cambridge, MA: Harvard University Press, 2015), 129.

147. According to the *Oxford English Dictionary*, the word "barber" has an extensive association with medical practice: "Formerly the barber was also a regular practitioner in surgery and dentistry. The Company of Barber-surgeons was incorporated by Edward IV. in 1461; under Henry VIII. the title was altered to 'Company of Barbers and Surgeons,' and barbers were restricted to the practice of dentistry; in 1745 they were divided into two distinct corporations."

148. Twain, *Pudd'nhead Wilson*, 130.

149. "Iowa Republican Losses: Another Prominent Man Withdraws from the Party," *New York Times*, October 19, 1891, 4.

150. "Old Mistresses Apologue, 25 June 1745," *Founders Online*, National Archives, https://founders.archives.gov/documents/Franklin/01-03-02-0011. Original source: *The Papers of Benjamin Franklin*, vol. 3, *January 1, 1745, through June 30, 1750*, ed. Leonard W. Labaree (New Haven, CT: Yale University Press, 1961), 27–31.

151. Display ad 90 (no title), *New York Times*, August 11, 1919, 17.

*Chapter 2 • The Pre-*Roe *Back-Alley Rhetorical Medical Encounter*

1. Miller, *The Worst of Times*, 108.

2. Miller, *The Worst of Times*, 95–103.

3. Miller, *The Worst of Times*, 114.

4. "Statement of Edgar B. Keemer Jr. M.D.," National Association for the Repeal of Abortion Laws, Box 1, Folder 5, Schlesinger Library, Harvard University, Cambridge, MA.

5. Ross, "African American Women and Abortion."

6. "Statement of Edgar B. Keemer." In his 1980 autobiography, Keemer discussed this speech, but when he recalls the contents of his address, he does not refer to Mrs. X having two back-alley abortions. Rather he writes, "Besides the seven children, she had two catheter and two coat-hanger, kitchen table abortions with hot water 'sterility.' There were serious complications on both occasions." Ed Keemer, *Confessions of a Pro-life Abortionist* (Detroit, MI: Vinco Press, 1980), 220. However, in the Michigan affiliate NARAL collection at the Schlesinger Library cited in the above footnote, there are several scripts of his speech–some printed on his personal letterhead that refer to Mrs. X's abortion as a "back-alley" procedure.

7. "Statement of Edgar B. Keemer."

8. "Statement of Edgar B. Keemer."

9. Edgar B. Keemer Jr., "Looking Back at Luenbach: 296 Non-hospital Abortions," *Journal of the National Medical Association* 62, no. 4 (1970): 291–293; Edgar B. Keemer Jr., "Update on Abortion in Michigan," *Journal of the National Medical Association* 64, no.6 (1972): 518–519; Edgar B. Keemer Jr., "Involuntary Sterilization," *Journal of the American Medical Association* 225, no. 13 (1973): 1658–1658.

10. Mitchell F. Rice and Woodrow Jones Jr., *Public Policy and the Black Hospital: From Slavery to Segregation to Integration* (Westport, CT: Greenwood Press, 1994); Harriet A. Washington, Robert B. Baker, Ololade Olakanmi, Todd L. Savitt, Elizabeth A. Jacobs, Eddie Hoover, and Matthew K. Wynia, "Segregation, Civil Rights, and Health Disparities: The Legacy of African American Physicians and Organized Medicine, 1910–1968," *Journal of the National Medical Association* 101, no. 6 (2009): 513–527.

11. J. Johnson, "The Skeleton on the Couch."

12. When it came to providing criminalized abortions, Keemer was deeply trusted; the Michigan Clergy Consultation services frequently referred patients to him. Following Keemer's statement, law professor Cyril C. Means Jr. took the podium, also engaging a back-alley appeal: "The threat of prosecution of physicians ministering to the poor in public hospitals is so pervasive that poor women know their only recourse is to back alley operators. . . . [I]t is Dr. Keemer's courage in rendering the veil of hypocrisy and secrecy, and his open commitment to equalization of this opportunity for treatment for rich and poor alike, make his statement this morning so unique." Cyril C. Means Jr., "Statement at a Press Conference of the National Association for Repeal of Abortion Laws, Hotel Sonesta, Washington D.C." (1971), National Association for Repeal of Abortion Laws, Box 1 Folder 5 (1971), Schlesinger Library, Harvard University, Cambridge, MA.

13. Nathan Stormer, *Signs of Pathology: U.S. Medical Rhetoric on Abortion, 1800s–1960s* (University Park: Pennsylvania State University Press, 2015), 139.

14. Solinger, *Beggars and Choosers*, 56.

15. Katie L. Gibson, "The Rhetoric of *Roe v. Wade*: When the (Male) Doctor Knows Best," *Southern Communication Journal* 73, no. 4 (2008): 316.

16. Jane Ward, "Don't Have an Abortion," *Reader's Digest*, August 1941, 17–21.

17. Patterson and Hall, "Abortion, Moral Maturity and Civic Journalism," 94.

18. Molly Margaret Kessler, *Stigma Stories: Rhetoric, Lived Experience, and Chronic Illness* (Columbus: Ohio University Press, 2022), 8.

19. Ward, "Don't Have an Abortion," 17.

20. Kenneth Burke, *A Grammar of Motives* (Berkeley: University of California Press, 1945), 59–61.

21. As a few guiding examples, see Nancy Ainsworth-Vaugn, "The Discourse of Medical Encounters," in *The Handbook of Discourse Analysis*, ed. Deborah Schiffrin, Deborah Tannen, and Heidi E. Hamilton (Malden, MA: Blackwell, 2005): 454; Barbara F. Sharf, "Physician-Patient Communication as Interpersonal Rhetoric: A Narrative Approach," *Health Communication* 2, no. 4 (1990): 217–231; Howard Waitzkin, *The Politics of Medical Encounters: How Patients and Doctors Deal with Social Problems* (New Haven, CT: Yale University Press, 1991).

22. Nancy Ainsworth-Vaughn identifies the provider centrism of "ritualized phases" in P. S. Byrne and B. E. L. Long, *Doctors Talking to Patients* (London: Department of Health and Social Security, 1976) as a germinal source for this perspective.

23. Patricia Geist and Jennifer Dreyer, "The Demise of Dialogue: A Critique of Medical Encounter Ideology," *Western Journal of Communication* 57, no. 2 (1993): 233–246. See also Waitzkin, *The Politics of Medical Encounters*; Richard L. Street Jr., "Communication in Medical Encounters: An Ecological Perspective," in *The Routledge Handbook of Health Communication* (New York: Routledge, 2003), 77–104.

24. Ben Anderson, *Encountering Affect: Capacities, Apparatuses, Conditions* (New York: Routledge, 2017), 80.

25. Deborah Lupton, "Toward the Development of Critical Health Communication Praxis," *Health Communication* 6, no. 1 (1994): 58.

26. Dána-Ain Davis, "Obstetric Racism: The Racial Politics of Pregnancy, Labor, and Birthing," *Medical Anthropology* 38, no. 7 (2019): 560–573.

27. Loretta J. Ross, "Teaching Reproductive Justice: An Activist's Approach," in *Black Women's Liberatory Pedagogies: Resistance, Transformation, and Healing within and beyond the Academy*, ed. Olivia N. Perlow, Durene I. Wheeler, Sharon L. Bethea, and BarBara M. Scott (London: Palgrave Macmillan, 2018), 159–180.

28. Leandra Hinojosa Hernández and Marleah Dean, "'I Felt Very Discounted': Negotiation of Caucasian and Hispanic/Latina Women's Bodily Ownership and Expertise in Patient-Provider Interactions," in *Interrogating Gendered Pathologies*, ed. Erin Clark and Michelle F. Eble (Louisville: University Press of Colorado, 2020), 101–120.

29. Kirt Wilson, "The Racial Contexts of Public Address: Interpreting Violence during the Reconstruction Era," in *The Handbook of Rhetoric and Public Address*, ed. Shawn J. Parry-Giles and J. Michael Hogan (Malden, MA: Wiley Blackwell, 2010), 213.

30. Rhetorical encounters also have the capacity for generative possibility, especially when figuring the relationship between the state, citizens, and the definitional contours of criminality. While this study focuses squarely on medical encounters publicly presented as dehumanizing, I am heartened by work such as Caitlin Frances Bruce, *Painting Publics: Transnational Legal Graffiti Scenes as Spaces for Encounter* (Philadelphia: Temple University Press, 2019) that demonstrates how encounters offer "plural, multiple spaces among publics" (7).

31. Sara Ahmed, *Strange Encounters: Embodied Others in Post-coloniality* (London: Routledge, 2000), 8.

32. Cynthia Gordon, "Framing and Positioning," in *The Handbook of Discourse Analysis*, 2nd ed., ed. Deborah Tannen, Heidi E. Hamilton, and Deborah Schiffrin (Malden, MA: Wiley Blackwell, 2015): 328.

33. Reagan, *When Abortion Was a Crime*.

34. Ward, "Don't Have an Abortion," 17.

35. Ward, "Don't Have an Abortion," 17.

36. Ward, "Don't Have an Abortion," 18.

37. Ahmed, *Strange Encounters*, 6.

38. See Gieryn, "Boundary-Work and the Demarcation of Science from Non-science"; Charles Allen Taylor, *Defining Science: A Rhetoric of Demarcation* (Madison: University of Wisconsin Press, 1996); Colleen Derkatch, *Bounding Biomedicine: Evidence and Rhetoric in the New Science of Alternative Medicine* (Chicago: University of Chicago Press, 2019).

39. Ward, "Don't Have an Abortion," 18, emphasis added.

40. Lay, *Rhetoric of Midwifery*; Smith-Rosenberg, *Disorderly Conduct*.

41. Judy Z. Segal, *Health and the Rhetoric of Medicine* (Carbondale: Southern Illinois University Press, 2005), 39.

42. Ward, "Don't Have an Abortion," 19.

43. Michel Foucault, *Birth of the Clinic: An Archaeology of Medical Perception*, trans. A. M. Sheridan Smith (New York: Vintage Books, 1973/1994), 31.

44. Jennifer Edwell, Sarah Ann Singer, and Jordynn Jack, "Healing Arts: Rhetorical *Techne* as Medical (Humanities) Intervention," *Technical Communication Quarterly* 27, no. 1 (2018): 51.

45. Ward, "Don't Have an Abortion," 17.

46. Edwell, Singer, and Jack, "Healing Arts," 52.

47. Gutierrez-Romine, *From Back-Alley to the Border,* 114.

48. Robin E. Jensen, "From Barren to Sterile: The Evolution of a Mixed Metaphor," *Rhetoric Society Quarterly* 45, no. 1 (2015): 25–46. Both Jensen and I respond to Leah Ceccarelli's call for analyses attentive to how metaphoric vehicles mix and to what rhetorical effect. See Leah Ceccarelli, "Neither Confusing Cacophony nor Culinary Complements: A Case Study of Mixed Metaphors for Genomic Science," *Written Communication* 21, no. 1 (2004): 92–105.

49. Clark's treatment of Hunter and the Minneapolis abortion mill was published over the course of several issues between 1912 to 1915.

50. Daniel R. Bergsmark, "Minneapolis, the Mill City," *Economic Geography* 3, no. 3 (1927): 391–396; Eugene V. Smalley, "The Flour-Mills of Minneapolis," *Century,* May 1886, 37–47, https://babel.hathitrust.org/cgi/pt?id=coo.31924079633354&seq=57.

51. "Minneapolis Flour Milling Boom," Minnesota Historical Society, https://www.mnhs.org/millcity/learn/history/flour-milling.

52. Emily Martin, *The Woman in the Body: A Cultural Analysis of Reproduction* (Boston: Beacon Press, 2001).

53. Sam Clark, "A Minneapolis Abortion Mill," *Jim Jam Jems* (April 1912): 12–24, Social Welfare History Archives, University of Minnesota, Minneapolis, MN.

54. Clark, "A Minneapolis Abortion Mill," 15.

55. Smalley, "The Flour-Mills of Minneapolis."

56. Clark, "A Minneapolis Abortion Mill," 15.

57. Reagan, *When Abortion Was a Crime,* 23.

58. Clark, "A Minneapolis Abortion Mill," 13.

59. Clark, "A Minneapolis Abortion Mill," 18–19.

60. Harper, *The Ethos of Black Motherhood,* 5.

61. Clark, "A Minneapolis Abortion Mill," 25–26, emphasis added.

62. *Oxford English Dictionary,* "Racket, noun," s.v., https://www.oed.com/dictionary/racket_n2?tab=meaning_and_use#27254590.

63. B. B. Tolnai, "The Abortion Racket," *Forum* 94 (1935): 176.

64. Tolnai, "The Abortion Racket," 176.

65. Ahmed, *The Cultural Politics of Emotion,* 84.

66. Stormer, *Articulating Life's Memory,* 33–35.

67. Tolnai, "The Abortion Racket," 179.

68. Tolnai, "The Abortion Racket," 177.

69. Jason Chambers, "Presenting the Black Middle Class: John H. Johnson and *Ebony* Magazine, 1945–1974," in *Historicizing Lifestyle: Mediating Taste, Consumption and Identity from the 1900s to 1970s,* ed. David Bell and Joanna Hollows (Burlington, VT: Ashgate, 2006), 61.

70. Korey Bowers Brown, "Souled Out: 'Ebony' Magazine in an Age of Black Power, 1965–1975" (PhD diss., Howard University, 2010).

71. "The Abortion Menace," *Ebony* 6 (January 1951): 24.

72. "The Abortion Menace," 24.
73. "The Abortion Menace," 24, emphasis added.
74. "The Abortion Menace," 21.
75. "The Abortion Menace," 24.
76. Gutierrez-Romine, *From Back-Alley to the Border,* 111.
77. Gutierrez-Romine, *From Back-Alley to the Border,* 115.
78. Rickie Solinger, *The Abortionist: A Woman Against the Law* (Berkeley: University of California Press, 1996).
79. Gutierrez-Romine, *From Back-Alley to the Border,* 115–116.
80. Gutierrez-Romine, *From Back-Alley to the Border,* 116.
81. Jerome E. Bates, "The Abortion Mill: An Institutional Study," *Journal of Criminal Law, Criminology, and Police Science* 45, no. 2 (1954): 157.
82. Bates, "The Abortion Mill," 157.
83. Bates, "The Abortion Mill," 157.
84. Bates, "The Abortion Mill," 157–158.
85. "The Abortion Menace," 24, emphases added.
86. Hallsby, "Recanonizing Rhetoric."
87. For a thorough database tracking film and television representations of abortion, see Gretchen Sisson, Stephanie Herold, and Katrina Kimport, Abortion Onscreen Database, Advancing New Standards in Reproductive Health (ANSIRH), University of California, San Francisco (2022), abortiononscreen.org.
88. "Discussion Guide: 'Abortion and the Law,'" Association for the Study of Abortion, Bill Baird Papers, Box 398, Folder 17, Schlesinger Library, Harvard University, Cambridge, MA.
89. "Abortion and the Law" (script), *CBS Reports,* Florynce Kennedy Papers, Box 9, Folder 4, Schlesinger Library, Harvard University, Cambridge, MA.
90. By "public vocabulary," I draw upon Condit's terminology: "the acceptable words, myths, and characterizations used for warranting social behavior in a community." Condit, *Decoding Abortion Rhetoric,* 228.
91. "Abortion and the Law," 3.
92. "Abortion and the Law," 3.
93. "Abortion and the Law," 3.
94. "Abortion and the Law," emphasis added.
95. "Abortion and the Law," 7.
96. "Abortion and the Law," 7.
97. I thank Leslie Reagan for this helpful reminder. See Larry W. Stephenson, "History of Cardiac Surgery," in *Surgery,* ed. Jeffrey A. Norton, Philip S. Barie, R. Randal Bollinger, Alfred E. Chang, Stephen F. Lowry, Sean J. Mulvihill, Harvey I. Pass, and Robert W. Thompson (New York: Springer, 2008) 1471–1479.
98. Solinger, *Beggars and Choosers,* 60.
99. "Abortion and the Law," 10.
100. "Abortion and the Law," 10.
101. "Abortion and the Law," 10.
102. "Discussion Guide: 'Abortion and the Law.'"
103. "Discussion Guide: 'Abortion and the Law.'"
104. *Society for Humane Abortion Newsletter* 1, no. 4 (December 1965), Society for

Humane Abortion Newsletters, 1965–1973 MC 289, Box 1, Folder 4, Schlesinger Library, Harvard University, Cambridge, MA.

105. Although this cartoon predated the emergence of James Q. Wilson and George L. Kelling's broken windows theory in a 1982 *Atlantic Monthly* article, a theory of criminology linking visible disorder to higher rates of criminality and even poor public health outcomes, I argue that a proto–broken window logic could be seen in this image. The implementation of broken windows theory in policing has led to significant racial disparities. See Jonathan Oberman and Kendea Johnson, "The Never Ending Tale: Racism and Inequality in the Era of Broken Windows Policing," *Cardozo Law Review* 37, no. 3 (2016): 1075–1092.

106. Larry Howe, "Abortion and the Law: California Report" (December 1966), Society for Humane Abortion MC289, Box 3, Folder 40, Schlesinger Library, Harvard University, Cambridge, MA.

107. Howe, "Abortion and the Law: California Report," 1-1-1.

108. Howe, "Abortion and the Law: California Report," 1-1-1.

109. Howe, "Abortion and the Law: California Report," 2-2-2.

110. Howe, "Abortion and the Law: California Report," 2-2-2.

111. Howe, 'Abortion and the Law: California Report," 2-2-2.

112. Richards, *Euthenics.*

113. Patricia Hill Collins, *Black Feminist Thought: Knowledge, Consciousness, and the Politics of Empowerment* (New York: Routledge, 2022).

114. Harper, *The Ethos of Black Motherhood*, 57.

115. Larry Howe, "Critique of the Script: Abortion and the Law: California Report" (December 1966), Society for Humane Abortion MC289, Box 3, Folder 40, Schlesinger Library, Harvard University, Cambridge, MA.

116. Howe, "Critique of the Script: Abortion and the Law."

117. Joffe, *Doctors of Conscience.*

118. Diane Schulder and Florynce Kennedy, *Abortion Rap: Testimony by Women Who Have Suffered the Consequences of Restrictive Abortion Laws* (New York: McGraw-Hill, 1971).

119. Tasha N. Dubriwny, "Consciousness-Raising as Collective Rhetoric: The Articulation of Experience in the Redstockings' Abortion Speak-Out of 1969," *Quarterly Journal of Speech* 91, no. 4 (2005): 395–422.

120. "Redstockings Abortion Speakout," Redstockings Women's Liberation Archives for Action (Mach 21, 1969), Archive.org, https://archive.org/details/RedstockingsAbortionSpeakoutNewYork1969March21.

121. "Redstockings Abortion Speakout."

122. Robert Hall, "Abortions on Demand," *Newsweek*, January 13, 1970, in National Abortion Rights Action League State Affiliate Printed Material Collection, 1969–1989, PR-3, New York Folder, Schlesinger Library, Harvard University, Cambridge, MA.

123. Lucinda Cisler, "Abortion Law Repeal (Sort of): A Warning to Women," in Papers of the National Abortion Rights Action League, MC 313, Box, 4 Folder 3 Schlesinger Library, Harvard University, Cambridge, MA.

124. *The First American Symposium on Office Abortion: The Proceedings of the Symposium on Office Abortion Procedures, San Francisco, May 16, 1970*, Society for Human Abortion, SHA Publications MC 289, Box 1, Folder 6, Schlesinger Library, Harvard University, Cambridge MA, 1.

125. Patricia Maginnis, "Opening Remarks at the First American Symposium on Office Abortion," *The Proceedings of the Symposium on Office Abortion Procedures, San Francisco, May 16, 1970*, Society for Human Abortion, SHA Publications MC 289, Box 1, Folder 6, Schlesinger Library, Harvard University, Cambridge MA, 1–2.

126. Patricia T. Maginnis, *Abortee's Songbook* (1969), Society for Humane Abortion, Papers of the Society for Humane Abortion, MC 289, Box 1, Folder 6, Schlesinger Library, Harvard University, Cambridge, MA.

127. Lana Clarke Phelan, "Luncheon Address," in *Proceedings of the Symposium on Office Abortion Procedures* (1970), Papers of the Society for Humane Abortion, MC 289, Box 1, Folder 6, Schlesinger Library, Harvard University, Cambridge, MA, 43.

128. "Luncheon Address," 44.

129. *The Proceedings of the Symposium on Office Abortion Procedures*, 48.

130. Nelson, "'Abortions under Community Control.'"

131. Darrel Enck-Wanzer, "Health and Hospitals," in *The Young Lords: A Reader*, ed. Darrel Enck-Wanzer (New York: New York University Press, 2010), 188.

132. Enck-Wanzer, "Health and Hospitals," 198. Gloria Cruz's article was originally published in the July 31, 1970, issue of *Palante*.

133. Enck-Wanzer, "Health and Hospitals," 198.

134. While Keemer was by no means the only physician providing abortions in Detroit, or the only physician arrested for having done so in this city, I am comfortable claiming the anonymized Detroit physician in the *Detroit Free Press* article was, indeed, Edgar Keemer. Keemer's 1980 autobiography *and* this article retell a formative story about a daughter of local clergy, for whom Keemer denied an abortion who subsequently drowned despite being an all-star swimmer: "What I'm going to tell you is true," he said. "Early in my practice I was approached by the daughter of a leading minister. He was a great conservative—a big morality man. I was young—just starting out. She begged—pleaded with me, but I thought I couldn't do anything. I advised her to go home and face her father. Three days later she drowned. She was a good swimmer. . . . The only death I feel responsible for was that first one—when I refused." Compare this to the entire second chapter of Keemer's autobiography, where he wrote about perhaps the most formative moment in his career that solidified his moral obligation to provide illegal abortions. He similarly wrote of the daughter of a very conservative preacher for whom he denied an abortion because he was concerned about medical ethics. Keemer's wife, physician Dr. Bea Keemer, came back from church just days after they denied her the procedure: "They said it was accidental drowning but we know it wasn't an accident, don't we? . . . She was an expert swimmer, Keemer. They said she won a prize in high school." Keemer gave the young woman the name Margie X and dedicated his entire autobiography to her. See Keemer, *Confessions*, 23–34.

135. Helen Fogel, "I've Performed Hundreds of Abortions," *Detroit Free Press*, December 7, 1969, NARAL State Affiliates Michigan Printed Material, PR-3, Michigan Folder, Schlesinger Library, Harvard University, Cambridge, MA.

136. Fogel, "I've Performed Hundreds of Abortions."

137. Fogel, "I've Performed Hundreds of Abortions."

138. Fogel, "I've Performed Hundreds of Abortions."

139. Fogel, "I've Performed Hundreds of Abortions."

140. Fogel, "I've Performed Hundreds of Abortions."

141. Fogel, "I've Performed Hundreds of Abortions."

142. "Appeal Denial for the *People of the State of Michigan v. Robert Stanley Nixon*," National Abortion Rights Action League, State Affiliate Printed Material Collection, 1969–1989, PR-3, Michigan Folder, Schlesinger Library, Harvard University, Cambridge, MA. The state of Michigan found him guilty of violating MCLA 750.14; MSA 28. 204: "Any person who shall willfully administer to any pregnant woman any medicine, drug, substance, or thing whatever—or shall employ any instrument or other means whatever, with intent to thereby to procure the miscarriage of any such woman, unless the same shall have been necessary to preserve the life of such woman, shall be guilt of a felony."

143. "Appeal Denial for the *People of the State of Michigan v. Robert Stanley Nixon*," 3.

144. "Appeal Denial for the *People of the State of Michigan v. Robert Stanley Nixon*," 4.

145. "Appeal Denial for the *People of the State of Michigan v. Robert Stanley Nixon*."

146. "Appeal Denial for the *People of the State of Michigan v. Robert Stanley Nixon*."

147. "Appeal Denial for the *People of the State of Michigan v. Robert Stanley Nixon*," 8. See also Murillo, "*Espanta Cigüeñas*," for a discussion of how *People v. Belous* is embedded with what in the United States would be framed as "back-alley logics."

148. "Appeal Denial for the *People of the State of Michigan v. Robert Stanley Nixon*," 7, emphasis added.

149. "Appeal Denial for the *People of the State of Michigan v. Robert Stanley Nixon*," 7.

150. "Appeal Denial for the *People of the State of Michigan v. Robert Stanley Nixon*," 8.

151. Robert E. Johnson, "Legal Abortion: Is It Genocide or Blessing in Disguise?," *Jet Magazine Archive* 43, no. 24 (March 22, 1973): 12–51. Cynthia Greenlee notes that this image could have been staged.

152. Cynthia R. Greenlee, "T. R. M. Howard: Civil Rights Rabble-Rouser, Abortion Provider," *Dissent*, May 16, 2013, https://www.dissentmagazine.org/blog/t-r-m-howard-civil-rights-rabble-rouser-abortion-provider/.

153. Greenlee, "T. R. M. Howard."

154. Johnson, "Legal Abortion."

155. Johnson, "Legal Abortion," 14.

156. "Women's Health Consumer's Union to Combat behind-the Scenes Anti-abortion Conspiracy" (March 23, 1973) Florynce Kennedy Papers MC 555 Reproductive Rights, Research, Press Releases, Schlesinger Library, Harvard University, Cambridge, MA.

157. "Women's Health Consumers Union."

158. Mediclinic, "Ambulatory Surgical Clinics," Florynce Kennedy Papers MC 555 Reproductive Rights, Research, Press Releases, Schlesinger Library, Harvard University, Cambridge, MA.

159. Mediclinic, "Ambulatory Surgical Clinics."

160. Mediclinic, "Ambulatory Surgical Clinics."

161. Mediclinic, "Ambulatory Surgical Clinics," 2.

162. Mediclinic, "Ambulatory Surgical Clinics," 2.

163. Specifically, I draw upon Hasian, Condit, and Lucaites's argument that "the law exists as part of an evolving rhetorical culture . . . the range of linguistic usages available to those who would address a historically particular audience as a public . . . Rhetorical cultures evolve by adapting to changing social, political, and economic

exigencies, and the law is an inevitable branch of such a culture." Marouf Hasian Jr., Celeste Michelle Condit, and John Louis Lucaites, "The Rhetorical Boundaries of 'the Law': A Consideration of the Rhetorical Culture of Legal Practice and the Case of the 'Separate but Equal' Doctrine," *Quarterly Journal of Speech* 82, no. 4 (1996): 326–327.

164. Gibson, "The Rhetoric of *Roe v. Wade*."

*Chapter 3 • The Post-*Roe *Visceral Public Memory of Back-Alley Abortion*

1. Miller, *The Worst of Times*, 12.
2. Miller, *The Worst of Times*, 40, 41, 46.
3. Roberta Brandes-Gratz, "Never Again," *Ms.*, April 1973, 44–49. I am electing not to reprint the iconic image of Gerri Santoro here to avoid fetishizing the image. You can find it at Amanda Arnold, "How a Harrowing Photo of One Woman's Death Became an Iconic Pro-choice Symbol," *Vice*, October 26, 2016, https://www.vice.com/en/article/evgdpw/how-a-harrowing-photo-of-one-womans-death-became-an-iconic-pro-choice-symbol. Illustration by Julia Kuo. Warning: Graphic and upsetting visual representation of death.
4. Arnold, "How a Harrowing Photo."
5. Sara Hayden, "Revitalizing the Debate between <Life> and <Choice>: The 2004 March for Women's Lives," *Communication and Critical/Cultural Studies* 6, no. 2 (2009): 126.
6. Karyn Sandlos, "Unifying Forces: Rhetorical Reflections on a Pro-choice Image," in *Transformations: Thinking through Feminism*, ed. Sara Ahmed, Jane Kilby, Celia Lury, Maureen McNeil, and Beverly Skeggs (London: Routledge, 2000), 85. Scholarship surrounding the cultural and rhetorical fetal images is vast, although somewhat outside of the scope of this chapter. For excellent exemplars, see Rosalind Pollack Petchesky, "Fetal Images: The Power of Visual Culture in the Politics of Reproduction," *Feminist Studies* 13, no. 2 (1987): 263–292; Carole Stabile, "Shooting the Mother," in *The Visible Woman: Imaging Technologies, Gender, and Science* (New York: New York University Press, 1998): 171–97; Janelle S. Taylor, *The Public Life of the Fetal Sonogram: Technology, Consumption, and the Politics of Reproduction* (New Brunswick, NJ: Rutgers University Press, 2008); Monica J. Casper, *The Making of the Unborn Patient: A Social Anatomy of Fetal Surgery* (New Brunswick, NJ: Rutgers University Press, 1998); Margarete Sandelowski, "Separate, but Less Unequal: Fetal Ultrasonography and the Transformation of Expectant Mother/Fatherhood," *Gender & Society* 8, no. 2 (1994): 230–245; Karen Newman, *Fetal Positions: Individualism, Science, Visuality* (Stanford, CA: Stanford University Press, 1996); Barbara Duden, *Disembodying Women: Perspectives on Pregnancy and the Unborn* (Cambridge, MA: Harvard University Press, 1993); Lynn Marie Morgan and Meredith W. Michaels, eds., *Fetal Subjects, Feminist Positions* (Philadelphia: University of Pennsylvania Press, 1999); Valerie Hartouni, "Fetal Exposures: Abortion Politics and the Optics of Allusion," *Camera Obscura: Feminism, Culture, and Media Studies* 10, no. 2 (1992): 130–149; Sara Dubow, *Ourselves Unborn: A History of the Fetus in Modern America* (Oxford: Oxford University Press, 2010).
7. *Leona's Sister Gerri*, directed by Jane Gilooly (Ho-Ho-Kus, NJ: New Day Films, 1994).
8. Larson, *What It Feels Like*, 4.
9. Combahee River Collective, "The Combahee River Collective Statement."

10. Rocío R. García, "'We're Not All Anti-choices': How Controlling Images Shape Latina/x Feminist Abortion Advocacy," *Sociological Perspectives* 65, no. 6 (2022): 1208. I follow García's labeling of Rosie Jiménez's positionality. She has been described in various writings as Mexican American, Chicana, and Latina. I cite García's specificity and often engage in the term "Mexican-origin" to recognize that, in Josue David Cisernos's words, "a number of ethnic identifiers have been used to refer to Latina American people or their descendants who live in the United States. These terms include Latino, Hispanic, Chicano, Latin, Spanish, and many others. Such identifiers are often deployed monolithically to refer to all people of Latin American descent and thus can be rife with inaccuracies and fraught with dangers of homogenization or essentialism." Josue David Cisneros, *The Border Crossed Us: Rhetorics of Borders, Citizenship, and Latina/o Identity* (Tuscaloosa: University of Alabama Press, 2013), x. Relatedly, I will sometimes refer to Rosie Jiménez as "Rosie" not because I am claiming any intimate familiarity with her, but rather to balance my naming in this section with the subsequent analysis of Becky Bell, whose story involves her parents and requires first-name reference for precision.

11. Johanna Schoen, *Abortion after "Roe"* (Chapel Hill: University of North Carolina Press, 2015).

12. Marita Sturken, *Tangled Memories: The Vietnam War, the AIDS Epidemic, and the Politics of Remembering* (University of California Press, 1997), 3.

13. Condit, *Decoding Abortion Rhetoric.*

14. Stormer, *Articulating Life's Memory.*

15. Stormer, *Articulating Life's Memory*, xiii.

16. Stormer, *Signs of Pathology*, 76.

17. Greg Dickinson, Carole Blair, and Brian L. Ott, eds., *Places of Public Memory: The Rhetoric of Museums and Memorials* (Tuscaloosa: University of Alabama Press, 2010).

18. Stormer, *Articulating Life's Memory.*

19. Thomas R. Dunn, "Remembering 'a Great Fag': Visualizing Public Memory and the Construction of Queer Space," *Quarterly Journal of Speech* 97, no. 4 (2011): 439.

20. Jane E. Hodgson, "The Law, the AMA, and Partial-Birth Abortion," *Journal of the American Medical Association* 281, no. 1 (July 7, 1999): 24, emphasis added.

21. Stormer, "A Likely Past."

22. It is important to provide context regarding figure 3.1. This photograph was captured at a protest event organized by Rise Up 4 Abortion Rights held in front of the US Supreme Court on January 22, 2022. I feature Mridula Amin's photograph because it represents a juxtaposition of "Never go back" language with a portrait of Gerri Santoro as exemplary of back-alley memory work. It is crucial to note that Rise Up 4 Abortion Rights makes use of back-alley abortion language on their website and has also been criticized by a pro-abortion coalition for its financial structure, use of coat hanger imagery, perpetuation of anti-Blackness, anti-queer and anti-trans language, and exclusion of sex workers. The statement is linked through the article Anna Merlan, "The Abortion Rights Group Other Activists Want Nothing to Do With," *Vice*, August 4, 2022, https://www.vice.com/en/article/the-abortion-rights-group-other-activists-want-nothing-to-do-with/.

23. Melody Rose, *Safe, Legal, and Unavailable? Abortion Politics in the United States* (Washington, DC: CQ Press, 2007).

24. Dubriwny, "Consciousness-Raising as Collective Rhetoric."

25. Dickinson, Blair, and Ott, *Places of Public Memory*, 7.

26. Emily Winderman, "(Never) Going Back: Black Feminist Impatience for a Post-*Dobbs* Future," *Women & Language* 46, no. 1 (2023): 287.

27. Ersula Ore and Matthew Houdek, "Lynching in Times of Suffocation: Toward a Spatiotemporal Politics of Breathing," *Women's Studies in Communication* 43, no. 4 (2020): 444.

28. Nelson, *Women of Color and the Reproductive Rights Movement*. Khiara M. Bridges argues that "wealth is a condition for privacy rights and that, lacking wealth, poor mothers do not have any privacy rights." Bridges makes an apt comparison to the role of poll taxes and literacy tests that informally disenfranchised Black men protected by the Fifteenth Amendment. She thus concludes that lack of ability to fund abortion equates with an *informal disenfranchisement* of privacy rights, wherein "a group that has been formally bestowed with a right is stripped of that very right by techniques that the Court has held to be consistent with the Constitution." Khiara M. Bridges, *The Poverty of Privacy Rights* (Palo Alto, CA: Stanford University Press, 2017), 12–13.

29. Kendall Phillips, introduction to *Framing Public Memory*, ed. Kendall Phillips (Tuscaloosa: University of Alabama Press, 2004), 4.

30. Schulder and Kennedy, *Abortion Rap*. For an in-depth analysis of Florynce Kennedy's rhetorical work in *Abramowicz v. Lefkowitz*, see Randolph, *Florynce "Flo" Kennedy*, 168–185.

31. Emily Winderman and Brittany Knutson, "Florynce Kennedy's Cultivation of Reproductive Expertise in *Abramowicz v. Lefkowitz* and *Abortion Rap*," *Rhetoric Society Quarterly* 53, no. 2 (2023): 262–277.

32. Sarah Weddington, *A Question of Choice: The Lawyer Who Won "Roe v. Wade"* (New York: Putnam Press, 1992), 151.

33. Phillips, introduction to *Framing Public Memory*, 7–9.

34. "Do You Want to Return to the Butchery of Back-Alley Abortion?," *Goldflower*, April 1975, Marie Kochaver Women's Movement Collection SW0358, Box 1, Folder 4, University of Minnesota Social Welfare History Archives, Minneapolis, MN.

35. National Abortion Rights Action League, "Introduction to Debating," in *NARAL Literature*, 1973–75, MC 313 Box 1, Folder 21, Schlesinger Library, Harvard University, Cambridge, MA.

36. Roberta Brandes Gratz, "She Had a Name. She Had a Family. She Was Leona's Sister Gerri," *Ms.*, November/December 1995, 72–74. Brandes Gratz notes how Leona ultimately became an abortion rights activist.

37. Sandlos, "Rhetorical Reflections on a Pro-choice Image," 85.

38. Arnold, "How a Harrowing Photo."

39. Carmen Rios, "Daring to Remember: Tell Us Your Story of Life before *Roe*," *Ms.*, July 2, 2018, https://msmagazine.com/2018/07/02/daring-remember-tell-us-story-life-roe/.

40. J. Johnson, "A Man's Mouth," 2.

41. Places of public memory have been crucial to providing a collective site for witnessing and reflection on a past deemed worthy of remembrance. On the one hand, anti-abortion activists have produced places of public memory to craft memorials to the "unborn," humanizing the fetus as grievable. See Allison L. Rowland, *Zoetropes and the*

Politics of Humanhood (Columbus: The Ohio State University Press, 2020). On the other hand, spaces of public memory such as "back-alley abortion" draw upon the imagined *bas-fonds* that I explicated in chapter 1 and become cultural repositories of experiences, events, and accompanying effects that mold and negotiate scenes of ongoing rhetorical invention.

42. Here, I am specifically discussing appeals to rhetorical vision that are more fully explicated in chapter 1.

43. Ashley Noel Mack, Carli Bershon, Douglas D. Laiche and Melissa Navarro, "Between Bodies and Institutions: Gendered Violence as Co-constitutive," *Women's Studies in Communication* 41, no. 2 (2018): 95–99.

44. National Institutes of Health, National Cancer Institute, "Viscera (Code c28287)," *NCI Thesaurus*, https://ncit.nci.nih.gov/ncitbrowser/ConceptReport.jsp?dictionary=NCI_Thesaurus&version=22.04d&ns=ncit&code=C28287.

45. Johnson, "A Man's Mouth," 4.

46. Johnson, "A Man's Mouth," 4.

47. Ahmed, *Cultural Politics of Emotion*.

48. Dickinson, Blair, and Ott, *Places of Public Memory*.

49. Stormer, *Articulating Life's Memory*, 41.

50. Karma R. Chávez, "The Body: An Abstract and Actual Rhetorical Concept," *Rhetoric Society Quarterly* 48, no. 3 (2018): 245.

51. Sturken, *Tangled Memories*, 220.

52. Reagan, *When Abortion Was a Crime*.

53. Barbara Winslow, *Revolutionary Feminists: The Women's Liberation Movement in Seattle* (Durham, NC: Duke University Press), 51.

54. Winslow, *Revolutionary Feminists*, 55. According to Winslow, this recollection stemmed from a 1992 interview between her and Nina Harding (n22).

55. Linda Averill, "How We Won Abortion Rights," Freedom Socialist Party, April 2004, https://socialism.com/fs-article/how-we-won-abortion-rights/.

56. Randolph, *Florynce "Flo" Kennedy*, 175.

57. Merle Hoffman, *Intimate Wars: The Life and Times of the Woman Who Brought Abortion from the Back-Alley to the Boardroom* (New York: Feminist Press at City University of New York, 2012), 152–153.

58. Stormer, *Signs of Pathology*.

59. Hortense J. Spillers, "Mama's Baby Papa's Maybe: An American Grammar Book," *Diacritics* 17, no. 2 (1987): 65–81.

60. Lisa A. Flores, *Deportable and Disposable: Public Rhetoric and the Making of the "Illegal" Immigrant* (University Park: Pennsylvania State University Press, 2020), 13.

61. Patricia Hill Collins, "It's All in the Family: Intersections of Gender, Race, and Nation," *Hypatia* 13, no. 3 (1998), 66.

62. Stormer, *Articulating Life's Memory*.

63. Condit, *Decoding Abortion Rhetoric*, 44.

64. Sara Hayden, "Family Metaphors and the Nation: Promoting a Politics of Care through the Million Mom March," *Quarterly Journal of Speech* 89, no. 3 (2003): 199. Hayden's article draws upon the work of George Lakoff, who articulates family metaphors to the nation in *Moral Politics: What Conservatives Know That Liberals Don't* (Chicago: University of Chicago Press, 1996).

65. Shui-yin Sharon Yam, "Citizenship Discourse in Hong Kong: The Limits of Familial Tropes," *Quarterly Journal of Speech* 104, no. 1 (2018): 4.

66. Barbie Zelizer, *About to Die: How Images Move the Public* (New York: Oxford University Press, 2010), 173–217.

67. Mariana Ortega, "Being Lovingly, Knowingly Ignorant: White Feminism and Women of Color," *Hypatia* 21, no. 3 (2006): 56–74.

68. Bessel van der Kolk, *The Body Keeps the Score: Brain, Mind, and Body in the Healing of Trauma* (New York: Random House, 2015).

69. Victoria Gómez Betancourt, "Rosie and Me: Remembering the Hyde Amendment's First Victim," *Rewire News Group*, October 3, 2017, https://rewirenewsgroup.com/article/2017/10/03/rosie-remembering-hyde-amendments-first-victim/.

70. Condit, *Decoding Abortion Rhetoric*, 114.

71. Goodwin, *Policing the Womb*, 66.

72. Khiara Bridges, *The Poverty of Privacy Rights* (Palto Alto, CA: Stanford University Press), 14.

73. García, "We're Not All Anti-choices," 1224.

74. Sarah De Los Santos Upton, "Neplanta Activism and Coalition Building: Locating Identity and Resistance in the Cracks between Worlds," *Women's Studies in Communication* 42, no. 2 (2019), 135.

75. Leandra Hinojosa Hernández and Sarah De Los Santos Upton, *Challenging Reproductive Control and Gendered Violence in the Américas: Intersectionality, Power, and Struggles for Rights* (Lanham, MD: Lexington, 2018), 9–14; See also Jessica Enoch, "Survival Stories: Feminist Historiographic Approaches to Chicana Rhetorics of Sterilization Abuse," *Rhetoric Society Quarterly* 35, no. 3 (2005): 5–30.

76. Catalina (Kathleen) M. de Onís, "Lost in Translation: Challenging (White, Monolingual Feminism's) <Choice> with *Justicia Reproductiva*," *Women's Studies in Communication* 38 (2015): 1–19; Nelson, *Women of Color and the Reproductive Rights Movement.*

77. Ellen Frankfort, *Rosie: The Investigation of a Wrongful Death* (New York: Dial Press, 1979).

78. García, "We're Not All Anti-choices," 1209

79. Frankfort, *Rosie: The Investigation*, 18.

80. Frankfort, *Rosie: The Investigation*, 19.

81. Sarah De Los Santos Upton, Carlos A. Tarin, and Leandra H. Hernández, "Construyendo Conexiones para los Niños: Environmental Justice, Reproductive Feminicidio, and Coalitional Possibility in the Borderlands," *Health Communication* 37, no. 9 (2022): 1242.

82. Murillo, "*Espanta Cigüeñas*," 796. See also Chávez, *The Borders of AIDS*.

83. Frankfort, *Rosie: The Investigation*, 19.

84. Murillo, "*Espanta Cigüeñas*"; and Reagan, *When Abortion Was a Crime.*

85. Frankfort, *Rosie: The Investigation*, 28.

86. Frankfort, *Rosie: The Investigation*, 36.

87. Frankfort, *Rosie: The Investigation*, 48. As Lila Burns described, her Planned Parenthood did not perform abortions. Rather, they would refer to four MDs who performed the procedure in McAllen (49).

88. Frankfort, *Rosie: The Investigation*, 19.

89. Lina-Maria Murillo, "A View from the Northern Border: Abortions before *Roe v. Wade*," *Bulletin of the History of Medicine* 97, no. 1 (2023): 38.

90. Frankfort, *Rosie: The Investigation*, 34.

91. Frankfort, *Rosie: The Investigation*, 29.

92. Frankfort, *Rosie: The Investigation*, 137.

93. Frankfort, *Rosie: The Investigation*, 50.

94. Frankfort, *Rosie: The Investigation*, 89.

95. Frankfort, *Rosie: The Investigation*, 89–90.

96. Frankfort, *Rosie: The Investigation*, 90.

97. Frankfort, *Rosie: The Investigation*, 91.

98. Frankfort, *Rosie: The Investigation*, 91.

99. Murillo, "*Espanta Cigüeñas*," 804.

100. Frankfort, *Rosie: The Investigation*, 92.

101. Isabel Molina Guzmán and Angharad N. Valdivia, "Brain, Brow, and Booty: Latina Iconicity in U.S. Popular Culture," *Communication Review* 7, no. 2 (2004): 212.

102. Frankfort, *Rosie: The Investigation*, 99.

103. Frankfort, *Rosie: The Investigation*, 152.

104. Kelly O'Donnell and Naomi Rogers, "Revisiting the History of Abortion in the Wake of the *Dobbs* Decision," *Bulletin of the History of Medicine* 97, no. 1 (2023): 1.

105. Frankfort, *Rosie: The Investigation*, 139.

106. O'Donnell and Rogers, "Revisiting the History," 2. The authors note (and the back of the book confirms) that Frankfort and Kissling pledged 5 percent of their book's royalties to the new Rosie Jiménez Fund to support low-income people seeking abortions in Texas.

107. Coalition for Reproductive Freedom, "En el 3 de Octubre, 1977 Rosie Jimenez murio de un aborto ilegal tal como ocurre con la vida de tantas mujeres cada ano," Northeastern University Digital Repository (October 1982), http://hdl.handle.net/2047/D20260044; Coalition for Reproductive Freedom, "On October 3, 1977 Rosie Jimenez Died from an Illegal, Back-Alley Abortion," Northeastern University Digital Repository (October 1982), http://hdl.handle.net/2047/D20247237.

108. Silliman et al., *Undivided Rights*, 39–40.

109. de Onís, "Lost in Translation," 9.

110. de Onís, "Lost in Translation," 9.

111. This poster helps illuminate why it comes as little surprise that "while R2N2 saw the link between women's oppression and ending racism, it was not always successful at putting its politics into practice, nor was it equipped to deal with racism within its organizations" (Silliman et al., *Undivided Rights*, 39–41). Owing to these dynamics, R2N2 fractured in 1981 and ultimately dissolved. Although I do not claim that this poster *caused* any dissolution on its own, I do see the rhetoric itself as symptomatic of these fraught coalitional dynamics.

112. Brian S. Amsden, "Performing Maturity in the Parental Consent and Notification Judicial Bypass Procedure," *Communication and Critical/Cultural Studies* 12, no. 1 (2015): 1–18.

113. Jenna Vinson, *Embodying the Problem: The Persuasive Power of the Teen Mother* (New Brunswick, NJ: Rutgers University Press, 2018), 10.

114. Fixmer-Oraiz, *Homeland Maternity*, 113.

115. Heather Brook Adams, "Rhetorics of Unwed Motherhood and Shame," *Women's Studies in Communication* 40, no. 1 (2017): 91–110. For some firsthand discussions related to the inability to access abortion and the physical and psychological toll maternity homes took before *Roe*, see Schulder and Kennedy, *Abortion Rap*.

116. Fixmer-Oraiz, *Homeland Maternity*, 115; Vinson, *Embodying the Problem*, 11; Kristin Luker, *Dubious Conceptions: The Politics of Teenage Pregnancy* (Cambridge, MA: Harvard University Press, 1997).

117. Heather Brook Adams, *Enduring Shame: A Recent History of Unwed Pregnancy and Righteous Reproduction* (Columbia: University of South Carolina Press, 2022), 151.

118. Vinson, *Embodying the Problem*, 12.

119. Collins, "It's All in the Family," 65.

120. Marcia D. Greenberger and Katherine Connor, "Parental Notice and Consent for Abortion: Out of Step with Family Law Principles and Policies," *Family Planning Perspectives* 23, no. 1 (1991): 31–35.

121. Harper, *The Ethos of Black Motherhood*, 39.

122. Seth Dowland, "'Family Values' and the Formation of a Christian Right Agenda," *Church History* 78, no. 3 (2009): 608.

123. "Focus on the Family Historical Timeline," Focus on the Family, accessed May 7, 2024, https://www.focusonthefamily.com/about/historical-timeline/.

124. Fixmer-Oraiz, *Homeland Maternity*, 137–138.

125. *Abortion Denied: Shattering Young Women's Lives*, produced by Eleanor Smeal and Toni Carabillo (Arlington County, Virginia: Fund for the Feminist Majority, 1990).

126. In 1973, Edelin was convicted by an all-white, mostly Catholic jury of ending a twenty-four-week pregnancy after the *Roe* decision had been handed down. While the legality of the abortion itself was not contested by the prosecution, the jury was convinced by the prosecution's arguments regarding fetal personhood, even though no such standard existed at the time. As his 2013 obituary remarked, jurors "made racial slurs against Dr. Edelin 'more than once' before closing arguments." Robert D. McFadden, "Kenneth C. Edelin, Doctor at Center of Landmark Abortion Case, Dies at 74," *New York Times*, December 30, 2013, https://www.nytimes.com/2013/12/31/us/kenneth-c-edelin-physician-at-center-of-landmark-abortion-case-dies-at-74.html; See also Schoen, *Abortion after "Roe,"* for an in-depth analysis of Edelin's case.

127. *Coroner's Report of Rebecca Suzanne Bell*, in Research and Writing for Becky Bell Video re: Parental Consent, October 3, 1988, Toni Carabillo / Judith Meuli Papers, Box 37, Folder 14, Schlesinger Library, Harvard University, Cambridge, MA.

128. "Coroner's Report," 5.

129. Robin E. Jensen and Ghanima Almuaili, "Abortion and Miscarriage Are Synonyms: Substandard Gynecological Care in the Wake of Abortion's Criminalization," *Women & Language* 46, no. 1 (2023): 267–273.

130. J. C. Willke, "Becky Bell Did Not Die from an Induced Abortion," *National Right to Life News*, October 2, 1990, Papers of Teresa Vaughn, Box 3 Folder 12 MC 1170, Schlesinger Library, Harvard University, Cambridge, MA.

131. Connie M. Pratt, "Should State Require That Parents Be Notified before a Minor Child Undergoes an Abortion Yes: Parents Have Every Right to be Involved in Decision,"

Colorado Springs Gazette-Telegraph, January 22, 1994, B7; James A. Miller, "In Indiana and Maryland, a Tale of Two Abortions," *Baltimore Sun*, February 14, 1991, https://www.baltimoresun.com/news/bs-xpm-1991-02-15-1991046187-story.html.

132. Juan José Campanella, "Public Law 106: The Becky Bell Story," season 1, episode 3, *Lifestories: Families in Crisis*, written by Bruce Harmon, aired August 15, 1992, in broadcast syndication, HBO.

133. Wanda S. Pillow, *Unfit Subjects: Education Policy and the Teen Mother, 1972–2002* (New York: Routledge, 2004).

134. Harper, *The Ethos of Black Motherhood*, 37–38.

135. See Adams, *Enduring Shame*, for an in-depth examination of the rhetorical capacities of shame as articulated to unwed motherhood.

136. Child Custody Protection Act, H.R. 3682, 105th Cong. §2, (1998), https://www.congress.gov/bill/105th-congress/house-bill/3682.

137. Child Custody Protection Act, H5524.

138. Child Custody Protection Act, H5530.

139. Child Custody Protection Act, H5538.

140. Child Custody Protection Act, H5538.

141. *Spirit of '73: Rock for Choice*, Sony Music, 1995, compact disc.

142. Price, "What Is Reproductive Justice?," 352.

143. Price, "What Is Reproductive Justice?," 351–352. During a speech at the March for Women's Lives, Ross notably remarked, "But nobody works alone so I'm going to call out the names of the sisters who did work. That's the way I want to use my time. Malika Redman, Deanna West, Luce Alvarez Martinez, Nancy Kotto, Rosalida Valacios, Nakenji Ture, Rosalynn Satchel, Dázon Dixon." Loretta Ross, "Speech at the 2004 March for Women's Lives," April 25, 2004, Washington, DC, C-SPAN, 02:36:15, https://www.c-span.org/video/?181451-1/march-womens-lives. Sara Hayden argues that the event rearticulated the ideograph of <choice>. Hayden, "Revitalizing the Debate."

144. Tyne Daly, "Speech at the 2004 March for Women's Lives on Becky Bell," April 25, 2004, Washington, DC, C-SPAN, 02:40:31, https://www.c-span.org/video/?181451-1/march-womens-lives.

145. Charlene Ortiz, "Speech at the 2004 March for Women's Lives on Rosie Jiménez," April 25, 2004, Washington, DC, C-SPAN, 02:43:30, https://www.c-span.org/video/?181451-1/march-womens-lives.

Chapter 4 • Kermit Gosnell and the Anti-abortion Uptake of Back-Alley Abortion

1. "*Whole Woman's Health v. Hellerstedt*," Center for Reproductive Rights, accessed May 7, 2024, https://www.reproductiverights.org/case/whole-womans-health-v-hellerstedt.

2. Some representative examples include discourse from anti-abortion and abortion rights journalists and activists: William Saletan, "The Back Alley: What Happened to the Women," *Slate*, February 16, 2011, https://slate.com/news-and-politics/2011/02/kermit-gosnell-and-abortion-clinic-regulation-did-pro-choice-politics-protect-him.html; James Taranto, "Back-Alley Abortion Never Ended: The Kermit Gosnell Murder Trial Challenges a Traditional Defense of Abortion," *Wall Street Journal*, April 18, 2013, https://www.wsj.com/articles/SB10001424127887324493704578429431398819380; Rich

Lowry, "Return of the Back Alley," *National Review*, February 4, 2011, https://www.nationalreview.com/2011/02/return-back-alley-rich-lowry/; Josh Levs, "Gosnell Horror Fuels Fight for Abortion Laws," CNN, May 14, 2013, https://www.cnn.com/2013/05/12/us/abortion-trial-significance/index.html.

3. Report of the Grand Jury, *In re* County Investigating Grand Jury XXIII, Misc. No. 0009901–2008. (First Jud. Dist. of PA, January 21, 2011), http://perma.cc/7QD3-B8KE.

4. To be sure, journalists have made this argument. See Nora Caplan-Bricker, "The Kermit Gosnell Effect: How His Gruesome Trial Is Helping Anti-abortion Legislation in Far-Away States," *New Republic*, April 30, 2013, https://newrepublic.com/article/113052/kermit-gosnell-trial-how-pro-lifers-are-using-him-pass-new-laws. This chapter differs by examining the discursive and affective pathways that enabled the Gosnell case's back-alley abortion framing to experience regressive uptake.

5. Linda Greenhouse and Reva B. Siegel, "*Casey* and the Clinic Closings: When 'Protecting Health' Obstructs Choice," *Yale Law Journal* 549 (2015): 1428.

6. Schoen, *Abortion after "Roe,"* 93–118; Carole Joffe, "Commentary: Abortion Provider Stigma and Mainstream Medicine," *Women & Health* 54, no. 7 (2014): 666–671.

7. Schoen, *Abortion after "Roe,"* 24.

8. Schoen, *Abortion after "Roe,"* 95, 110.

9. Schoen, *Abortion after "Roe,"* 110.

10. Schoen, *Abortion after "Roe,"* 96.

11. Marshall H. Medoff, "State Abortion Politics and TRAP Abortion Laws," *Journal of Women, Politics & Policy* 33 (2012): 239–262.

12. Medoff, "State Abortion Politics," 241.

13. Schoen, *Abortion after "Roe,"* 25.

14. Bonnie S. Jones, Sara Daniel, and Lindsay K. Cloud, "State Law Approaches to Facility Regulation of Abortion and Other Office Interventions," *American Journal of Public Health* 108 (2018): 486–492.

15. Jones, Daniel, and Cloud, "State Law Approaches," 491. See also Schoen, *Abortion after "Roe,"* 44–45. As Schoen explains, local building codes and zoning ordinances often required "certificates of need." These procedures alongside "unsympathetic inspectors" would frequently place blocks in the way of clinic openings.

16. Nancy F. Berglas and Sarah C. M. Roberts, "The Development of Facility Standards for Common Outpatient Procedures and Implications for the Context of Abortion," *BMC Health Services Research* 18, no. 212 (2018), https://doi.org/10.1186/s12913-018-3048-3.

17. Rebecca J. Mercier, Mara Buchbinder, and Amy Bryant, "TRAP Laws and the Invisible Labor of US Abortion Providers," *Critical Public Health* 26, no. 1 (2016): 77–87.

18. Abortion Control Act of 1982 No. 138 1982 Pa Laws 476 (Codified at 18 Pa Cons. Stat. Ann. § 3201–3220), 3208.

19. Abortion Control Act of 1982, 3202.

20. Lucy Perkins, "How a Supreme Court Case from Pennsylvania Changed Abortion Access across the Country," WESA NPR, September 7, 2018, https://www.wesa.fm/politics-government/2018-09-07/how-a-supreme-court-case-from-pennsylvania-changed-abortion-access-across-the-country.

21. Macarena Sáez, "Commentary on *Planned Parenthood of Southeastern Pennsylvania v. Casey*," in *Feminist Judgments: Rewritten Opinions of the United States Supreme*

Court, ed. Kathryn M. Stanchi, Linda L. Berger, and Bridget J. Crawford (New York: Cambridge University Press, 2016), 361–365.

22. Sáez, "Commentary," 362.

23. Akiba Solomon, "The Personal Is Political: That's the Challenge; *Roe v. Wade* and a Black Nationalist Womanist Writer," *Dissent* 60, no. 1 (2013): 61, 63.

24. Dána Ain Davis, *Reproductive Injustice* (New York: New York University Press, 2019).

25. W. E. B. Du Bois and Isabel Eaton, *The Philadelphia Negro: A Social Study*, Publications of the University of Pennsylvania, Series in Political Economy and Public Law, no. 14 (Philadelphia: Published for the University, 1899), 6, https://catalog.hathitrust.org/Record/001263090. Du Bois's book has been republished four times.

26. Du Bois and Eaton, *The Philadelphia Negro*, 25.

27. Du Bois and Eaton, *The Philadelphia Negro*, 28–31.

28. Marcus Anthony Hunter, "Black Philly after *The Philadelphia Negro*," *Contexts* 13, no. 1 (2014): 27.

29. Marvin J. H. Lee, Kruthika Reddy, Junad Chowdhury, Nishant Kumar, Peter A. Clark, Papa Ndao, Stacy J. Suh, and Sara Song, "Overcoming a Legacy of Mistrust: African Americans' Mistrust of Medical Profession," *Journal of Healthcare Ethics & Administration* 4, no. 1 (2018): 19.

30. David C. Humphrey, "Dissection and Discrimination: The Social Origins of Cadavers in America, 1760–1915," *Bulletin of the NY Academy of Medicine* 49, no. 9 (1973): 823; Vanessa Northington Gamble, "Under the Shadow of Tuskegee: African Americans and Healthcare," *American Journal of Public Health* 87 (1997): 1773–1778.

31. Humphrey, "Dissection and Discrimination," 823.

32. Patricia A. Turner, *I Heard It through the Grapevine: Rumor in African-American Culture* (Berkeley: University of California Press, 1993).

33. Emily A. Largent, "Public Health, Racism, and the Lasting Impact of Hospital Segregation," *Public Health Reports* 133, no. 6 (2018): 715–720.

34. Vanessa Northington Gamble, *Making a Place for Ourselves: The Black Hospital Movement, 1920–1945* (Oxford: Oxford University Press, 1995), 11.

35. Elliott M. Rudwick, "A Brief History of Mercy-Douglass Hospital in Philadelphia," *Journal of Negro Education* 20, no. 1 (1951): 57.

36. Gamble, *Making a Place*, xi.

37. Harley F. Etienne, *Pushing Back the Gates: Neighborhood Perspectives on University-Driven Revitalization in West Philadelphia* (Philadelphia: Temple University Press, 2012).

38. Etienne, *Pushing Back the Gates*, 18.

39. Etienne, *Pushing Back the Gates*, 18–19.

40. *Brotherly Love: Health of Black Men and Boys in Philadelphia*, City of Philadelphia, March 14, 2019, https://www.phila.gov/media/20190314105459/Brotherly-Love_Health-Of-Black-Men-And-Boys_3_19.pdf.

41. Elizabeth J. Brown, Daniel Polsky, Corentin M. Barbu, Jane W. Seymour, and David Grande, "Racial Disparities in Geographic Access to Primary Care in Philadelphia," *Health Affairs* 35, no. 8 (2016): 1374–1381.

42. Report of the Grand Jury, 1, emphasis added.

43. Julia Kristeva, *Powers of Horror* (New York: Columbia University Press, 1980), 4.

44. Ellis, "'Doctors Don't Kill Babies! Monsters Do!,'" 80.

45. Kendall R. Phillips, *A Place of Darkness: The Rhetoric of Horror in Early American Cinema* (Austin: University of Texas Press, 2018), 2, 19.

46. Marina Levina and Diem-My T. Bui, "Introduction: Toward a Comprehensive Monster Theory in the 21st Century," in *Monster Culture in the 21st Century: A Reader*, ed. Marina Levina and Diem-My T. Bui (New York: Bloomsbury, 2013), 5.

47. Bernadette Marie Calafell, *Monstrosity, Performance, and Race in Contemporary Culture* (New York: Peter Lang, 2015), 6.

48. William Ian Miller, *Anatomy of Disgust* (Cambridge, MA: Harvard University Press, 1997), 187.

49. Report of the Grand Jury, 89.

50. Chelsea Conaboy, "Doctor's Long Tumble to Jail," *Philadelphia Inquirer*, January 23, 2011, http://articles.philly.com/2011-01-23/news/27044753_1_abortion-clinic-methadone-clinic-abortion-practice.

51. Report of the Grand Jury, 38.

52. Report of the Grand Jury, 88.

53. Report of the Grand Jury, 25.

54. Report of the Grand Jury, 32. In addition to the laundry list of charges brought against Gosnell, he was also charged with "corrupting the morals of a minor."

55. Report of the Grand Jury, 88.

56. Report of the Grand Jury, 61.

57. Report of the Grand Jury, 62.

58. Report of the Grand Jury, 24.

59. Report of the Grand Jury, 90.

60. Report of the Grand Jury, 27.

61. Niall Scott, "The Monstrous Metallic in Medicine and Horror Cinema," *Medicina nei Secoli: Journal of History of Medicine and Medical Humanities* 26, no. 1 (2014): 317.

62. Report of the Grand Jury, 223.

63. Report of the Grand Jury, 115.

64. Report of the Grand Jury, 223.

65. I would be remiss if I did not acknowledge the complex status of psychologist Harvey Karman throughout the history of criminalized abortion. While Karman developed the revolutionary cannula, *Jet* magazine described troubling accusations that Karman performed "illegal abortions on a group of women, mostly Black, before television cameras. . . . Dr. Karman denies performing the abortions." See "Medic Denies Performing TV Abortions on Blacks," *Jet Magazine Archive* 45, no. 3 (January 4, 1973): 13. For a nuanced exploration of how Harvey Karman was at times celebrated and other times vilified in the changing landscape of criminalized abortion, medical boundaries, and feminist self-help, see Bibia Pavard, "The 'Karman Method' and the Boundaries of Self-Help: Itinerary of an Abortion Technology," *Gender & History* (2024): 1–18.

66. Scott, "The Monstrous Metallic," 317.

67. Report of the Grand Jury, 45, emphasis mine.

68. Report of the Grand Jury, 2.

69. Report of the Grand Jury, 20.

70. Report of the Grand Jury, 46.

71. Bennett, *Banning Queer Blood*; Marina Levina, *Pandemics and the Media* (New York: Peter Lang, 2012).

72. Report of the Grand Jury, 46–48.

73. Report of the Grand Jury, 48.

74. Report of the Grand Jury, 46.

75. Report of the Grand Jury, 50

76. Report of the Grand Jury, 48–49.

77. Report of the Grand Jury, 77.

78. Zornitsa Keremidchieva, "Locating Argument's Location: The Stasis of Jurisdiction and the Establishment of the First Meridian of the United States," in *Local Theories of Argument*, ed. Dale Hample (London: Routledge, 2021): 242.

79. Report of the Grand Jury, 170.

80. Report of the Grand Jury, 168.

81. Report of the Grand Jury, 143, italic emphasis in original, underlining is my addition to demonstrate how the DOH punctuated Gosnell's practices.

82. Report of the Grand Jury, 162.

83. Report of the Grand Jury, 190.

84. Report of the Grand Jury, 175.

85. Report of the Grand Jury, 192.

86. Edbauer, "Unframing Models of Public Distribution," 20.

87. Kimberly K. Emmons, "Uptake and the Biomedical Subject," in *Genre in a Changing World*, ed. Charles Bazerman, Adair Bonini, and Débora Figueiredo (Anderson, SC: Parlor Press, 2009), 139–160.

88. Emmons, "Uptake and the Biomedical Subject," 140, emphasis added.

89. *Oxford English Dictionary*, 2nd. ed. (1989), s.v., "uptake."

90. Here, I draw upon Carolyn R. Miller's formulation of genre as social action, where she argues that "a rhetorically sound definition of genre must be centered not on the substance or the form of discourse but on the action it is used to accomplish." (151) See Carolyn R. Miller, "Genre as Social Action," *Quarterly Journal of Speech* 70, no. 2 (1984): 151–167.

91. Amy D. Propen and Mary Lay Schuster, "Understanding Genre through the Lens of Advocacy: The Rhetorical Work of the Victim Impact Statement," *Written Communication* 27, no. 1 (2010): 5.

92. Propen and Schuster, "Understanding Genre," 9.

93. Jon Hurdle and Trip Gabriel, "Philadelphia Abortion Doctor Guilty of Murder in Late-Term Procedures," *New York Times*, May 13, 2013, https://www.nytimes.com/2013/05/14/us/kermit-gosnell-abortion-doctor-found-guilty-of-murder.html

94. J. N. Salters, "Are All the Women Still White? Kermit Gosnell, 'Back Alley' Abortions, and the Politics of Motherhood," *Feminist Wire*, May 23, 2013, https://thefeministwire.com/2013/05/are-all-the-women-still-white-kermit-gosnell-back-alley-abortions-and-the-politics-of-motherhood/.

95. Hernández and Upton, *Challenging Reproductive Control*, 39.

96. Charmaine Yoest, "How Science, State Laws, and Exposure Are Driving the Pro-life Comeback," *Medium*, July 16, 2015, https://medium.com/2015-index-of-culture-and-opportunity/abortion-rate-total-abortions-563778596c02.

97. Julie Rovner, "A Sharper Abortion Debate after Gosnell Verdict," NPR, May 14,

2013, https://www.npr.org/sections/health-shots/2013/05/14/183911268/a-sharper-abortion-debate-after-gosnell-verdict.

98. Their perception has absolutely no grounding in reality. In addition to Hernández and Upton's news framing analysis that indicated frequent invocation of Gosnell, my own LexisNexis search revealed that the case received copious and impassioned coverage within the Philadelphia metropolitan area beginning with the clinic's raid in 2010 and continuing to the final sentencing of Pearl Gosnell in 2013. Nonetheless, a collective sticking point for anti-abortion activists has been a concern with a lack of coverage for the Gosnell case. Fox News political analyst Kirsten Powers accused "mainstream" news outlets of radio silence on the Gosnell case, asserting that the *New York Times* ran a tucked-away story on the first day of the trial and nothing more. In an appeal to a wide range of ideological affiliations, Powers trumpeted, "You don't have to oppose abortion rights to find late-term abortion abhorrent or to find the Gosnell trial eminently newsworthy. This is not about being 'pro-choice' or 'pro-life.' It's about basic human rights." Kirsten Powers, "Philadelphia Abortion Clinic Horror: Column," *USA Today*, April 11, 2013, https://www.usatoday.com/story/opinion/2013/04/10/philadelphia-abortion-clinic-horror-column/2072577/. One day later, Irin Carmon of *Slate* tracked coverage from feminist news to more mainstream news, showing sustained coverage of the Gosnell case. Irin Carmon, "There Is No Gosnell Cover Up," *Slate*, April 12, 2013, https://www.salon.com/2013/04/12/there_is_no_gosnell_coverup/.

99. Ann McElhinney and Phelim McAleer, "Gosnell Movie," Indigogo, https://www.indiegogo.com/projects/gosnell-movie. The funding campaign has since closed.

100. "The Man Who Interviewed Gosnell: Five Takeaways," *PA Family*, September 4, 2018, https://pafamily.org/2018/09/04/gosnelldocumentary/.

101. Mari Boor Tonn, "Donning Sackcloth and Ashes: *Webster v. Reproductive Health Services* and Moral Agony in Abortion Rights Rhetoric," *Communication Quarterly* 44, no. 3 (1996): 266.

102. Tonn, "Donning Sackcloth and Ashes," 267.

103. Levs, "Gosnell Horror Fuels Fight for Abortion Laws."

104. Silvie Colman and Ted Joyce, "Regulating Abortion: Impact on Patients and Providers in Texas," *Journal of Policy Analysis and Management* 30, no. 4 (2011): 775–797.

105. Brief of the Governors of Texas, Alabama, Arkansas, Iowa, Kentucky, Louisiana, Maine, Mississippi, Nebraska, and South Dakota as Amici Curiae in Support of the Respondents, Whole Woman's Health v. Hellerstedt, 579 U.S. 582 (2016) (No. 15-274), 3, https://gov.texas.gov/uploads/files/press/HB2_02032016.pdf.

106. Brief of the Governors, 7.

107. Ted Cruz, "Cruz, Cornyn Lead Coalition Filing Amicus Brief in Support of Texas HB 2," Cruz.Senate.Gov, February 3, 2016, https://www.cruz.senate.gov/newsroom/press-releases/cruz-cornyn-lead-coalition-filing-amicus-brief-in-support-of-texas-hb-2. Brief of Amici Curiae Bipartisan Group of 174 United States Senators and Members of the United States House of Representatives in Support of the Respondents," *Whole Woman's Health*.

108. Ken Paxton, "Texas Defends Important Women's Health Protections at US Supreme Court," Website of Ken Paxton, Attorney General of Texas, March 2, 2016, https://www.texasattorneygeneral.gov/news/releases/texas-defends-important-womens-health-protections-us-supreme-court.

109. *Whole Woman's Health.*

110. Jen Kinney, "West Philly Abortion Doctor's 'House of Horrors' Listed for Sheriff's Sale. Anti-Choice Activists Want to Buy It," WHYY-PBS, September 13, 2019, https://whyy.org/articles/kermit-gosnells-west-philly-house-of-horrors-could-be-bought-by-anti-abortion-group/.

111. Kinney, "West Philly Abortion."

112. Amy G. Bryant and Jonas Swartz, "Why Crisis Pregnancy Centers Are Legal but Unethical," *AMA Journal of Ethics* 20, no. 3 (2018): 269–277; another statement: Andrea Swartzendruber, Abigail English, Katherine Blumoff Greenberg, Pamela J. Murray, Matt Freeman, Krishna Upadhya, Tina Simpson, Elizabeth Miller, and John Santelli, "Crisis Pregnancy Centers in the United States: Lack of Adherence to Medical and Ethical Practice Standards; A Joint Position Statement of the Society for Adolescent Health and Medicine and the North American Society for Pediatric and Adolescent Gynecology," *Journal of Pediatric and Adolescent Gynecology* 32, no. 6 (2019): 563–566.

113. AlphaCare is a crisis pregnancy center according to the website crisispregnancycentermap.com. This website is part of a project from Andrea Swartzendruber, assistant professor of epidemiology and biostatistics at the University of Georgia.

114. Jay Hobbs, "Meet the New Tenants One Wall Away from Gosnell's Shuttered Clinic," *National Right to Life News Today*, January 11, 2016, https://nrlc.org/nrlnewstoday/2016/01/meet-the-new-tenants-one-wall-away-from-gosnells-shuttered-clinic/.

115. For an excellent consideration of how the Gosnell case was taken up in anti-abortion journalistic coverage after *Whole Woman's Health v. Hellerstedt*, see Hernández and Upton, *Challenging Reproductive Control.*

Conclusion

1. Audra Heinrichs, "HBO Max's *The Janes* Is a Crystal Ball, a Time Machine, and a Warning," *Jezebel*, June 8, 2022, https://jezebel.com/hbo-max-s-the-janes-is-a-crystal-ball-a-time-machine-1848977528.

2. Lauren Berlant, "The Subject of True Feeling: Pain, Privacy, and Politics," in *Cultural Studies and Political Theory*, ed. Jodi Dean (Ithaca, NY: Cornell University Press, 2018), 42–61.

3. Beth Galton and Dana Goodyear, "The Tools and Tactics the Desperate Used to End Unwanted Pregnancies," *Washington Post*, February 10, 2023, https://www.washingtonpost.com/photography/2023/02/10/tools-tactics-desperate-used-end-unwanted-pregnancies/.

4. Ryan Mitchell, "'Whatever Happened to Our Great Gay Imaginations? The Invention of Safe Sex and the Visceral Imagination," *Quarterly Journal of Speech* 107, no. 1 (2021): 26–48.

5. Joffe, *Doctors of Conscience.*

6. Stormer, *Articulating Life's Memory.*

7. Gutierrez-Romine, *From Back-Alley to the Border.*

8. Kalifa, *Vice, Poverty, and Crime.*

9. "Mifepristone (Oral Route)," Mayo Clinic, accessed January 3, 2023, https://www.mayoclinic.org/drugs-supplements/mifepristone-oral-route/side-effects/drg-20067123.

10. Carrie N. Baker, "We Heart: The Giant Abortion Pill Snow Drawing at Sun-

dance, Celebrating Reproductive Autonomy," *Ms.*, January 25, 2023, https://msmagazine.com/2023/01/25/abortion-pill-sundance-film-festival/.

11. Abbe R. Gluck, "The Mifepristone Case and the Legitimacy of the FDA," *JAMA* 329, no. 24 (2023): 2121–2122.

12. Planned Parenthood, "Protest Tips: It's Our Fight, Let's Do It Right," accessed July 4, 2024, https://www.plannedparenthoodaction.org/rightfully-ours/bans-off-our-bodies/protest-tips-lets-do-it-right.

13. Magdalene Taylor, "Can We Stop with the Coat Hanger Imagery," *Mel Magazine* (2022), https://melmagazine.com/en-us/story/coat-hanger-abortion-meme.

14. "Activists Call for Demonstrations Protesting the Sale of Chemical Abortion Pills at Neighborhood Pharmacies," *Standard Newswire*, February 4, 2023, http://standardnewswire.com/news/9464819017.html, emphasis added.

15. Robin E. Jensen, "Improving upon Nature: The Rhetorical Ecology of Chemical Language, Reproductive Endocrinology, and the Medicalization of Infertility," *Quarterly Journal of Speech* 101, no. 2 (2015): 329–353.

16. "Walgreens Statement on Mifepristone," Walgreens Boots Alliance, March 6, 2023, https://news.walgreens.com/press-center/walgreens-statement-on-mifepristone.htm; Emily Olson, "California Will Cut Ties with Walgreens over the Company's Plan to Drop Abortion Pills," NPR, March 7, 2023, https://www.npr.org/2023/03/07/1161590750/california-walgreens-mifepristone-abortion-pill.

17. "US Supreme Court Maintains Abortion Pill Access but Threatens to Undermine Access to Medical Care for All Patients," Gender Justice, June 13, 2024, https://www.genderjustice.us/scotus-maintains-abortion-pill-access/.

18. Johanna Schoen, "Between Choice and Coercion: Women and the Politics of Sterilization in North Carolina, 1929–1975," *Journal of Women's History* 13, no. 1 (2001): 132–156.

19. Natalie Fixmer-Oraiz, "No Going Back: The Struggle for a Post-*Roe* Reproductive Justice," *Quarterly Journal of Speech* 108, no. 4 (2022): 426–430.

20. Berkley Conner, "Menstrual Histories, Reproductive Futures," *Women & Language* 46, no. 1 (2023): 309–313.

21. Ross, "Reproductive Justice as Intersectional," 292.

22. Winderman, "(Never) Going Back," 285.

23. Logan Rae Gomez, "Temporal Containment and the Singularity of Anti-Blackness: Saying Her Name in and across Time,' *Rhetoric Society Quarterly* 51, no. 3 (2021): 188.

24. Tamika L. Carey, "Necessary Adjustments: Black Women's Rhetorical Impatience," *Rhetoric Review* 39, no. 3 (2020): 270, 273.

25. Carey, "Necessary Adjustments," 273.

26. Roberts, *Killing the Black Body*; Goodwin, *Policing the Womb*.

27. Carey, "Necessary Adjustments."

28. Winderman and Knutson, "Florynce Kennedy's Cultivation."

29. Randolph, *Florynce "Flo" Kennedy*, 168.

30. Lauren Rankin, *Bodies on the Line: At the Front Lines of the Fight to Protect Abortion in America* (Berkeley, CA: Counterpoint, 2022).

31. Elaine Chan, Yelena Korotkaya, Vadim Osadchiy, and Aparna Sridhar, "Patient Experiences at California Crisis Pregnancy Centers: A Mixed-Methods Analysis of

Online Crowd-Sourced Reviews, 2010–2019," *Southern Medical Journal* 115, no. 2 (2022): 144–151.

32. Anna Sikoa and Farah Zahra, "Nosocomial Infections," National Library of Medicine, last modified January 23, 2023, https://www.ncbi.nlm.nih.gov/books/NBK559312/.

33. Kelly M. Hoffman, Sophie Trawalter, Jordan R. Axt, M. Normal Oliver, "Racial Bias in Pain Assessment and Treatment Recommendations, and False Beliefs about Biological Differences between Blacks and Whites," *PNAS* 113, no. 16 (2016): 4296–4301.

34. Oluwafunmilayo Akinlade, "Taking Black Pain Seriously," *New England Journal of Medicine* 303, no. 68 (2020), https://www.nejm.org/doi/full/10.1056/NEJMpv2024759.

35. Raquel M. Robvais. "We Are No Longer Invisible." *POROI* 15, no. 1 (2020), https://doi.org/10.13008/2151-2957.1296.

36. The following are just a sampling of studies that have confirmed Akinlade's assertions: Karen O. Anderson, Carmen R. Green, and Richard Payne, "Racial and Ethnic Disparities in Pain: Causes and Consequences of Unequal Care," *Journal of Pain* 10, no. 12 (2009): 1187–1204; Vence L. Bonham, "Race, Ethnicity, and Pain Treatment: Striving to Understand the Causes and Solutions to the Disparities in Pain Treatment," *Journal of Law, Medicine & Ethics* 29, no. 1 (2001): 52–68; Alexie Cintron and R. Sean Morrison, "Pain and Ethnicity in the United States: A Systematic Review," *Journal of Palliative Medicine* 9, no. 6 (2006): 1454–1473; Charles S. Cleeland, Rene Gonin, Luis Baez, Patrick Loehrer, and Kishan J. Pandya, "Pain and Treatment of Pain in Minority Patients with Cancer: The Eastern Cooperative Oncology Group Minority Outpatient Pain Study," *Annals of Internal Medicine* 127, no. 9 (1997): 813–816; Harold P. Freeman and Richard Payne, "Racial Injustice in Health Care," *New England Journal of Medicine* 342, no. 14 (2000): 1045–1047; Monika K. Goyal, Nathan Kuppermann, Sean D. Cleary, Stephen J. Teach, and James M. Chamberlain, "Racial Disparities in Pain Management of Children with Appendicitis in Emergency Departments," *JAMA Pediatrics* 169, no. 11 (2015): 996–1002; Carmen R. Green, Karen O. Anderson, Tamara A. Baker, Lisa C. Campbell, Sheila Decker, Roger B. Fillingim, Donna A. Kaloukalani Kathryn E. Lasch, Cynthia Myers, Raymond C. Tate, et al., "The Unequal Burden of Pain: Confronting Racial and Ethnic Disparities in Pain," *Pain Medicine* 4, no. 3 (2003): 277–294; Vickie L. Shavers, Alexis Bakos, and Vanessa B. Sheppard, "Race, Ethnicity, and Pain among the US Adult Population," *Journal of Health Care for the Poor and Underserved* 21, no. 1 (2010): 177–220; Brian D. Smedley, Adrienne Y. Stith, Alan R. Nelson, *Unequal Treatment: Confronting Racial and Ethnic Disparities in Health Care* (Washington, DC: National Academies Press, 2013); Knox H. Todd, Christi Deaton, Anne P. D'adamo, and Leon Goe, "Ethnicity and Analgesic Practice," *Annals of Emergency Medicine* 35, no. 1 (2000): 11–16.

37. Jensen and Almuaili, "Abortion and Miscarriage are Synonyms."

38. Harper, *The Ethos of Black Motherhood*, 5.

39. The entire interview quoted in this paragraph can be found at Jericka Duncan, Rachel Bailey, Cassandra Gauthier, and Hilary Cook, "Brittany Watts, Ohio Woman Charged with Felony after Miscarriage at Home, Describes Shock of Her Arrest," CBS News, January 26, 2024, https://www.cbsnews.com/news/brittany-watts-the-ohio-woman-charged-with-a-felony-after-a-miscarriage-talks-shock-of-her-arrest/.

40. Solinger, *Beggars and Choosers*.

41. Gibson, "The Rhetoric of *Roe v. Wade*."

42. Ross, "Reproductive Justice as Intersectional," 299.

43. Rachel Bloom-Pojar and Maria Barker, "The Role of Confianza in Community-Engaged Work for Reproductive Justice," *Reflections* 20, no. 2 (2020): 91.

44. "Congresswomen Share Personal Stories of Abortion in Hopes of Bringing Change to Policy Conversation," NBC News, September 29, 2021, https://www.nbcnews.com/now/video/congresswomen-share-personal-stories-of-abortion-ahead-of-testimony-on-the-hill-122316869731.

Manuscript Collections

"Abortion and the Law" (script). *CBS Reports* (aired April 5, 1965). Florynce Kennedy Papers, Box 9, Folder 4, Schlesinger Library, Harvard University, Cambridge, MA.

"Appeal Denial for the *People of the State of Michigan v. Robert Stanley Nixon*" (August 23, 1972). National Abortion Rights Action League, State Affiliate Printed Material Collection, 1969–1989, PR-3, Michigan Folder, Schlesinger Library, Harvard University, Cambridge, MA.

Cisler, Lucinda. "Abortion Law Repeal (Sort of): A Warning to Women" (1970). Papers of the National Abortion Rights Action League, MC 313, Box 4, Folder 3, Schlesinger Library, Harvard University, Cambridge, MA.

Clark, Sam. "A Minneapolis Abortion Mill." *Jim Jam Jems* (April 1912): 12–24. Social Welfare History Archives, University of Minnesota, Minneapolis, MN.

Coalition for Reproductive Freedom. "En el 3 de Octubre, 1977 Rosie Jimenez murio de un aborto ilegal tal como ocurre con la vida de tantas mujeres cada ano." Northeastern University Digital Repository (October 1982). http://hdl.handle.net/2047/D20260044.

Coalition for Reproductive Freedom. "On October 3, 1977 Rosie Jimenez Died from an Illegal, Back-Alley Abortion." Northeastern University Digital Repository (October 1982). http://hdl.handle.net/2047/D20247237.

Coroner's Report of Rebecca Suzanne Bell. Research and Writing for Becky Bell Video re: Parental Consent (October 3, 1988). Toni Carabillo / Judith Meuli Papers, Box 37, Folder 14, Schlesinger Library, Harvard University, Cambridge, MA.

Discussion guide: "Abortion and the Law" (n.d.). Association for the Study of Abortion, Bill Baird Papers, Box 398, Folder 17, Schlesinger Library, Harvard University, Cambridge, MA.

"Do You Want to Return to the Butchery of Back-Alley Abortion?" *Goldflower*, April 1975. Marie Kochaver Women's Movement Collection, SW0358, Box 1, Folder 4, University of Minnesota Social Welfare History Archives, Minneapolis, MN.

The First American Symposium on Office Abortion: The Proceedings of the Symposium on Office Abortion Procedures, San Francisco, May 16, 1970. Society for Human Abortion, SHA Publications MC 289, Box 1, Folder 6, Schlesinger Library, Harvard University, Cambridge, MA.

Fogel, Helen. "I've Performed Hundreds of Abortions." *Detroit Free Press*, December 7, 1969. NARAL State Affiliates Michigan Printed Material, PR-3, Michigan Folder, Schlesinger Library, Harvard University, Cambridge, MA.

Hall, Robert. "Abortions on Demand." *Newsweek*, January 13, 1970. National Abortion Rights Action League State Affiliate Printed Material Collection, 1969–1989, PR-3, New York Folder, Schlesinger Library, Harvard University, Cambridge, MA.

Howe, Larry. "Abortion and the Law: California Report" (December 1966). Society for Humane Abortion, MC289, Box 3, Folder 40, Schlesinger Library, Harvard University, Cambridge, MA.

Howe, Larry. "Critique of the Script: Abortion and the Law: California Report" (December 1966). Society for Humane Abortion, MC289, Box 3, Folder 40, Schlesinger Library, Harvard University, Cambridge, MA.

Maginnis, Patricia T. *The Abortee's Songbook* (1969). Society for Humane Abortion, MC289, Box 1, Folder 6, Schlesinger Library, Harvard University, Cambridge, MA.

Maginnis, Patricia T. "Opening Remarks at the First American Symposium on Office Abortion," *The Proceedings of the Symposium on Office Abortion Procedures, San Francisco, May 16, 1970*. Society for Human Abortion, SHA Publications MC 289, Box 1, Folder 6, Schlesinger Library, Harvard University, Cambridge MA, 1–2.

Means, Cyril C., Jr. "Statement at a Press Conference of the National Association for Repeal of Abortion Laws, Hotel Sonesta, Washington D.C." (October 4, 1971). National Association for Repeal of Abortion Laws, Box 1, Folder 5, Schlesinger Library, Harvard University, Cambridge, MA.

Mediclinic. "Ambulatory Surgical Clinics" (1973). Florynce Kennedy Papers MC 555 Reproductive Rights, Research, Press Releases, Schlesinger Library, Harvard University, Cambridge, MA.

National Abortion Rights Action League. "Introduction to Debating" (n.d. [1973–1975]). NARAL Literature, 1973–75, MC 313 Box 1, Folder 21, Schlesinger Library, Harvard University, Cambridge, MA.

Phelan, Lana Clarke. "Luncheon Address." In *Proceedings of the Symposium on Office Abortion Procedures* (May 16, 1970). Papers of the Society for Humane Abortion, MC 289, Box 1, Folder 6, Schlesinger Library, Harvard University, Cambridge, MA.

"Redstockings Abortion Speakout." Redstockings Women's Liberation Archives for Action (March 21, 1969). Archive.org. https://archive.org/details/Redstockings AbortionSpeakoutNewYork1969March21.

Society for Humane Abortion Newsletter 1, no. 4 (December 1965). Society for Humane Abortion Newsletters, 1965–1973, MC 289, Box 1, Folder 4, Schlesinger Library, Harvard University, Cambridge, MA.

"Statement of Edgar B. Keemer Jr. M.D." (October 4, 1971). National Association for the Repeal of Abortion Laws, Box 1, Folder 5, Schlesinger Library, Harvard University, Cambridge, MA.

Willke, J. C. "Becky Bell Did Not Die from an Induced Abortion." *National Right to Life News*, October 2, 1990. Papers of Teresa Vaughn, Box 3, Folder 12, Schlesinger Library, Harvard University, Cambridge, MA.

"Women's Health Consumer's Union to Combat behind-the-Scenes Anti-abortion Conspiracy" (March 23, 1973). Florynce Kennedy Papers MC 555 Reproductive

Rights, Research, Press Releases, Schlesinger Library, Harvard University, Cambridge, MA.

Newspapers and Magazines

Baltimore Sun
Colorado Springs Gazette-Telegraph
Ebony
Jet
Jezebel
Ms.
New York Times
Playboy
Washington Post

Governmental Documents

Abortion Control Act of 1982 No. 138 1982 Pa Laws 476 (Codified at 18 Pa Cons. Stat. Ann. § 3201-3220).
Child Custody Protection Act, H.R. 3682, 105th Cong. §2, (1998). https://www.congress.gov/bill/105th-congress/house-bill/3682.
Report of the Grand Jury, *In re* County Investigating Grand Jury XXIII, Misc. No. 0009901–2008. (First Jud. Dist. of PA, January 21, 2011). http://perma.cc/7QD3-B8KE.

Books, Book Chapters, Articles, and Online Materials

"The Abortion Menace." *Ebony* 6 (January 1951).
"Activists Call for Demonstrations Protesting the Sale of Chemical Abortion Pills at Neighborhood Pharmacies." *Standard Newswire*, February 4, 2023, http://www.standardnewswire.com/news/8952918865.html.
Adams, Heather Brook. *Enduring Shame: A Recent History of Unwed Pregnancy and Righteous Reproduction*. Columbia: University of South Carolina Press, 2022.
Adams, Heather Brook. "Rhetorics of Unwed Motherhood and Shame." *Women's Studies in Communication* 40, no. 1 (2017): 91–110.
Ahmed, Sara. *Cultural Politics of Emotion*. Edinburgh: Edinburgh University Press, 2004.
Ahmed, Sara. *Living a Feminist Life*. Durham, NC: Duke University Press, 2017.
Ahmed, Sara. *Strange Encounters: Embodied Others in Post-coloniality*. London: Routledge, 2000.
Ainsworth-Vaugn, Nancy. "The Discourse of Medical Encounters." In *The Handbook of Discourse Analysis*, edited by Deborah Schiffrin, Deborah Tannen, and Heidi E. Hamilton, 453–469. Malden, MA: Blackwell, 2005.
Akinlade, Oluwafunmilayo. "Taking Black Pain Seriously." *New England Journal of Medicine* 303, no. 68 (2020). https://www.nejm.org/doi/full/10.1056/NEJMpv2024759.
Allen, Michelle. "From Cesspool to Sewer: Sanitary Reform and the Rhetoric of Resistance, 1848–1880." *Victorian Literature and Culture* 30, no. 2 (2002): 383–402.
"Alley Improvement Association, Washington D.C." In *Organizing Black America: An*

Encyclopedia of African American Associations, edited by Nina Mjagkij, 25. New York: Routledge, 2010.

Anderson, Ben. *Encountering Affect: Capacities, Apparatuses, Conditions*. New York: Routledge, 2017.

Anderson, Karen O., Carmen R. Green, and Richard Payne. "Racial and Ethnic Disparities in Pain: Causes and Consequences of Unequal Care." *Journal of Pain* 10, no. 12 (2009): 1187–1204.

Amsden, Brian S. "Performing Maturity in the Parental Consent and Notification Judicial Bypass Procedure." *Communication and Critical/Cultural Studies* 12, no. 1 (2015): 1–18.

Anzaldúa, Gloria. *Borderlands: The New Mestiza—La Frontera*. Vol. 3. San Francisco: Aunt Lute Books, 1987.

Arnold, Amanda. "How a Harrowing Photo of One Woman's Death Became an Iconic Pro-choice Symbol." *Vice*, October 26, 2016. https://www.vice.com/en/article/evgdpw/how-a-harrowing-photo-of-one-womans-death-became-an-iconic-pro-choice-symbol.

Badour, Christal L., and Thomas G. Adams. "Contaminated by Trauma: Understanding Links Between Self-Disgust, Mental Contamination, and Post-traumatic Stress Disorder." In *The Revolting Self*, 127–149. New York: Routledge, 2018.

Balaji, Murali. "Racializing Pity: The Haiti Earthquake and the Plight of 'Others.'" *Critical Studies in Media Communication* 28, no. 1 (2011): 50–67.

Baker, Carrie N. "We Heart: The Giant Abortion Pill Snow Drawing at Sundance, Celebrating Reproductive Autonomy." *Ms.*, January 25, 2023. https://msmagazine.com/2023/01/25/abortion-pill-sundance-film-festival/.

Barnes, David S. *The Great Stink of Paris and the Nineteenth-Century Struggle against Filth and Germs*. Baltimore: John Hopkins University Press, 2006.

Bashford, Alison. *Purity and Pollution: Gender, Embodiment, and Victorian Medicine*. Studies in Gender History. London: Palgrave Macmillan, 1998.

Bates, Jerome E. "The Abortion Mill: An Institutional Study." *Journal of Criminal Law, Criminology, and Police Science* 45, no. 2 (1954): 157.

Beisel, Nicola, and Tamara Kay. "Abortion, Race, and Gender in Nineteenth-Century America." *American Sociological Review* 69 (2004): 498–518.

Bell, Amy Helen. "Abortion Crime Scene Photography in London, 1950–1968." *Social History of Medicine* 30, no. 3 (2017): 661–684.

Bennett, Jeffrey A. *Banning Queer Blood: Rhetorics of Citizenship, Contagion, and Resistance*. Tuscaloosa: University of Alabama Press, 2015.

Berglas, Nancy F., and Sarah C. M. Roberts. "The Development of Facility Standards for Common Outpatient Procedures and Implications for the Context of Abortion." *BMC Health Services Research* 18, no. 212 (2018). https://doi.org/10.1186/s12913-018-3048-3.

Bergsmark, Daniel R. "Minneapolis, the Mill City." *Economic Geography* 3, no. 3 (1927): 391–396.

Berland, Lauren, "The Subject of True Feeling: Pain, Privacy, and Politics." In *Cultural Studies and Political Theory*, edited by Jodi Dean, 42–61. Ithaca, NY: Cornell University Press, 2018.

Bessette, Jean. "Queer Rhetoric in Situ." *Rhetoric Review* 35, no. 2 (2016): 148–164.

Betancourt, Victoria Gómez. "Rosie and Me: Remembering the Hyde Amendment's First Victim." *Rewire News Group*. October 3, 2017. https://rewirenewsgroup.com/article/2017/10/03/rosie-remembering-hyde-amendments-first-victim/.

Biehler, Dawn Day. *Pests in the City: Flies, Bedbugs, Cockroaches, and Rats*. Seattle: University of Washington Press, 2013.

Bloom-Pojar, Rachel, and Maria Barker. "The Role of Confianza in Community-Engaged Work for Reproductive Justice." *Reflections* 20, no. 2 (2020): 84–101.

Bonham, Vence L. "Race, Ethnicity, and Pain Treatment: Striving to Understand the Causes and Solutions to the Disparities in Pain Treatment." *Journal of Law, Medicine & Ethics* 29, no. 1 (2001): 52–68.

Borchert, James. *Alley Life in Washington: Family, Community, Religion, and Folklife in the City, 1850–1970*. Vol. 82. Champaign: University of Illinois Press, 1982.

Brandes Gratz, Roberta. "Never Again." *Ms.*, April 1973.

Brandes Gratz, Roberta. "She Had a Name. She Had a Family. She Was Leona's Sister Gerri." *Ms.*, November/December 1995.

Bremner, Robert H. *From the Depths: The Discovery of Poverty in the United States*. New Brunswick, NJ: Transaction, 1956.

Brennan, Teresa. *The Transmission of Affect*. Ithaca, NY: Cornell University Press, 2004.

Bridges, Khiara M. *The Poverty of Privacy Rights*. Palo Alto, CA: Stanford University Press, 2017.

Briggs, Laura. *How All Politics Became Reproductive Politics: From Welfare Reform to Foreclosure to Trump*. Oakland: University of California Press, 2017.

Briggs, Laura. *Reproducing Empire: Race, Sex, Science, and U.S. Imperialism in Puerto Rico*. Berkeley: University of California Press, 2002.

Brodie, Janet Farrell. *Contraception and Abortion in Nineteenth-Century America*. Ithaca, NY: Cornell University Press, 1994.

"Brotherly Love: Health of Black Men and Boys in Philadelphia." City of Philadelphia, March 14, 2019. https://www.phila.gov/media/20190314105459/Brotherly-Love_Health-Of-Black-Men-And-Boys_3_19.pdf.

Brown, Elizabeth J., Daniel Polsky, Corentin M. Barbu, Jane W. Seymour, and David Grande. "Racial Disparities in Geographic Access to Primary Care in Philadelphia." *Health Affairs* 35, no. 8 (2016): 1374–1381.

Brown, Korey Bowers. "Souled Out: 'Ebony' Magazine in an Age of Black Power, 1965–1975." PhD diss. Howard University, 2010.

Brown, Lori A. *Contested Spaces: Abortion Clinics, Women's Shelters, and Hospitals: Politicizing the Female Body*. New York: Routledge, 2016.

Bruce, Caitlin Frances. *Painting Publics: Transnational Legal Graffiti Scenes as Spaces for Encounter*. Philadelphia: Temple University Press, 2019.

Bryant, Amy G., and Jonas Swartz. "Why Crisis Pregnancy Centers Are Legal but Unethical." *AMA Journal of Ethics* 20, no. 3 (2018): 269–277.

Buntline, Ned. *Mysteries and Miseries of New York: A Story of Real Life*. New York: W. F. Burgess, 1849.

Burke, Kenneth. *A Grammar of Motives*. Berkeley: University of California Press, 1945.

Burns, Lisa M. "Ellen Axson Wilson: A Rhetorical Reassessment of a Forgotten First Lady." In *Inventing a Voice: The Rhetoric of American First Ladies of the Twentieth Century*, edited by Molly Meijer Wertheimer, 79–102. Lanham, MD: Rowman & Littlefield, 2004.

Byrne, P. S., and B. E. L. Long. *Doctors Talking to Patients.* London: Department of Health and Social Security, 1976.

Calafell, Bernadette Marie. *Monstrosity, Performance, and Race in Contemporary Culture.* New York: Peter Lang, 2015.

Campanella, Juan José. *Lifestories: Families in Crisis.* Season 1, episode 3, "Public Law 106: The Becky Bell Story." Bruce Harmon, writer. Aired August 15, 1992, in broadcast syndication. HBO.

Caplan-Bricker, Nora. "The Kermit Gosnell Effect: How His Gruesome Trial Is Helping Anti-abortion Legislation in Far-Away States." *New Republic*, April 30, 2013. https://newrepublic.com/article/113052/kermit-gosnell-trial-how-pro-lifers-are-using-him-pass-new-laws.

Carey, Tamika L. "Necessary Adjustments: Black Women's Rhetorical Impatience." *Rhetoric Review* 39, no. 3 (2020): 269–286.

Casper, Monica J. *The Making of the Unborn Patient: A Social Anatomy of Fetal Surgery.* New Brunswick, NJ: Rutgers University Press, 1998.

Ceccarelli, Leah. "Neither Confusing Cacophony nor Culinary Complements: A Case Study of Mixed Metaphors for Genomic Science." *Written Communication* 21, no. 1 (2004): 92–105.

Chambers, Jason. "Presenting the Black Middle Class: John H. Johnson and *Ebony* Magazine, 1945–1974." In *Historicizing Lifestyle: Mediating Taste, Consumption and Identity from the 1900s to 1970s*, edited by David Bell and Joanna Hollows, 54–69. Burlington, VT: Ashgate, 2006.

Chambers, Robert. *The Book of Days: A Miscellany of Popular Antiquities in Connection with the Calendar, Including Anecdote, Biography, and History Curiosities of Literature and Oddities of Human Life and Character.* London: W&R Chambers, 1863.

Chan, Elaine, Yelena Korotkaya, Vadim Osadchiy, and Aparna Sridhar. "Patient Experiences at California Crisis Pregnancy Centers: A Mixed-Methods Analysis of Online Crowd-Sourced Reviews, 2010–2019." *Southern Medical Journal* 115, no. 2 (2022): 144–151.

Charland, Maurice. "Constitutive Rhetoric: The Case of the *Peuple Québécois.*" *Quarterly Journal of Speech* 73, no. 2 (1987): 133–150.

Chávez, Karma R. "The Body: An Abstract and Actual Rhetorical Concept." *Rhetoric Society Quarterly* 48, no. 3 (2018): 242–250.

Chávez, Karma R. *The Borders of AIDS: Race, Quarantine, and Resistance.* Seattle: University of Washington Press, 2021.

Cintron, Alexie, and R. Sean Morrison. "Pain and Ethnicity in the United States: A Systematic Review." *Journal of Palliative Medicine* 9, no. 6 (2006): 1454–1473.

Cisneros, Josue David. *The Border Crossed Us: Rhetorics of Borders, Citizenship, and Latina/o Identity.* Tuscaloosa: University of Alabama Press, 2013.

Clark-Lewis, Elizabeth. *Living In, Living Out: African American Domestics in Washington D.C., 1910–1940.* Washington, DC: Smithsonian Institution Press, 1994.

Cleeland, Charles S., Rene Gonin, Luis Baez, Patrick Loehrer, and Kishan J. Pandya.

"Pain and Treatment of Pain in Minority Patients with Cancer: The Eastern Cooperative Oncology Group Minority Outpatient Pain Study." *Annals of Internal Medicine* 127, no. 9 (1997): 813–816.

Cobrin, Alain. *The Foul and the Fragrant: Odor and the French Social Imagination.* Cambridge, MA: Harvard University Press, 2006.

Cohen, Jeffrey Jerome. Introduction to *Monster Theory: Reading Culture.* Minneapolis: University of Minnesota Press, 1996.

Collins, Patricia Hill. *Black Feminist Thought: Knowledge, Consciousness, and the Politics of Empowerment.* New York: Routledge, 2022.

Collins, Patricia Hill. "It's All in the Family: Intersections of Gender, Race, and Nation." *Hypatia* 13, no. 3 (1998): 62–82.

Colman, Silvie, and Ted Joyce. "Regulating Abortion: Impact on Patients and Providers in Texas." *Journal of Policy Analysis and Management* 30, no. 4 (2011): 775–797.

Combahee River Collective. "The Combahee River Collective Statement." In *Home Girls: A Black Feminist Anthology*, edited by Barbara Smith, 264–274. New Brunswick, NJ: Rutgers University Press, 1983.

Conaboy, Chelsea. "Doctor's Long Tumble to Jail." *Philadelphia Inquirer*, January 23, 2011. http://articles.philly.com/2011-01-23/news/27044753_1_abortion-clinic-methadone-clinic-abortion-practice.

Condit, Celeste Michelle. *Decoding Abortion Rhetoric: Communicating Social Change.* Champaign: University of Illinois Press, 1992.

"Congresswomen Share Personal Stories of Abortion in Hopes of Bringing Change to Policy Conversation," NBC News, September 29, 2021. https://www.nbcnews.com/now/video/congresswomen-share-personal-stories-of-abortion-ahead-of-testimony-on-the-hill-122316869731.

Conner, Berkley. "Menstrual Histories, Reproductive Futures." *Women & Language* 46, no. 1 (2023): 309–313.

Conquergood, Dwight. "Life in Big Red: Struggles and Accommodations in a Chicago Polyethnic Tenement." *Structuring Diversity: Ethnographic Perspectives on the New Immigration* (1992): 95–144.

Cooper, Brittney. "Intersectionality." In *The Oxford Handbook of Feminist Theory*, edited by Lisa Disch and Mary Hawkesworth, 385–406. New York: Oxford University Press, 2016.

Cooper, Thia. "Achieving Reproductive Justice." In *Taking It to the Streets: Public Theologies of Activism and Resistance*, edited by Jennifer Baldwin, 129–146. Lanham, MD: Lexington Books, 2018.

Cram, Emerson. "Archival Ambience and Sensory Memory: Generating Queer Intimacies in the Settler Colonial Archive." *Communication and Critical/Cultural Studies* 13, no. 2 (2016): 109–129.

Cram, Emerson. *Violent Inheritance: Sexuality, Land, and Energy in Making the North American West.* Berkeley: University of California Press, 2022.

Crenshaw, Kimberlé Williams. "Demarginalizing the Intersection of Race and Sex: A Black Feminist Critique of Antidiscrimination Doctrine, Feminist Theory, and Antiracist Politics." *University of Chicago Legal Forum* (1989): 139–167.

Cruz, Ted. "Cruz, Cornyn Lead Coalition Filing Amicus Brief in Support of Texas HB 2" (press release). Cruz.Senate.Gov. February 3, 2016. https://www.cruz.senate.gov

/newsroom/press-releases/cruz-cornyn-lead-coalition-filing-amicus-brief-in-support-of-texas-hb-2.

Daly, Tyne. "Speech at the 2004 March for Women's Lives on Becky Bell." April 25, 2004, Washington, DC. C-SPAN. 02:40:31. https://www.c-span.org/video/?181451-1/march-womens-lives.

Davis, Angela. "Racism, Birth Control and Reproductive Rights." In *Women, Race and Class*. London: Women's Press; New York: Random House, 1982.

Davis, Dána-Ain. "Obstetric Racism: The Racial Politics of Pregnancy, Labor, and Birthing." *Medical Anthropology* 38, no. 7 (2019): 560–573.

Davis, Dána Ain. *Reproductive Injustice*. New York: New York University Press, 2019.

de Onís, Catalina (Kathleen) M. "Lost in Translation: Challenging (White, Monolingual Feminism's) <Choice> with *Justicia Reproductiva*." *Women's Studies in Communication* 38 (2015): 1–19.

de Onís, Catalina M. "Reproductive Justice as Environmental Justice: Contexts, Coalitions, and Cautions." In *The Routledge Companion to Motherhood*, 496–509. New York: Routledge, 2019.

Derkatch, Colleen. *Bounding Biomedicine: Evidence and Rhetoric in the New Science of Alternative Medicine*. Chicago: University of Chicago Press, 2019.

Derkatch, Colleen. "Method as Argument: Boundary Work in Evidence-Based Medicine." *Social Epistemology* 22, no. 4 (2008): 371–388.

Dickinson, Greg, Carole Blair, and Brian L. Ott. *Places of Public Memory: The Rhetoric of Museums and Memorials*. Tuscaloosa: University of Alabama Press, 2010.

Douglas, Mary. *Purity and Danger: An Analysis of Concept of Pollution and Taboo*. United Kingdom: Routledge, 1966.

Dowland, Seth. "'Family Values' and the Formation of a Christian Right Agenda." *Church History* 78, no. 3 (2009): 606–631.

Downing, Savannah Greer. "Toward Reproductive Justice Rhetorics of Care: State Senator Jen Jordan's Dissent of Georgia's Heartbeat Bill." *Quarterly Journal of Speech* 109, no. 4 (2023): 376–399.

Du Bois, W. E. B., and Isabel Eaton. *The Philadelphia Negro: A Social Study*. Publications of the University of Pennsylvania. Series in Political Economy and Public Law, no. 14. Philadelphia: Published for the University, 1899. https://catalog.hathitrust.org/Record/001263090.

Dubow, Sara. *Ourselves Unborn: A History of the Fetus in Modern America*. Oxford: Oxford University Press, 2010.

Dubriwny, Tasha. "Consciousness-Raising as Collective Rhetoric: The Articulation of Experience in the Redstockings' Abortion Speak-Out of 1969." *Quarterly Journal of Speech* 91, no. 4 (2005): 395–422.

Duden, Barbara. *Disembodying Women: Perspectives on Pregnancy and the Unborn*. Cambridge, MA: Harvard University Press, 1993.

Dudley-Shotwell, Hannah. *Revolutionizing Women's Healthcare: The Feminist Self-Help Movement in America*. New Brunswick, NJ: Rutgers University Press, 2020.

Duncan, Jericka, Rachel Bailey, Cassandra Gauthier, and Hilary Cook. "Brittany Watts, Ohio Woman Charged with Felony after Miscarriage at Home, Describes Shock of Her Arrest." *CBS News*, January 26, 2024. https://www.cbsnews.com/news/brittany

-watts-the-ohio-woman-charged-with-a-felony-after-a-miscarriage-talks-shock-of-her-arrest/.

Dunn, Thomas R. "Remembering 'a Great Fag': Visualizing Public Memory and the Construction of Queer Space." *Quarterly Journal of Speech* 97, no. 4 (2011): 435–460.

Edbauer, Jenny. "Unframing Models of Public Distribution: From Rhetorical Situation to Rhetorical Ecologies." *Rhetoric Society Quarterly* 35, no. 4 (2005): 5–24.

Edwell, Jennifer, Sarah Ann Singer, and Jordynn Jack. "Healing Arts: Rhetorical *Techne* as Medical (Humanities) Intervention." *Technical Communication Quarterly* 27, no. 1 (2018): 50–63.

Ellis, Cassidy D. "'Doctors Don't Kill Babies! Monsters Do!': Using Performance and Personal Narrative to Identify the U.S. Abortion Monster." *Text and Performance Quarterly* 42, no. 1 (2022): 67–82.

Emmons, Kimberly K. "Uptake and the Biomedical Subject." In *Genre in a Changing World*, edited by Charles Bazerman, Adair Bonini, and Débora Figueiredo, 154–181. Anderson, SC: Parlor Press, 2009.

Enck-Wanzer, Darrel. "Health and Hospitals." In *The Young Lords: A Reader*, edited by Darrel Enck-Wanzer, 188–201. New York: New York University Press, 2010. *See also* Wanzer-Serrano, Darrel.

Enck-Wanzer, Darrel. "Trashing the System: Social Movement, Intersectional Rhetoric, and Collective Agency in the Young Lords Organization's Garbage Offensive." *Quarterly Journal of Speech* 92, no. 2 (2006): 183. *See also* Wanzer-Serrano, Darrel.

Endres, Danielle, and Samantha Senda-Cook. "Location Matters: The Rhetoric of Place in Protest." *Quarterly Journal of Speech* 97, no. 3 (2011): 259–260.

Enoch, Jessica. "Survival Stories: Feminist Historiographic Approaches to Chicana Rhetorics of Sterilization Abuse." *Rhetoric Society Quarterly* 35, no. 3 (2005): 5–30.

Etienne, Harley F. *Pushing Back the Gates: Neighborhood Perspectives on University-Driven Revitalization in West Philadelphia*. Philadelphia: Temple University Press, 2012.

Fair, Freda L. "Surveilling Social Difference: Black Women's 'Alley Work' in Industrializing Minneapolis." *Surveillance & Society* 15, no. 5 (2017): 655–675.

Feld, Stephen. "Places Sensed, Senses Placed: Toward a Sensuous Epistemology of Environments." In *Empire of the Senses: The Sensual Culture Reader*, edited by David Howes, 179–191. Oxford: Berg, 2005.

Finnegan, Cara A. "Doing Rhetorical History of the Visual: The Photograph and the Archive." In *Defining Visual Rhetorics*, edited by Charles A. Hill and Marguerite Helmers, 195–214. Mahwah, NJ: Lawrence Erlbaum, 2003.

Fixmer-Oraiz, Natalie. *Homeland Maternity: US Security Culture and the New Reproductive Regime*. Champaign: University of Illinois Press, 2019.

Fixmer-Oraiz, Natalie. "No Going Back: The Struggle for a Post-*Roe* Reproductive Justice." *Quarterly Journal of Speech* 108, no. 4 (2022): 426–430.

Fixmer-Oraiz, Natalie, and Shui-yin Sharon Yam. "Queer(ing) Reproductive Justice." *Oxford Encyclopedia of Queer Studies and Communication*, edited by Isaac West, Emerson Cram. Frederick Dhanens, Pamela Lannutti, and Gust A. Yep, 713–731. New York: Oxford University Press, 2024.

Fleury, Sonia. "Brazil's Health-Care Reform: Social Movements and Civil Society." *Lancet* 377, no. 9779 (2011): 1724–1725.

Flores, Lisa A. *Deportable and Disposable: Public Rhetoric and the Making of the "Illegal" Immigrant.* University Park: Pennsylvania State University Press, 2020.

"Focus on the Family Historical Timeline." Focus on the Family. Accessed May 7, 2024. https://www.focusonthefamily.com/about/historical-timeline/.

Foucault, Michel. *Birth of the Clinic: An Archaeology of Medical Perception.* Translated by A. M. Sheridan Smith. New York: Vintage Books, 1973/1994.

Frank, Gillian. "The Miseries and Heartbreak of Backstreet Abortions: Before and after *Roe*." *NursingClio,* March 28, 2017. https://nursingclio.org/2017/03/28/the-miseries-and-heartbreak-of-backstreet-abortions-before-and-after-roe/#footnote1.

Frankfort, Ellen. *Rosie: The Investigation of a Wrongful Death.* New York: Dial Press, 1979.

Freeman, Harold P., and Richard Payne. "Racial Injustice in Health Care." *New England Journal of Medicine* 342, no. 14 (2000): 1045–1047.

Galton, Beth, and Dana Goodyear. "The Tools and Tactics the Desperate Used to End Unwanted Pregnancies." *Washington Post,* February 10, 2023. https://www.washingtonpost.com/photography/2023/02/10/tools-tactics-desperate-used-end-unwanted-pregnancies/.

Gamble, Vanessa Northington. *Making a Place for Ourselves: The Black Hospital Movement, 1920–1945.* Oxford: Oxford University Press, 1995.

Gamble, Vanessa Northington. "Under the Shadow of Tuskegee: African Americans and Healthcare." *American Journal of Public Health* 87 (1997): 1773–1778.

García, Rocío R. "'We're Not All Anti-choices': How Controlling Images Shape Latina/x Feminist Abortion Advocacy." *Sociological Perspectives* 65, no. 6 (2022): 1208–1227.

Geist, Patricia, and Jennifer Dreyer. "The Demise of Dialogue: A Critique of Medical Encounter Ideology." *Western Journal of Communication* 57, no. 2 (1993): 233–246.

Gibson, Katie L. "The Rhetoric of *Roe v. Wade*: When the (Male) Doctor Knows Best." *Southern Communication Journal* 73, no. 4 (2008): 312–331.

Gieryn, Thomas F. "Boundary-Work and the Demarcation of Science from Non-science: Strains and Interests in Professional Ideologies of Scientists." *American Sociological Review* (1983): 781–795.

Gluck, Abbe R. "The Mifepristone Case and the Legitimacy of the FDA." *JAMA* 329, no. 24 (2023): 2121–2122.

Goffman, Erving. *Stigma: Notes on the Management of a Spoiled Identity.* New York: Simon & Schuster, 1963.

Gomez, Logan Rae. "Temporal Containment and the Singularity of Anti-Blackness: Saying Her Name in and across Time." *Rhetoric Society Quarterly* 51, no. 3 (2021): 182–192.

Goode, Keisha, and Barbara Katz Rothman. "African American Midwifery, a History and a Lament." *American Journal of Economics and Sociology* 76, no. 1 (2017): 65–94.

Goodwin, Michele. *Policing the Womb: Invisible Women and the Criminalization of Motherhood.* New York: Cambridge University Press, 2020.

Gordon, Cynthia. "Framing and Positioning." In *The Handbook of Discourse Analysis,* 2nd ed., edited by Deborah Tannen, Heidi E. Hamilton, and Deborah Schiffrin, 324–345. Malden, MA: Wiley Blackwell, 2015.

Gould, Deborah B. *Moving Politics: Emotion and ACT UP's Fight against AIDS.* Chicago: University of Chicago Press, 2009.

Goyal, Monika K., Nathan Kuppermann, Sean D. Cleary, Stephen J. Teach, and James M. Chamberlain. "Racial Disparities in Pain Management of Children with Appendicitis in Emergency Departments." *JAMA Pediatrics* 169, no. 11 (2015): 996–1002.

Graybill, Lela. "The Forensic Eye and the Public Mind: The Bertillon System of Crime Scene Photography." *Cultural History* 8, no. 1 (2019): 94–119.

Green, Carmen R., Karen O. Anderson, Tamara A. Baker, Lisa C. Campbell, Sheila Decker, Roger B. Fillingim, Donna A. Kaloukalani, Kathryn E. Lasch, Cynthia Myers, Raymond C. Tate, et al. "The Unequal Burden of Pain: Confronting Racial and Ethnic Disparities in Pain." *Pain Medicine* 4, no. 3 (2003): 277–294.

Green, Constance McLaughlin. *The Secret City: A History of Race Relations in the Nation's Capital*. Princeton, NJ: Princeton University Press, 1967.

Greenberger, Marcia D., and Katherine Connor. "Parental Notice and Consent for Abortion: Out of Step with Family Law Principles and Policies." *Family Planning Perspectives* 23, no. 1 (1991): 31–35.

Greenhouse, Linda, and Reva B. Siegel. "*Casey* and the Clinic Closings: When 'Protecting Health' Obstructs Choice." *Yale Law Journal* 549 (2015): 1428–1480.

Gutierrez-Romine, Alicia. *From Back-Alley to the Border: Criminal Abortion in California: 1920–1969*. Lincoln: University of Nebraska Press, 2020.

Guzmán, Isabel Molina, and Angharad N. Valdivia. "Brain, Brow, and Booty: Latina Iconicity in U.S. Popular Culture." *Communication Review* 7, no. 2 (2004): 205–221.

Hahner, Leslie A. *To Become an American: Immigrants and Americanization Campaigns of the Early Twentieth Century*. East Lansing: Michigan State University Press, 2017.

Hall, Stuart. "Lecture 8: Culture, Resistance, and Struggle." In *Cultural Studies 1983: A Theoretical History*, edited by Jennifer Daryl Slack and Lawrence Grossberg, 180–206. Durham, NC: Duke University Press, 2016.

Halliday, Stephen. "Death and Miasma in Victorian London: An Obstinate Belief." *British Medical Journal* 323, no. 7327 (2001): 1469–1471.

Hallsby, Atilla. "Recanonizing Rhetoric: The Secret *in* and *of* Discourse." *Journal for the History of Rhetoric* 25, no. 3 (2022): 346–370.

Hamilakis, Yannis. *Archaeology and the Senses: Human Experience, Memory, and Affect*. New York: Cambridge University Press, 2014.

Hardeman, Rachel R., Tongtan Chantarat, Morrison Luke Smith, David C. Van Riper, and Dara D. Mendez. "Association of Residence in High–Police Contact Neighborhoods with Preterm Birth among Black and White Individuals in Minneapolis." *JAMA Network Open* 4, no. 12 (2021): e2130290–e2130290.

Harper, Kimberly C. *The Ethos of Black Motherhood in America: Only White Women Get Pregnant*. Lanham, MD: Lexington Books, 2020.

Hartouni, Valerie. "Fetal Exposures: Abortion Politics and the Optics of Allusion." *Camera Obscura: Feminism, Culture, and Media Studies* 10, no. 2 (1992): 130–149.

Hasian, Marouf, Jr., Celeste Michelle Condit, and John Louis Lucaites. "The Rhetorical Boundaries of 'the Law': A Consideration of the Rhetorical Culture of Legal Practice and the Case of the 'Separate but Equal' Doctrine." *Quarterly Journal of Speech* 82, no.4 (1996): 323–342.

Hawhee, Debra. "Looking into Aristotle's Eyes: Toward a Theory of Rhetorical Vision." *Advances in the History of Rhetoric* 14, no. 2 (2011): 139–165.

Hawhee, Debra. *Rhetoric in Tooth and Claw: Animals, Language, Sensation.* Chicago: University of Chicago Press, 2017.

Hawhee, Debra. "Rhetoric's Sensorium." *Quarterly Journal of Speech* 101, no. 1 (2014): 2–17.

Hawhee, Debra, and Christa J. Olson. "Pan-historiography: The Challenges of Writing History across Time and Space." In *Theorizing Histories of Rhetoric,* 90–105. Carbondale: Southern Illinois University Press, 2013.

Hayden, Sara. "Family Metaphors and the Nation: Promoting a Politics of Care through the Million Mom March." *Quarterly Journal of Speech* 89, no. 3 (2003): 196–215.

Hayden, Sara. "Revitalizing the Debate between <Life> and <Choice>: The 2004 March for Women's Lives." *Communication and Critical/Cultural Studies* 6, no. 2 (2009): 111–131.

Hayes, Heather Ashley. "Doing Rhetorical Studies in Situ: The Nomad Citizen in Jordan." *Advances in the History of Rhetoric* 20, no. 2 (2017): 167.

Heinrichs, Audra. "HBO Max's *The Janes* Is a Crystal Ball, a Time Machine, and a Warning." *Jezebel,* June 8, 2022. https://jezebel.com/hbo-max-s-the-janes-is-a-crystal-ball-a-time-machine-1848977528.

Heller, Heidi. "Minneapolis 'Alleywalkers' and the Campaign to End Prostitution." Minneapolis Project, July 1, 2024. https://historyapolis.com/2014/07/01/minneapolis-alleywalkers-and-the-campaign-to-end-prostitution/index.html.

Hernández, Leandra Hinojosa, and Marleah Dean. "'I Felt Very Discounted': Negotiation of Caucasian and Hispanic/Latina Women's Bodily Ownership and Expertise in Patient-Provider Interactions." In *Interrogating Gendered Pathologies,* edited by Erin Clark and Michelle F. Eble, 101–120. Louisville: University Press of Colorado, 2020.

Hernández, Leandra Hinojosa, and Sarah De Los Santos Upton. *Challenging Reproductive Control and Gendered Violence in the Américas: Intersectionality, Power, and Struggles for Rights.* Lanham, MD: Lexington, 2018.

Hernández, Leandra Hinojosa, and Sarah De Los Santos Upton. "Reproductive Justice and the Post-*Roe* Landscape: Chicana Feminisms, Coraje, and Collective Solidarity." *Journal of Autoethnography* 4, no. 4 (2023): 577–585.

Hobbs, Jay. "Meet the New Tenants One Wall Away from Gosnell's Shuttered Clinic." *National Right to Life News Today,* January 11, 2016. https://www.nationalrighttolifenews.org/2016/01/meet-the-new-tenants-one-wall-away-from-gosnells-shuttered-clinic/.

Hoberman, John. *Black and Blue: The Origins and Consequences of Medical Racism.* Berkeley: University of California Press, 2012.

Hodgson, Jane E. "The Law, the AMA, and Partial-Birth Abortion." *Journal of the American Medical Association* 281, no. 1 (July 7, 1999): 23–24.

Hoffman, Kelly M., Sophie Trawalter, Jordan R. Axt, and M. Normal Oliver. "Racial Bias in Pain Assessment and Treatment Recommendations, and False Beliefs about Biological Differences between Blacks and Whites." *PNAS* 113, no. 16 (2016): 4296–4301.

Hoffman, Merle. *Intimate Wars: The Life and Times of the Woman Who Brought Abortion from the Back-Alley to the Boardroom.* New York: Feminist Press at City University of New York, 2012.

Hsu, Hsuan L. *The Smell of Risk: Environmental Disparities and Olfactory Aesthetics.* New York: New York University Press, 2020.

Humphrey, David C. "Dissection and Discrimination: The Social Origins of Cadavers in America, 1760–1915." *Bulletin of the NY Academy of Medicine* 49, no. 9 (1973): 819–827.

Hunter, Marcus Anthony. "Black Philly after *The Philadelphia Negro.*" *Contexts* 13, no. 1 (2014): 26–31.

Jacob Riis: Revealing "How the Other Half Lives." Library of Congress. Accessed April 23, 2020, https://www.loc.gov/exhibits/jacob-riis/writer.html.

Jasinski, James. "A Constitutive Framework for Rhetorical Historiography: Toward an Understanding of the Discursive (Re)constitution of the 'Constitution' in the *Federalist Papers.*" In *Doing Rhetorical History: Concepts and Cases,* edited by Kathleen J. Turner, 72–92. Tuscaloosa: University of Alabama Press, 1998.

Jenkins, J. Foster. *Relations of the War to Medical Science: The Annual Address Delivered Before the Westchester County (N.Y.) Medical Society, June 16, 1863.* New York: Baillière Brothers, 1863. http://resource.nlm.nih.gov/62730350R.

Jensen, Robin E. "An Ecological Turn in Rhetoric of Health Scholarship: Attending to the Historical Flow and Percolation of Ideas, Assumptions, and Arguments." *Communication Quarterly* 63, no. 5 (2015): 522–526.

Jensen, Robin E. "From Barren to Sterile: The Evolution of a Mixed Metaphor." *Rhetoric Society Quarterly* 45, no. 1 (2015): 25–46.

Jensen, Robin E. "Improving Upon Nature: The Rhetorical Ecology of Chemical Language, Reproductive Endocrinology, and the Medicalization of Infertility." *Quarterly Journal of Speech* 101, no. 2 (2015): 329–353.

Jensen, Robin E. *Infertility: Tracing the History of a Transformative Term.* University Park: Pennsylvania State University Press, 2016.

Jensen, Robin E. "Using Science to Argue for Sexual Education in US Public Schools: Dr. Ella Flagg Young and the 1913 'Chicago Experiment.'" *Science Communication* 29, no. 2 (2007): 217–241.

Jensen, Robin E., and Ghanima Almuaili. "Abortion and Miscarriage Are Synonyms: Substandard Gynecological Care in the Wake of Abortion's Criminalization." *Women & Language* 46, no. 1 (2023): 267–273.

Jesse, Margaret Jay. *Female Physicians in American Literature: Abortion in 19th Century Literature.* London: Routledge, 2023.

Joffe, Carole E. "Commentary: Abortion Provider Stigma and Mainstream Medicine." *Women & Health* 54, no. 7 (2014): 666–671.

Joffe, Carole E. *Doctors of Conscience: The Struggle to Provide Abortion before and after "Roe v. Wade."* New York: Beacon Press, 1995.

Johnson, Jenell. *American Lobotomy: A Rhetorical History.* Ann Arbor: University of Michigan Press, 2014.

Johnson, Jenell. "'A Man's Mouth Is His Castle': The Midcentury Fluoridation Controversy and the Visceral Public." *Quarterly Journal of Speech* 102, no. 1 (2016): 1–20.

Johnson, Jenell. "The Skeleton on the Couch: The Eagleton Affair, Rhetorical Disability, and the Stigma of Mental Illness." *Rhetoric Society Quarterly* 40, no. 5 (2010): 459–478.

Johnson, Robert E. "Legal Abortion: Is It Genocide or Blessing in Disguise?" *Jet Magazine Archive* 43, no. 24 (March 22, 1973): 12–51.

Jones, Bonnie S., Sara Daniel, and Lindsay K. Cloud. "State Law Approaches to Facility Regulation of Abortion and Other Office Interventions." *American Journal of Public Health* 108 (2018): 486–492.

Kalifa, Dominique. *Vice, Crime, and Poverty: How the Western Imagination Invented the Underworld.* New York: Columbia University Press, 2019.

Kaplan, Laura. *The Story of Jane: The Legendary Underground Feminist Abortion Service.* Chicago: University of Chicago Press, 1995.

Kearns, Gerry. "Cholera, Nuisances and Environmental Management in Islington, 1830–55." *Medical History* 35, no. S11 (1991): 94–125.

Kearns, Gerry. "Private Property and Public Health Reform in England 1830–1870." *Social Science & Medicine* 26, no. 1 (1988): 187–199.

Keemer, Edgar B., Jr. *Confessions of a Pro-life Abortionist.* Detroit, MI: Vinco Press, 1980.

Keemer, Edgar B., Jr. "Looking Back at Luenbach: 296 Non-hospital Abortions." *Journal of the National Medical Association* 62, no. 4 (1970): 291–293.

Keemer, Edgar B., Jr. "Involuntary Sterilization." *Journal of the American Medical Association* 225, no. 13 (1973): 1658–1658.

Keemer, Edgar B., Jr. "Update on Abortion in Michigan." *Journal of the National Medical Association* 64, no. 6 (1972): 518–519.

Kelly, Casey Ryan, and Kristen Hoerl. "Shaved or Saved? Disciplining Women's Bodies." *Women's Studies in Communication* 43, no. 1 (2020): 1–22.

Kennerly, Michele. "Getting Carried Away: How Rhetorical Transport Gets Judgment Going." *Rhetoric Society Quarterly* 40 no. 3 (2010): 269–291.

Kerber, Linda. "The Republican Mother: Women and the Enlightenment—an American Perspective." *American Quarterly* 28, no. 2 (1976): 187–205.

Keremidchieva, Zornitsa. "Locating Argument's Location: The Stasis of Jurisdiction and the Establishment of the First Meridian of the United States." In *Local Theories of Argument*, edited by Dale Hample, 241–246. London: Routledge, 2021.

Kessler, Molly Margaret. *Stigma Stories: Rhetoric, Lived Experience, and Chronic Illness.* Columbus: Ohio University Press, 2022.

Kiechle, Melanie. *Smell Detectives: An Olfactory History of Nineteenth-Century Urban America.* Seattle: University of Washington Press, 2017.

King, Miriam, and Steven Ruggles. "American Immigration, Fertility, and Race Suicide at the Turn of the Century." *Journal of Interdisciplinary History* 20, no. 3 (1990): 347–369.

Kinney, Jen. "West Philly Abortion Doctor's 'House of Horrors' Listed for Sheriff's Sale: Anti-Choice Activists Want to Buy It." WHYY-PBS, September 13, 2019. https://whyy.org/articles/kermit-gosnells-west-philly-house-of-horrors-could-be-bought-by-anti-abortion-group/.

Krall, Madison A. "Regulatory Rhetoric and Mediated Health Narratives: Justifying Oversight in the Sherri Chessen Finkbine Thalidomide Story." *Rhetoric of Health & Medicine* 6, no. 3 (2023): 304–334.

Kristeva, Julia. *Powers of Horror.* New York: Columbia University Press, 1980.

Kumar, Anuradha, Leila Hessini, and Ellen M. H. Mitchell. "Conceptualising Abortion Stigma." *Culture, Health, and Society* 11, no. 6 (2009): 625–639.

Lakoff, George. *Moral Politics: What Conservatives Know That Liberals Don't*. Chicago: University of Chicago Press, 1996.

Lamp, Kathleen S. "Rhetoric in Situ." *Advances in the History of Rhetoric* 20, no. 2 (2017): 118–120.

Largent, Emily A. "Public Health, Racism, and the Lasting Impact of Hospital Segregation." *Public Health Reports* 133, no. 6 (2018): 715–720.

Larson, Stephanie R. *What It Feels Like: Visceral Rhetoric and the Politics of Rape Culture*. University Park: Pennsylvania State University Press, 2021.

Lay, Mary M. *The Rhetoric of Midwifery: Gender, Knowledge, and Power*. New Brunswick, NJ: Rutgers University Press, 2000.

Lee, Joel. "Odor and Order: How Caste Is Inscribed in Space and Sensoria." *Comparative Studies of South Asia, Africa, and the Middle East* 37, no. 3 (2017): 470–90.

Lee, Marvin J. H., Kruthika Reddy, Junad Chowdhury, Nishant Kumar, Peter A. Clark, Papa Ndao, Stacy J. Suh, and Sara Song. "Overcoming a Legacy of Mistrust: African Americans' Mistrust of Medical Profession." *Journal of Healthcare Ethics & Administration* 4, no. 1 (2018): 16–40.

Leona's Sister Gerri, directed by Jane Gilooly. Ho-Ho-Kus, NJ: New Day Films, 1994.

Levina, Marina. *Pandemics and the Media*. New York: Peter Lang, 2012.

Levina, Marina, and Diem-My T. Bui. "Introduction: Toward a Comprehensive Monster Theory in the 21st Century." In *Monster Culture in the 21st Century: A Reader*, ed. Marina Levina and Diem-My T. Bui, 1–14. New York: Bloomsbury, 2013.

Levs, Josh. "Gosnell Horror Fuels Fight for Abortion Laws." CNN, May 14, 2013. https://www.cnn.com/2013/05/12/us/abortion-trial-significance/index.html.

Lowry, Rich. "Return of the Back Alley." *National Review*, February 4, 2011. https://www.nationalreview.com/2011/02/return-back-alley-rich-lowry/.

Luker, Kristin. *Abortion and the Politics of Motherhood*. Berkeley: University of California Press, 1984.

Luker, Kristin. *Dubious Conceptions: The Politics of Teenage Pregnancy*. Cambridge, MA: Harvard University Press, 1997.

Luna, Zakiya. *Reproductive Rights as Human Rights: Women of Color and the Fight for Reproductive Justice*. New York: New York University Press, 2020.

Lupton, Deborah. "Toward the Development of Critical Health Communication Praxis." *Health Communication* 6, no. 1 (1994): 55–67.

Mack, Ashley Noel, Carli Bershon, Douglas D. Laiche, and Melissa Navarro. "Between Bodies and Institutions: Gendered Violence as Co-constitutive." *Women's Studies in Communication* 41, no. 2 (2018): 95–99.

Mahar, William J. *Behind the Burnt Cork Mask: Early Blackface Minstrelsy and Antebellum American Popular Culture*. Champaign: University of Illinois Press, 1999.

Makagon, Daniel. "Sloths in the Streets." In *The Urban Communication Reader*, edited by G. Burd, S. J. Drucker, and G. Gumpers, 141–158. Cresskill, NJ: Hampton Press, 2007.

Martin, Emily. *The Woman in the Body: A Cultural Analysis of Reproduction*. Boston: Beacon Press, 2001.

McElhinney, Ann, and Phelim McAleer. "Gosnell Movie." Indiegogo, https://www.indiegogo.com/projects/gosnell-movie.

McGee, Michael Calvin. "Text, Context, and the Fragmentation of Contemporary Culture." *Western Journal of Speech Communication* 54 (1990): 274–289.

"Medic Denies Performing TV Abortions on Blacks." *Jet Magazine Archive* 45, no. 3 (January 4, 1973): 13.

Medoff, Marshall H. "State Abortion Politics and TRAP Abortion Laws." *Journal of Women, Politics & Policy* 33 (2012): 239–262.

Mercier, Rebecca J., Mara Buchbinder, and Amy Bryant. "TRAP Laws and the Invisible Labor of US Abortion Providers." *Critical Public Health* 26, no. 1 (2016): 77–87.

Merlan, Anna. "The Abortion Rights Group Other Activists Want Nothing to Do With." *Vice*, August 4, 2022. https://www.com/en/article/the-abortion-rights-group-other-activists-want-nothing-to-do-with/.

Middleton, Michael, Aaron Hess, Danielle Endres, and Samantha Senda-Cook. *Participatory Critical Rhetoric: Theoretical and Methodological Foundations for Studying Rhetoric in Situ*. Lanham, MD: Lexington Books, 2015.

"Mifepristone (Oral Route)." Mayo Clinic. Accessed January 3, 2023. https://www.mayoclinic.org/drugs-supplements/mifepristone-oral-route/side-effects/drg-20067123?.

Milbauer, Barbara. *The Law Giveth: Legal Aspects of the Abortion Controversy*. New York: Atheneum, 1983.

Miller, Carolyn R. "Genre as Social Action." *Quarterly Journal of Speech* 70, no. 2 (1984): 151–167.

Miller, Patricia G. *The Worst of Times: Illegal Abortion—Survivors, Practitioners, Coroners, Cops, and the Children of Women Who Died Talk about Its Horrors*. New York: Harper Collins, 1994.

Miller, William Ian. *Anatomy of Disgust*. Cambridge, MA: Harvard University Press, 1997.

"Minneapolis Flour Milling Boom." Minnesota Historical Society. https://www.mnhs.org/millcity/learn/history/flour-milling.

Mitchell, Peta. "Contagion, Virology, Autoimmunity: Derrida's Rhetoric of Contamination." *Parallax* 23, no. 1 (2017): 77–93.

Mitchell, Ryan. "'Whatever Happened to Our Great Gay Imaginations?' The Invention of Safe Sex and the Visceral Imagination." *Quarterly Journal of Speech* 107, no. 1 (2021): 26–48.

Mohr, James C. *Abortion in America: The Origins and Evolution of National Policy*. Oxford: Oxford University Press, 1979. Ebook.

Moody, Howard. "Abortion: A Woman's Right and Legal Problem." *Christianity and Crisis* (1971): 340–341.

Moody, Howard. "Abortion: Woman's Right and Legal Problem." *Theology Today* 28, no. 3 (1971): 337–346.

Morantz, Regina Markell. "Introduction: From Art to Science; Women Physicians in American Medicine, 1600–1980." In *In Her Own Words: Oral Histories of Women Physicians*, edited by Regina Markell Morantz, Cynthia Stodola Pomerleau, and Carol Hansen Fenichel, 3–44. Westport, CT: Greenwood Press, 1982.

Morgan, Lynn Marie, and Meredith W. Michaels. *Fetal Subjects, Feminist Positions*. Philadelphia: University of Pennsylvania Press, 1999.

Moss, Sandra W. *The Country Practitioner: Ellis P. Townsend's Brave Little Medical Journal*. Self-published, Xlibris, 2011.

Morales, Andrea C., Darren W. Dahl, and Jennifer J. Argo. "Amending the Law of

Contagion: A General Theory of Property Transference." *Journal of the Association for Consumer Research* 3, no. 4 (2018): 555–565.

Murillo, Lina-Maria. "*Espanta Cigüeñas*: Race and Abortion in the US-Mexico Borderlands." *Signs: Journal of Women in Culture and Society* 48, no. 4 (2023): 796.

Murillo, Lina-Maria. "A View from the Northern Border: Abortions before *Roe v. Wade*." *Bulletin of the History of Medicine* 97, no. 1 (2023): 30–38.

Nakayama, Thomas K., and Robert L. Krizek. "Whiteness: A Strategic Rhetoric." *Quarterly Journal of Speech* 81, no. 3 (1995): 291–309.

NARAL Pro-Choice America. "Statement on the Kermit Gosnell Conviction." May 13, 2013. https://www.prochoiceamerica.org/2013/05/13/statement-kermit-gosnell-verdict/.

Nash, Linda Lorraine. *Inescapable Ecologies: A History of Environment, Disease, and Knowledge*. Berkeley: University of California Press, 2006.

Nelson, Jennifer A. "'Abortions under Community Control': Feminism, Nationalism, and the Politics of Reproduction among New York City's Young Lords." *Journal of Women's History* 13, no. 1 (2001): 157–180.

Nelson, Jennifer A. *Women of Color and the Reproductive Rights Movement*. New York: New York University Press, 2003.

Newman, Karen. *Fetal Positions: Individualism, Science, Visuality*. Stanford, CA: Stanford University Press, 1996.

Norris, Alison, Danielle Bessett, Julia R. Steinberg, Megan L. Kavanaugh, Silvia De Zordo, and Davida Becker. "Abortion Stigma: A Reconceptualization of Constituents, Causes, and Consequences." *Women's Health Issues* 3 (2011): S49–54.

Nussbaum, Martha Craven. *Aristotle's "De Motu Animalium."* Princeton, NJ: Princeton University Press, 1985.

Oberman, Jonathan, and Kendea Johnson. "The Never Ending Tale: Racism and Inequality in the Era of Broken Windows Policing." *Cardozo Law Review* 37, no. 3 (2016): 1075–1092.

O'Donnell, Kelly, and Naomi Rogers. "Revisiting the History of Abortion in the Wake of the *Dobbs* Decision." *Bulletin of the History of Medicine* 97, no. 1 (2023): 1–10.

O'Gorman, Ned. "Aristotle's *Phantasia* in the *Rhetoric*: *Lexis*, Appearance, and the Epideictic Function of Discourse." *Philosophy & Rhetoric* 38, no. 1 (2005): 16–40.

Olasky, Marvin. "Advertising Abortion during the 1830s and 1840s: Madame Restell Builds a Business." *Journalism History* 13, no. 2 (1986): 49–55.

Olson, Emily. "California Will Cut Ties with Walgreens over the Company's Plan to Drop Abortion Pills." NPR, March 7, 2023. https://www.npr.org/2023/03/07/1161590750/california-walgreens-mifepristone-abortion-pill.

Ore, Ersula, and Matthew Houdek. "Lynching in Times of Suffocation: Toward a Spatiotemporal Politics of Breathing." *Women's Studies in Communication* 43, no. 4 (2020): 443–458.

Ortega, Mariana. "Being Lovingly, Knowingly Ignorant: White Feminism and Women of Color." *Hypatia* 21, no. 3 (2006): 56–74.

Ortiz, Charlene. "Speech at the 2004 March for Women's Lives on Rosie Jiménez." April 25, 2004, Washington, DC. C-SPAN. 02:43:30. https://www.c-span.org/video/?181451-1/march-womens-lives.

PA Family. "The Man Who Interviewed Gosnell: Five Takeaways." September 4, 2018. https://pafamily.org/2018/09/04/gosnelldocumentary/.

Parry-Giles, Shawn J., and Diane M. Blair. "The Rise of the Rhetorical First Lady: Politics, Gender Ideology, and Women's Voice, 1789–2002." *Rhetoric & Public Affairs* 5, no .4 (2002): 565–600.

Patterson, Maggie Jones, and Megan Williams Hall. "Abortion, Moral Maturity and Civic Journalism." *Critical Studies in Mass Communication* 15, no. 2 (1998): 91–115.

Pavard, Bibia. "The 'Karman Method' and the Boundaries of Self-Help: Itinerary of an Abortion Technology." *Gender & History* (2024): 1–18.

Paxton, Ken. "Texas Defends Important Women's Health Protections at U.S. Supreme Court." Website of Ken Paxton, Attorney General of Texas. March 2, 2016. https://www.texasattorneygeneral.gov/news/releases/texas-defends-important-womens-health-protections-us-supreme-court.

Penner, Louise. *Victorian Medicine and Social Reform: Florence Nightingale among the Novelists*. New York: Springer, 2010.

Perkins, Lucy. "How a Supreme Court Case from Pennsylvania Changed Abortion Access across the Country." WESA NPR, September 7, 2018. https://www.wesa.fm/politics-government/2018-09-07/how-a-supreme-court-case-from-pennsylvania-changed-abortion-access-across-the-country.

Petchesky, Rosalind Pollack. "Fetal Images: The Power of Visual Culture in the Politics of Reproduction." *Feminist Studies* 13, no. 2 (1987): 263–292.

Phillips, Kendall. Introduction to *Framing Public Memory*, edited by Kendall Phillips, 1–14. Tuscaloosa: University of Alabama Press, 2004.

Phillips, Kendall. *A Place of Darkness: The Rhetoric of Horror in Early American Cinema*. Austin: University of Texas Press, 2018.

Phyllis, Virtual Volunteer Storyteller. "I Had an Illegal Abortion before *Roe v. Wade*." Planned Parenthood, March 15, 2022. www.plannedparenthood.org/blog/i-had-an-illegal-abortion-before-roe-v-wade.

Pillow, Wanda S. *Unfit Subjects: Education Policy and the Teen Mother, 1972–2002*. New York: Routledge, 2004.

Pittman, Coretta. "Black Women Writers and the Trouble with Ethos: Harriet Jacobs, Billie Holiday, and Sister Souljah." *Rhetoric Society Quarterly* 37, no. 1 (2006): 43–70.

"The Playboy Panel: Religion and the New Morality." *Playboy*, June 1967.

"Protest Tips: It's Our Fight, Let's Do It Right." Planned Parenthood. Accessed July 4, 2024. https://www.plannedparenthoodaction.org/rightfully-ours/bans-off-our-bodies/protest-tips-lets-do-it-right.

Poovey, Mary. *Making a Social Body: British Cultural Formation, 1830–1864*. Chicago: University of Chicago Press, 1995.

Prasch, Allison M. "Obama in Selma: Deixis, Rhetorical Vision, and the 'True Meaning of America.'" *Quarterly Journal of Speech* 105, no. 1 (2019): 42–67.

Price, Kimala. "What Is Reproductive Justice? How Women of Color Activists Are Redefining the Pro-choice Paradigm." *Meridians* 19 (2020): 340–362.

Propen, Amy D., and Mary Lay Schuster. "Understanding Genre through the Lens of Advocacy: The Rhetorical Work of the Victim Impact Statement." *Written Communication* 27, no. 1 (2010): 3–35.

Ramsey, Shawn D. "Gustave Le Bon, Rhetoric as Mass Contagion, and 19th Century

Rhetoric." *Celt: A Journal of Culture, English Language Teaching & Literature* 17, no. 2 (2017): 230–249.

Randolph, Sherie M. *Florynce "Flo" Kennedy: The Life of a Black Feminist Radical.* Chapel Hill: University of North Carolina Press, 2015.

Rankin, Lauren. *Bodies on the Line: At the Front Lines of the Fight to Protect Abortion in America.* Berkeley, CA: Counterpoint, 2022.

Rayner, Geof. "Conventional and Ecological Public Health." *Public Health* 123, no. 9 (2009): 587–591.

Reagan, Leslie J. "Crossing the Border for Abortions: California Activists, Mexican Clinics, and the Creation of a Feminist Health Agency in the 1960s." *Feminist Studies* 26, no. 2 (2000): 323–348.

Reagan, Leslie J. *Dangerous Pregnancies: Mothers, Disabilities, and Abortion in Modern America.* Los Angeles: University of California Press, 2012.

Reagan, Leslie J. *When Abortion Was a Crime: Women, Medicine, and the Law in the United States, 1867–1973.* Los Angeles: University of California Press, 1997.

Reel, Guy. *"National Police Gazette" and the Making of the Modern American Man, 1879–1906.* New York: Palgrave, 2006.

Rice, Mitchell F., and Woodrow Jones Jr. *Public Policy and the Black Hospital: From Slavery to Segregation to Integration.* Westport, CT: Greenwood Press, 1994.

Richards, Ellen H. *Euthenics: The Science of Controllable Environment—a Plea for Better Living Conditions as a First Step toward Higher Human Efficiency.* Boston: Whitcomb & Barrows, 1910.

Riis, Jacob A. *How the Other Half Lives: Studies among the Tenements of New York.* Mansfield Centre, CT: Martino, 2015.

Rios, Carmen. "Daring to Remember: Tell Us Your Story of Life before Roe." *Ms.*, July 2, 2018. https://msmagazine.com/2018/07/02/daring-remember-tell-us-story-life-roe/.

Roberts, Dorothy. *Killing the Black Body: Race, Reproduction, and the Meaning of Liberty.* New York: Vantage Books, 1997.

Robvais, Raquel M. "We Are No Longer Invisible," *POROI* 15, no. 1 (2020). https://doi.org/10.13008/2151-2957.1296.

Roosevelt, Theodore. *State Papers as Governor and President.* New York: Charles Scribner's Sons, 1925.

Root (@TheRoot)."These U.S. Reps Want to End the Hyde Amendment Now." Twitter, September 30, 2019. https://twitter.com/theroot/status/1178730705322418176.

Rose, Melody. *Safe, Legal, and Unavailable? Abortion Politics in the United States.* Washington, DC: CQ Press, 2007.

Ross, Loretta J. "African American Women and Abortion: A Neglected History." *Journal of Health Care for the Poor and Underserved* 3, no. 2 (1992): 274–284.

Ross, Loretta J., and Rickie Solinger. *Reproductive Justice: An Introduction.* Vol. 1. Berkeley: University of California Press, 2017.

Ross, Loretta J. "Reproductive Justice as Intersectional Feminist Activism." *Souls: A Critical Journal of Black Politics, Culture, and Society* 19, no. 3 (2017): 286–314.

Ross, Loretta J. "Speech at the 2004 March for Women's Lives." April 25, 2004, Washington, DC. C-SPAN. 02:35:57–02:37:45. https://www.c-span.org/video/?181451-1/march-womens-lives.

Ross, Loretta J. "Teaching Reproductive Justice: An Activist's Approach." In *Black*

Women's Liberatory Pedagogies: Resistance, Transformation, and Healing within and beyond the Academy, edited by Olivia N. Perlow, Durene I. Wheeler, Sharon L. Bethea, and BarBara M. Scott, 159–180. London: Palgrave Macmillan, 2018.

Rovner, Julie. "A Sharper Abortion Debate after Gosnell Verdict." NPR, May 14, 2013. https://www.npr.org/sections/health-shots/2013/05/14/183911268/a-sharper-abortion-debate-after-gosnell-verdict.

Rowland, Allison L. *Zoetropes and the Politics of Humanhood*. Columbus: The Ohio State University Press, 2020.

Rozin, Paul, Maureen Markwith, and Carol Nemeroff. "Magical Contagion Beliefs and Fear of AIDS 1." *Journal of Applied Social Psychology* 22, no. 14 (1992): 1081–1092.

Rudwick, Elliott M. "A Brief History of Mercy-Douglass Hospital in Philadelphia." *Journal of Negro Education* 20, no. 1 (1951): 50–66.

Ryan, April. "Black Women Leaders 'Mad as Hell' after Supreme Court Overturns Abortion Rights, Vow to 'Right.'" *Grio*, June 24, 2022. https://thegrio.com/2022/06/24/black-women-supreme-court-overturn-abortion/.

Sáez, Macarena. "Commentary on *Planned Parenthood of Southeastern Pennsylvania v. Casey*." In *Feminist Judgments: Rewritten Opinions of the United States Supreme Court*, edited by Kathryn M. Stanchi, Linda L. Berger, and Bridget J. Crawford, 361–365. New York: Cambridge University Press, 2016.

Saletan, William. "The Back Alley: What Happened to the Women." *Slate*, February 16, 2011. https://slate.com/news-and-politics/2011/02/kermit-gosnell-and-abortion-clinic-regulation-did-pro-choice-politics-protect-him.html.

Salters, J. N. "Are All the Women Still White? Kermit Gosnell, 'Back Alley' Abortions, and the Politics of Motherhood." *Feminist Wire*, May 23, 2013. https://thefeministwire.com/2013/05/are-all-the-women-still-white-kermit-gosnell-back-alley-abortions-and-the-politics-of-motherhood/.

Sandelowski, Margarete. "Separate, but Less Unequal: Fetal Ultrasonography and the Transformation of Expectant Mother/Fatherhood." *Gender & Society* 8, no. 2 (1994): 230–245.

Sandlos, Karyn. "Unifying Forces: Rhetorical Reflections on a Pro-choice Image." In *Transformations: Thinking through Feminism*, edited by Sara Ahmed, Jane Kilby, Celia Lury, Maureen McNeil, and Beverly Skeggs, 77–91. London: Routledge, 2000.

Savani, Krishna, Satishchandra Kumar, N. V. R. Naidu, and Carol S. Dweck, "Beliefs about Emotional Residue: The Idea That Emotions Leave a Trace in the Physical Environment." *Journal of Personality and Social Psychology* 101, no. 4 (2011): 684–701.

Schoen, Johanna. *Abortion after "Roe."* Chapel Hill: University of North Carolina Press, 2015.

Schoen, Johanna. "Between Choice and Coercion: Women and the Politics of Sterilization in North Carolina, 1929–1975." *Journal of Women's History* 13, no. 1 (2001): 132–156.

Schoen, Johanna. *Choice and Coercion: Birth Control, Sterilization, and Abortion in Public Health and Welfare*. Chapel Hill: University of North Carolina Press, 2005.

Schulder, Diane, and Florynce Kennedy. *Abortion Rap: Testimony by Women Who Have Suffered the Consequences of Restrictive Abortion Laws*. New York: McGraw-Hill, 1971.

Schülting, Sabine. *Dirt in Victorian Literature and Culture: Writing Materiality*. London: Routledge, 2016.

Schweitzer, Marlis. "Surviving the City: Press Agents, Publicity Stunts, and the Spectacle of the Urban Female Body." In *Performance and the City*, 133–151. London: Palgrave Macmillan, 2009.

Scott, Niall. "The Monstrous Metallic in Medicine and Horror Cinema." *Medicina nei Secoli: Journal of History of Medicine and Medical Humanities* 26, no. 1 (2014): 313–331.

Sedgwick, Eve Kosofsky. *Touching Feeling: Affect, Pedagogy, Performativity*. Durham, NC: Duke University Press, 2003.

Segal, Judy Z. *Health and the Rhetoric of Medicine*. Carbondale: Southern Illinois University Press, 2005.

"Sewer Connections to Private Houses." *Sanitary Engineer* 6 (1883): 531.

Sharf, Barbara F. "Physician-Patient Communication as Interpersonal Rhetoric: A Narrative Approach." *Health Communication* 2, no. 4 (1990): 217–231.

Shavers, Vickie L., Alexis Bakos, and Vanessa B. Sheppard. "Race, Ethnicity, and Pain among the US Adult Population." *Journal of Health Care for the Poor and Underserved* 21, no. 1 (2010): 177–220.

Shome, Raka. "Space Matters: The Power and Practice of Space." *Communication Theory* 13, no. 1 (2003): 39–56.

Shotwell, Alexis. *Against Purity: Living Ethically in Compromised Times*. Minneapolis: University of Minnesota Press, 2016.

Siegfried, Kate. "Making Settler Colonialism Concrete: Agentive Materialism and Habitational Violence in Palestine." *Communication and Critical/Cultural Studies* 17, no. 3 (2020): 267–284.

Sikoa, Anna, and Farah Zahra. "Nosocomial Infections." National Library of Medicine. Last modified January 23, 2023. https://www.ncbi.nlm.nih.gov/books/NBK559312/.

Silliman, Jael, Marlene Gerber Fried, Loretta Ross, and Elena R. Gutiérrez. *Undivided Rights: Women of Color Organize for Reproductive Justice*. Chicago: Haymarket, 2016.

Sinclair, George. "Actress' Ready-Press-Agent." *Green Book Album* 6 (August 1911): 368–372.

Singler, Charles A. "Alleys—Past and Present." *Cement Era: Devotes to Cement, Concrete and Related Machinery* 15, no. 3 (1917): 35.

Sisson, Gretchen, Stephanie Herold, and Katrina Kimport. "Abortion Onscreen Database." Advancing New Standards in Reproductive Health (ANSIRH), University of California, San Francisco (2022). abortiononscreen.org.

Smalley, Eugene V. "The Flour-Mills of Minneapolis." *Century*, May 1886, 37–47, https://babel.hathitrust.org/cgi/pt?id=coo.31924079633354&seq=57.

Smeal, Eleanor, and Tony Carabillo, prod. *Abortion Denied: Shattering Young Women's Lives*. Arlington County, VA: Fund for the Feminist Majority, 1990.

Smedley, Brian D., Adrienne Y. Stith, and Alan R. Nelson. *Unequal Treatment: Confronting Racial and Ethnic Disparities in Health Care*. Washington, DC: National Academies Press, 2013.

Smith-Rosenberg, Carroll. *Disorderly Conduct: Visions of Gender in Victorian America*. Oxford: Oxford University Press, 1986.

Solinger, Rickie. *The Abortionist: A Woman against the Law*. Berkeley: University of California Press, 1996.

Solinger, Rickie. *Beggars and Choosers: How the Politics of Choice Shapes Adoption, Abortion, and Welfare in the United States*. New York: Hill and Wang, 2001.

Solinger, Rickie. "'A Complete Disaster': Abortion and the Politics of Hospital Abortion Committees, 1950–1970," *Feminist Studies* 19, no. 2 (1993): 241–268.

Solinger, Rickie. *Pregnancy and Power: A Short History of Reproductive Politics in America.* New York: New York University Press, 2005.

Solomon, Akiba. "The Personal Is Political: That's the Challenge; *Roe v. Wade* and a Black Nationalist Womanist Writer." *Dissent* 60, no. 1 (2013): 60–63.

Southard, Belinda A. Stillion. *Militant Citizenship: Rhetorical Strategies of the National Woman's Party, 1913–1920.* Vol. 21. College Station: Texas A&M University Press, 2011.

Spillers, Hortense J. "Mama's Baby Papa's Maybe: An American Grammar Book." *Diacritics* 17, no. 2 (1987): 65–81.

Spirit of '73: Rock for Choice. 1995. Sony Music, compact disc.

Srebnick, Amy Gilman. *The Mysterious Death of Mary Rogers: Sex and Culture in Nineteenth-Century New York.* New York: Oxford University Press, 1995.

Stabile, Carole. "Shooting the Mother." In *The Visible Woman: Imaging Technologies, Gender, and Science,* 171–97. New York: New York University Press, 1998.

Stansell, Christine. *City of Women: Sex and Class in New York, 1789–1860.* Urbana: University of Illinois Press, 1987.

Stashower, Daniel. *The Beautiful Cigar Girl: Mary Rogers, Edgar Allan Poe, and the Invention of Murder.* London: Penguin Press, 2007.

Stephenson, Larry W. "History of Cardiac Surgery." In *Surgery,* edited by Jeffrey A. Norton, Philip S. Barie, R. Randal Bollinger, Alfred E. Chang, Stephen F. Lowry, Sean J. Mulvihill, Harvey I. Pass, and Robert W. Thompson, 1471–1479. New York: Springer, 2008.

Stewart, Kathleen. "Afterword: Worlding Refrains." In *The Affect Theory Reader,* edited by Melissa Gregg and Gregory J. Seigworth, 339–353. Durham, NC: Duke University Press, 2010.

Stormer, Nathan. *Articulating Life's Memory: U.S. Medical Rhetoric about Abortion in the Nineteenth Century.* Lanham, MD: Lexington Books, 2002.

Stormer, Nathan. "A Likely Past: Abortion, Social Data, and a Collective Memory of Secrets in 1950s America." *Communication and Critical/Cultural Studies* 7, no. 4 (2010): 337–359.

Stormer, Nathan. *Signs of Pathology: U.S. Medical Rhetoric on Abortion, 1800s–1960s.* University Park: Pennsylvania State University Press, 2015.

Street, Richard L., Jr. "Communication in Medical Encounters: An Ecological Perspective." In *The Routledge Handbook of Health Communication,* 77–104. New York: Routledge, 2003.

Sturken, Marita. *Tangled Memories: The Vietnam War, the AIDS Epidemic, and the Politics of Remembering.* Berkeley: University of California Press, 1997.

Swartzendruber, Andrea, Abigail English, Katherine Blumoff Greenberg, Pamela J. Murray, Matt Freeman, Krishna Upadhya, Tina Simpson, Elizabeth Miller, and John Santelli. "Crisis Pregnancy Centers in the United States: Lack of Adherence to Medical and Ethical Practice Standards; A Joint Position Statement of the Society for Adolescent Health and Medicine and the North American Society for Pediatric and Adolescent Gynecology." *Journal of Pediatric and Adolescent Gynecology* 32, no. 6 (2019): 563–566.

Taylor, Charles Allen. *Defining Science: A Rhetoric of Demarcation*. Madison: University of Wisconsin Press, 1996.
Taylor, Janelle S. *The Public Life of the Fetal Sonogram: Technology, Consumption, and the Politics of Reproduction*. New Brunswick, NJ: Rutgers University Press, 2008.
Taylor, Magdalene. "Can We Stop with the Coat Hanger Imagery." *Mel Magazine* (2022). https://melmagazine.com/en-us/story/coat-hanger-abortion-meme.
Todd, Knox H., Christi Deaton, Anne P. D'adamo, and Leon Goe. "Ethnicity and Analgesic Practice." *Annals of Emergency Medicine* 35, no. 1 (2000): 11–16.
Tolnai, B. B. "The Abortion Racket." *Forum* 94 (1935): 176–181.
Tonn, Mari Boor. "Donning Sackcloth and Ashes: *Webster v. Reproductive Health Services* and Moral Agony in Abortion Rights Rhetoric." *Communication Quarterly* 44, no. 3 (1996): 265–279.
Townsend, Ellis P. "Back Alley Obstetrics." *Medical Visitor* (1894): 206.
Tuan, Yi-Fu. *Space and Place: The Perspective of Experience*. Minneapolis: University of Minnesota Press, 1977.
Tunç, Tanfer Emin. "Unlocking the Mysterious Trunk: Nineteenth-Century American Criminal Abortion Narratives." In *Transcending Borders: Abortion in the Past and Present*, edited by Shannon Stettner, Katrina Ackerman, Kristin Burnett, Travis Hay, 35–52. London: Palgrave Macmillan, 2017.
Turner, Patricia A. *I Heard It through the Grapevine: Rumor in African-American Culture*. Berkeley: University of California Press, 1993.
Twain, Mark. *Pudd'nhead Wilson*. Cambridge, MA: Harvard University Press, 2015.
Twigg, Reginald. "The Performative Dimensions of Surveillance: Jacob Riis' *How the Other Half Lives*." *Text & Performance Quarterly* 12, no. 4 (1992): 305–328.
Upton, Sarah De Los Santos. "Nepantla Activism and Coalition Building: Locating Identity and Resistance in the Cracks between Worlds." *Women's Studies in Communication* 42, no. 2 (2019): 135–139.
Upton, Sarah De Los Santos, Carlos A. Tarin, and Leandra H. Hernández. "Construyendo Conexiones para los Niños: Environmental Justice, Reproductive Feminicidio, and Coalitional Possibility in the Borderlands." *Health Communication* 37, no. 9 (2022): 1242–1252.
"Urges Clean Alleys. J. M. Waldron Says Conditions Should Be Improved: Cites Menace to Health." *Washington Post*, July 27, 1910.
"U.S. Supreme Court Maintains Abortion Pill Access but Threatens to Undermine Access to Medical Care for All Patients." Gender Justice, June 13, 2024. https://www.genderjustice.us/scotus-maintains-abortion-pill-access/.
Valenti, Jessica. *The Purity Myth: How America's Obsession with Virginity Is Hurting Young Women*. Berkeley, CA: Seal Press, 2010.
van der Kolk, Bessel. *The Body Keeps the Score: Brain, Mind, and Body in the Healing of Trauma*. New York: Random House, 2015.
Vesely-Flad, Rima L. *Racial Purity and Dangerous Bodies: Moral Pollution, Black Lives, and the Struggle for Justice*. Minneapolis, MN: Fortress Press, 2017.
Vinson, Jenna. *Embodying the Problem: The Persuasive Power of the Teen Mother*. New Brunswick, NJ: Rutgers University Press, 2018.
Waitzkin, Howard. *The Politics of Medical Encounters: How Patients and Doctors Deal with Social Problems*. New Haven, CT: Yale University Press, 1991.

"Walgreens Statement on Mifepristone." Walgreens, March 6, 2023, https://news.walgreens.com/press-center/walgreens-statement-on-mifepristone.htm.

Wanzer-Serrano, Darrel. *The New York Young Lords and the Struggle for Liberation.* Philadelphia: Temple University Press, 2015. *See also* Enck-Wanzer, Darrel.

Ward, Jane. "Don't Have an Abortion." *Reader's Digest,* August 1941, 17–21.

Warren, Elizabeth. "America Can Never Go Back to the Era of Back-Alley Abortions." *Time,* January 21, 2018. https://www.warren.senate.gov/newsroom/op-eds/2018/01/21/time-op-ed-america-can-never-go-back-to-the-era-of-back-alley-abortions-1.

Washington, Harriet A., Robert B. Baker, Ololade Olakanmi, Todd L. Savitt, Elizabeth A. Jacobs, Eddie Hoover, and Matthew K. Wynia. "Segregation, Civil Rights, and Health Disparities: The Legacy of African American Physicians and Organized Medicine, 1910–1968." *Journal of the National Medical Association* 101, no. 6 (2009): 513–527.

Weber, Anne-Kathrin. "The Pitfalls of 'Love and Kindness': On the Challenges to Compassion/Pity as a Political Emotion." *Politics and Governance* 6, no. 4 (2018): 53–61.

Weddington, Sarah. *A Question of Choice: The Lawyer Who Won "Roe v. Wade."* New York: Putnam Press, 1992.

Weingarten, Karen. *Abortion in the American Imagination: Before Life and Choice, 1880–1940.* New Brunswick, NJ: Rutgers University Press, 2015.

Weller, Charles Frederick, and Eugenia Winston Weller. *Neglected Neighbors: Stories of Life in the Alleys, Tenements, and Shanties of the National Capital.* Philadelphia: J. C. Winston, 1909.

"*Whole Woman's Health v. Hellerstedt.*" Center for Reproductive Rights. Accessed May 7, 2024. https://www.reproductiverights.org/case/whole-womans-health-v-hellerstedt.

Williams, Raymond. *Marxism and Literature.* Oxford: Oxford University Press, 1977.

Wilson, Kirt. "The Racial Contexts of Public Address: Interpreting Violence during the Reconstruction Era." In *The Handbook of Rhetoric and Public Address,* edited by Shawn J. Parry-Giles and J. Michael Hogan, 205–228. Malden, MA: Wiley Blackwell, 2010.

Winderman, Emily. "(Never) Going Back: Black Feminist Impatience for a Post-*Dobbs* Future." *Women & Language* 46, no. 1 (2023): 285–291.

Winderman, Emily, and Brittany Knutson. "Florynce Kennedy's Cultivation of Reproductive Expertise in *Abramowicz v. Lefkowitz* and *Abortion Rap.*" *Rhetoric Society Quarterly* 53, no. 2 (2023): 262–277.

Winderman, Emily, Robert Mejia, and Brandon Rogers. "'All Smell Is Disease': Miasma, Sensory Rhetoric, and the Sanitary-Bacteriologic of Visceral Public Health." *Rhetoric of Health & Medicine* 2, no. 2 (2019): 115–146.

Winslow, Barbara. *Revolutionary Feminists: The Women's Liberation Movement in Seattle.* Durham, NC: Duke University Press.

Wright, Ian A., Peter J. Davies, Sophia J. Findlay, and Olof J. Jonasson. "A New Type of Water Pollution: Concrete Drainage Infrastructure and Geochemical Contamination of Urban Waters." *Marine and Freshwater Research* 62, no. 12 (2011): 1355–1361.

Yam, Shui-yin Sharon. "Citizenship Discourse in Hong Kong: The Limits of Familial Tropes." *Quarterly Journal of Speech* 104, no. 1 (2018): 1–21.

Yam, Shui-yin Sharon. "Visualizing Birth Stories from the Margin: Toward a Reproductive Justice Model of Rhetorical Analysis." *Rhetoric Society Quarterly* 50, no. 1 (2020): 19–34.

Yam, Shui-yin Sharon, and Natalie Fixmer-Oraiz. "Against Gender Essentialism: Reproductive Justice Doulas and Gender Inclusivity in Pregnancy and Birth Discourse." *Women's Studies in Communication* 46, no. 1 (2023): 1–22.

Yoest, Charmaine. "How Science, State Laws, and Exposure Are Driving the Pro-life Comeback." *Medium*, July 16, 2015. https://medium.com/2015-index-of-culture-and-opportunity/abortion-rate-total-abortions-563778596c02.

Zanjani, Zahra, Hamid Yaghubi, Ladan Fata, Mohammadreza Shaiiri, and Mohammad Gholami. "The Mediating Role of Fear of Contagion in Explaining the Relationship between Disgust Propensity and Fear of Contamination." *Iranian Journal of Psychiatry and Clinical Psychology* 23, no. 4 (2018): 454–465.

Zarefsky, David. "The Four Senses of Rhetorical History." In *Doing Rhetorical History: Concepts and Cases*, edited by Kathleen J. Turner, 19–32. Tuscaloosa: University of Alabama Press, 1998.

Zelizer, Barbie. *About to Die: How Images Move the Public*. New York: Oxford University Press, 2010.

INDEX

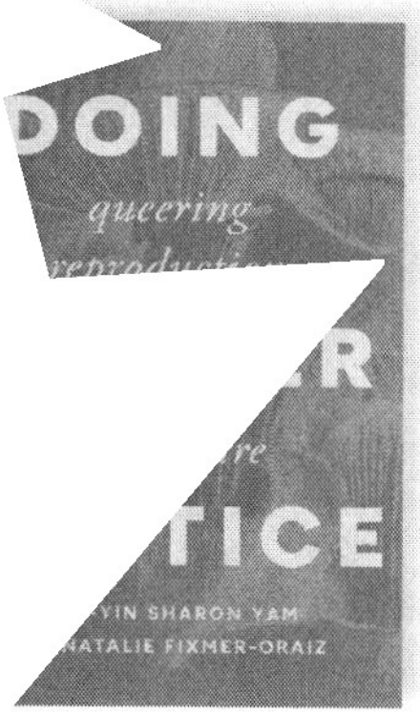

"*Doing Gender Justice* helps us imagine new spaces of possibility and coalition where all reproduction is valued."

—Zakiya Luna, author of *Reproductive Rights as Human Rights*

"Not only does Derkatch see the scam of wellness for what it is, she takes it apart and shows us exactly how it works. *Why Wellness Sells* is a deft, incisive analysis of a modern scourge."

—Carl Elliott, author of *Better Than Well*

"Dignified care is not only an ethical but also a rhetorical practice."

—Mary Lay Schuster, author of *The Victim's Voice in the Sexual Misconduct Crisis*